A Clinician's Survival Guide to Acute Medical Emergencies

T0294368

FOURTH EDITION

A Clinician's Survival Guide to Acute Medical Emergencies

RICHARD HARRISON, MD, FRCP

Consultant Physician, Salisbury District Hospital, United Kingdom

LYNDA DALY, RN, RM, RHV

Stockbridge, United Kingdom

ELSEVIER

First edition 2001
Second edition 2006
Third edition 2011, Third updated edition 2019

ISBN: 978-0-443-11219-5

Printed in India

Last digit is the print number: 9 8 7 6 5 4 3 2 1

Content Strategist: Andrae Akeh
Content Project Manager: Taranpreet Kaur
Design: Matthew Limbert
Marketing Manager: Deborah Watkins

To Clara Lotte and Emmeline Primrose

ABCDE	Mnemonic used for primary assessment (Airway, Breathing, Circulation, Disability, Exposure)
ACE	Angiotensin-converting enzyme
ACEI	Angiotensin-converting enzyme inhibitor
ACS	Acute coronary syndrome
ACVPU	AVPU plus new-onset confusion
ADH	Antidiuretic hormone
ADL	Activities of daily living
AED	Accident and Emergency Department
AF	Atrial fibrillation
AIDS	Acquired immunodeficiency syndrome
ALS	Advanced life support
ALT	Alanine transaminase
AMI	Acute myocardial infarction
AMTS	Abbreviated mental test score
APPT	Activated partial thromboplastin time
ASO	Antistreptolysin O
AST	Aspartate transaminase
AV node	Atrioventricular node
AVPU	Mnemonic for assessing conscious level (Alert, Voice, Pain, Unresponsive)
bd	Twice a day
BLS	Basic life support
BMI	Body mass index
BNP	B-natriuretic peptide
BP	Blood pressure
CABG	Coronary artery bypass grafting
CCDC	Consultant for communicable disease control
CCF	Congestive cardiac failure
CCU	Coronary care unit
CJD	Creutzfeldt–Jakob disease
CK	Creatinine kinase
CNS	Central nervous system
CO_2	Carbon dioxide
COHb	Carboxyhemoglobin
COPD	Chronic obstructive pulmonary disease
CPAP	Continuous positive airway pressure

CPR	Cardiopulmonary resuscitation
CRP	C-reactive protein
CSF	Cerebrospinal fluid
CT	Computed tomography
CTPA	CT pulmonary angiogram
CVA	Cerebrovascular accident
CVP	Central venous pressure
DC	Direct current (countershock)
DIC	Disseminated intravascular coagulopathy
DIGAMI	Diabetes Mellitus, Insulin Glucose Infusion in Acute Myocardial Infarction
DKA	Diabetic ketoacidosis
DNACPR	Do not attempt cardio-pulmonary resuscitation
DOACS	Direct acting oral anti-coagulants (also known as NOACs)
ECG	Electrocardiogram
ECT	Electroconvulsive therapy
EDTA	Ethylenediamine tetra-acetic acid
EMD	Electromechanical dissociation
ENT	Ear, Nose, and Throat
EPAP	Expiratory positive airway pressure
ERCP	Endoscopic retrograde cholangiopancreatogram
FBC	Full blood count
FFP	Fresh frozen plasma
FVC	Forced vital capacity
GHB	γ-Hydroxybutyric acid
GCS	Glasgow Coma Score
GI	Gastrointestinal
GKI	Glucose–potassium–insulin infusion
GTN	Glyceryl trinitrate
Hb	Haemoglobin
HbA$_{1c}$	Glycated haemoglobin
HBeAg	Hepatitis B e antigen
HBsAg	Hepatitis B surface antigen
HBV	Hepatitis B virus
HCO$_3$	Bicarbonate
HCV	Hepatitis C virus
HDU	High Dependency Unit
HIV	Human immunodeficiency virus
HONK	Hyperosmolar non-ketotic diabetic coma
HR	Heart rate
HUS	Haemolytic uremic syndrome

ICD	Implantable cardioverter-defibrillator
ICP	Intracranial pressure
IDDM	Insulin-dependent diabetes mellitus (i.e. Type I)
INR	International normalised ratio
IPAP	Inspiratory positive airway pressure
ITU	Intensive therapy unit
IV	Intravenous
JVP	Jugular venous pressure
KCCT	Kaolin cephalin clotting time
KCl	Potassium chloride
LFT	Liver function test
LMWH	Low-molecular-weight heparin
LP	Lumbar puncture
LTOT	Long-term oxygen therapy
LVF	Left ventricular failure
MCV	Mean corpuscular volume (size of the red cell)
MDAC	Multiple-dose activated charcoal
MDMA	3,4-Methylenedioxymethamphetamine
MDTB	Multidrug-resistant tuberculosis
MRC	Medical Research Council
MRI	Magnetic resonance imaging
MRSA	Methicillin-resistant *Staphylococcus aureus*
MSU	Midstream urine
MTS	Mental test score
NAPQI	*N*-acetyl-*p*-benzoquinoneimine
NG	Nasogastric
NEWS	National Early Warning Score
NIDDM	Non insulin-dependent diabetes mellitus (i.e. Type II)
NIV	Non-invasive ventilation
NSAIDs	Non-steroidal anti-inflammatory drugs
NSTEMI	Non-ST elevation myocardial infarction
NYHA	New York Heart Association
od	Once a day
PAAP	Personalised asthma action plan
PACI	Partial anterior circulation infarct
PCC	Prothrombin complex concentrate
PCI	Percutaneous coronary intervention
$p\text{CO}_2$	Carbon dioxide level (partial pressure)
PCR	Polymerase chain reaction
PE	Pulmonary embolism
PEA	Pulseless electrical activity

PERL	Pupils are equal and react to light
PFR	Peak flow rate
pH	A measure of acidity (low pH = high acidity)
PND	Paroxysmal nocturnal dyspnoea
pO_2	Oxygen level (partial pressure)
PPI	Proton pump inhibitor
p.r.n.	As required
PT	Prothrombin time
PVC	Polyvinyl chloride
qds	Four times a day
RR	Respiratory rate
rt-PA	Recombinant tissue plasminogen activator
SA node	Sinoatrial node
SARS	Severe acute respiratory syndrome
SBAR	Situation, Background, Assessment, Recommendation
SCD	Sudden cardiac death
SCRA	Synthetic cannabinoid receptor agonist
SHO	Senior house officer
SpO_2	Oxygen saturation
SOB	Shortness of breath
SRSV	Small round-structured virus
SSRI	Selective serotonin reuptake inhibitor
STEMI	ST elevation myocardial infarction
TACI	Total anterior circulation infarct
TB	Tuberculosis
tds	Three times a day
TIA	Transient ischaemic attack
TIPS	Transjugular intrahepatic portosystemic shunt
U&E	Urea and electrolytes
UTI	Urinary tract infection
VF	Ventricular fibrillation
VHF	Viral haemorrhagic fever
V/Q	Ventilation perfusion (isotope lung scan)
VT	Ventricular tachycardia
WCC	White cell count
WKS	Wernicke–Korsakoff syndrome

This book is a primer on acute medical care. It is designed for nurses, physician associates, medical students, and first-year doctors. In other words, anyone who is new to the challenges of emergency medical management. It aims to give the rationale behind the assessment and treatment of the conditions that you will encounter on the Acute Medical Unit. This is based on an understanding of the basic disease mechanisms, an understanding that is the key to a logical and systematic approach in dealing with what, at first sight, may appear dauntingly complex medical situations.

The outlook for these acute illnesses is often determined by our initial assessment and interventions–for this reason the book focuses on the management within the critical first 24 hours of admission.

Since the third edition, one of the major advances in the recognition and management of the acutely deteriorating patient has been widespread adoption of a standardised assessment method and documentation—NEWS2—based on every day clinical observations. The NEWS2 chart encourages the ABCDE approach to assessment and treatment. It provides clear thresholds for action, it simplifies the early identification of patients with sepsis and it encourages the correct use and monitoring of emergency oxygen therapy. Critically it also facilitates effective interprofessional communication.

Advice to the reader: refer to, and practice with, a NEWS2 observation chart, when reading the case histories. Have a BNF to hand to check drug doses and look up any unfamiliar drugs. Refer online to various scales and scoring systems to supplement the text. Refer to your own organisation's guidelines and protocols, for example on patient escalation, sepsis and COVID-19.

Please note the terms 0.9% saline, normal saline and isotonic saline refer to the same preparation. The terms dextrose infusion and glucose infusion mean the same thing and are used interchangeably.

The case histories are designed for illustrative purposes and are a composite of real case—updated where appropriate to emphasise the use of current guidelines.

Richard Harrison, MD, FRCP
Lynda Daly, RN, RM, RHV

CONTENTS

CHAPTER 1

Introduction: Immediate Assessment of the Critically Ill

This book is concerned with the recognition, assessment and management of acute medical patients during the first 24h of admission. The effectiveness of care during this time will have a major impact on both the immediate chances of survival and the long-term outlook. Delays in initiating treatment cost lives; this has long been known in acute myocardial infarction (the historical concept of 'door-to-needle' time) but is also the case in other conditions – notably, stroke and sepsis. The initial care of critically ill patients has to be targeted, timely and skilled.

To address this issue, the organisation of the medical care of critically ill patients has undergone a revolution in recent years. Interprofessional demarcation is being removed with the development of multidisciplinary teams. The clinicians within these teams have extended skills in the recognition and management of acutely ill medical patients. These teams have a number of overriding principles:

1. Core competencies in the management of the critically ill
2. Immediate access to appropriately skilled team members
3. Effective prioritisation – assessing and treating the sickest patients first
4. Emphasis on the immediate identification of patients who are critically ill, who are deteriorating or who are at risk of deterioration
5. Need to initiate appropriate corrective action and know whom to call for help and with what degree of urgency
6. Reduction in duplication of work such as multiple admission clerking

This process has been facilitated by the widespread adoption by the National Health Service (NHS) of the National Early Warning Score (NEWS and its successor NEWS2) based on simple clinical observations. NEWS identifies patients who require urgent intervention and who may need prompt detailed assessment from the medical staff or, increasingly, from a critical care team. Examples of such teams include medical emergency teams and nurse-led critical care outreach teams.

ABCDE: Immediate Assessment and Intervention

Immediate survival depends on urgent attention to the safety of the critically ill patient – the *A*irway, the *B*reathing, the *C*irculation. Subsequent progress depends on a more comprehensive assessment – by measuring *D*isability and *E*xposing the patient for detailed examination. This plan of immediate action based on the mnemonic ABCDE is a recurring theme in the book – emphasising the critical importance of urgent and effective resuscitation. Urgent initial treatment may have to proceed in the absence of a definite diagnosis. However, a detailed assessment will be necessary to make a comprehensive diagnosis and to plan subsequent management; this requires a history, an examination and an understanding of the underlying medical conditions. Each chapter therefore emphasises both the immediate safety of the patient and the nature, mechanisms and management of the underlying disease. The challenge for the clinician is to integrate this very technically demanding work with a humane and compassionate approach, combining modern clinical expertise with traditional caring skills.

This chapter gives an overview of the initial assessment and the early management, which will be necessary to ensure the patient's immediate survival. Fig. 1.1 provides a summary of the most urgent clinical observations – matched with the corrective interventions that may be necessary – and page references to relevant sections in the book. Detailed descriptions of resuscitation in specific conditions appear in later chapters.

It is important to develop a structured and systematic approach to immediate resuscitation. The focus should be on two fundamental issues: getting oxygen into the blood (*A*irway and *B*reathing) and getting blood (*C*irculation) to the brain and kidneys. The format for the initial assessment (Fig. 1.1) is based on the primary survey performed by first response teams such as the ambulance crew. It is found in the standard ABCDE system, in which the most important observations are performed first and the identified problems are rectified before moving on to the next stage. The primary survey is repeated when the patient is admitted to the ward; its structure ensures that the immediate safety of the patient continues to be addressed.

Subsequent progress is monitored from six physiological measurements obtained using standard clinical observations (the 'vital signs'):

Assessment	Possible interventions	Quick reference
Airway ☐ Clear ☐ Partial obstruction ☐ Obstruction ☐ Vomited & aspirated	Suction Chin lift/jaw thrust Guedel airway Bag, mask & valve Recovery position	105 ⎫ 113 ⎬ ABCDE 353 ⎭
Breathing ☐ Present ☐ Absent ☐ Rate	Oxygen	387 BLS 360 Oxygen 24 LVF
☐ 1 Normal ☐ 2 Deep ☐ 3 Shallow ☐ 4 Irregular	Bag, mask and valve	65 Asthma 84 COPD
☐ 5 Wheeze ☐ 6 Dyspnoea ☐ 7 Uneven chest movement ☐ 8 Unable to talk in full sentences	CPR	88 Pneumonia 258 PE
PFR ☐☐☐	Nebuliser	284 Self-harm 96 Pneumothorax
O₂ saturation ☐☐☐ on air ☐ on oxygen ☐	Physiotherapy Chest drain?	68 PFR 65 Oximetry
Circulation *Pulse* ☐ Present ☐ Absent ☐☐☐ Rate	CPR	386 CPR
☐ 1 ☐ 2 ☐ 3 ☐ 4 *Quality:* Reg Irreg Strong Weak	IV fluids	227 DKA 42 AF
Capillary refill ☐ <2 s ☐ >2 s		30 ⎫ 323 ⎬ Hypotension
Skin ☐ N ☐ P ☐ F ☐ B ☐ S ☐ C		351 Hypotensive collapse 367 Sepsis
Blood pressure ☐☐☐ / ☐☐☐		348 Shock 191 Acute abdomen
Temp ☐☐☐	Glucose	33 Acute chest pain
Blood loss (GI or haemoptysis) ☐☐☐ mL	IV antibotics	240 Hypoglycaemia 134 Meningitis 166 GI bleeding
Urine output ☐☐☐ 1st h ☐☐☐ 2nd h ☐☐☐ 3rd h	Fluid challenge	378 Acute kidney injury

FIGURE 1.1   Scheme for a structured approach to the initial assessment and early management of the critically ill patient. *ACVPU*, Alert, confusion, (reacts to) voice, pain, unresponsive; *AF*, atrial fibrillation; *BLS*, basic life support; *BP*, blood pressure; *COPD*, chronic obstructive pulmonary disease; *CPR*, cardio-pulmonary resuscitation; *CT*, computed tomography; *CVA*, cerebrovascular accident; *GCS*, Glasgow coma score; *GI*, gastrointestinal; *IV*, intravenous; *LVF*, left ventricular failure; *NG*, nasogastric; *PE*, pulmonary embolism; *PERL*, pupils equal and react to light; Skin: *N*, normal; *P*, pale; *F*, flushed: *B*, blue; *S*, sweaty; *C*, cold: *SpO₂*, oxygen saturation (oximeter); *TIA*, transient ischaemic attack.

Assessment		Possible interventions	Quick reference
Disability			
	A C V P U (□ □ □ □ □)	Secure airway	353 ABCDE
			332 Delirium
GCS	Eyes (4) Motor (6) Verbal (5) (□ □ □)	Correct hypotension (systolic >100)	365 Fluid challenge
BM Stix	<2 >30 (□ □ □□)	Oxygen	108 GCS
		Recovery position	112 ⎫ Coma 152 ⎭
Eyes	1.PERL 2.Dilated 3.Constricted R L (□ □) 4.Fixed	Glucose (Beware C-spine)	151 Seizures 240 Hypoglycaemia
Exposure			
Abdomen	Pain Y N (□ □)	NG intubation	
	1 2 3 (□ □ □) Soft Rigid Distended	Pain relief	93 ⎫ 126 ⎬ Aspiration 165 ⎭
Skin rash/ infected wounds	Y N (□ □)	Anaphylaxis ℞ • Adrenaline (epinephrine) • Steroids • Fluids	368 Anaphylaxis
CVA/TIA	Y N (□ □)		191 Acute abdomen
New deficit			
Speech	Y N (□ □)	Antibiotics Urgent CT	134 Meningitis
Facial palsy	Y N R L (□ □ □ □)	Hyperacute stroke pathway	117 Stroke
Weak arm Weak leg	(□ □ □ □) (□ □ □ □) Y N R L		

FIGURE 1.1, cont'd

- Respiratory rate   (**A**irway and **B**reathing)
- Oxygen saturation   (**A**irway and **B**reathing)
- Blood pressure   (**C**irculation)
- Pulse rate   (**C**irculation)
- Conscious level and new confusion   (**D**isability)
- Temperature   (**E**xposure)

Early Warning: Track and Trigger – NEWS and NEWS2

In response to the criticisms that critically ill medical patients are not recognised soon enough and that resuscitative measures are delayed, inadequate, or both, several tools have been developed that use the observation of vital signs to identify patients who are at risk. These tools, known as 'track and trigger' systems, are used to monitor progress (track) and provide specific criteria which, when met, trigger a call for assistance with a view for urgent corrective intervention. NEWS provides a 'common language' to describe the severity of an acutely unwell patient. The adoption of NEWS in all NHS emergency ambulance services and Accident and Emergency Departments therefore gives the acute admitting ward critical information on how a patient's condition is changing.

The aim is to prevent any patient from passing through an unrecognised yet potentially reversible period of instability and deterioration. The most common events preceding a cardiac arrest or transfer to an intensive therapy unit are a falling blood pressure and a reduction in the level of consciousness.

NEWS gives a weighted score to each of the six routine physiological observations. For example, a respiratory rate equal to or greater than 25 breaths/min scores 3 points whereas between 12 and 20 breaths/min scores 0. Scores from the observations at each point in time are added up, and the total (the aggregate score) is used to determine the action that the staff are required to take. An explicit protocol matches the aggregate score with the action that is required. The observations usually change together, so an active GI bleed, for example, raises the pulse and respiratory rate and drops the blood pressure. Adding up the scores rather than over-relying on a single parameter, such as the blood pressure, makes it much more likely that a significant deterioration will not be missed.

As the score increases, there is a graded escalation in the response. There are four grades of response – each representing a step change in outcome (mortality):

1. **Low** (NEWS 1–4)
   Response: Prompt assessment by a registered nurse, or equivalent, to increase observation frequency (to four hourly) or, if there is no improvement, to an escalation of care.
2. **A single score of 3 in any observation**
   Response: Urgent review by the ward doctor to determine the need to escalate care. Increase the frequency to hourly monitoring.
3. **Medium** (Total NEWS of 5–6)
   Response: This is the key trigger value for escalation. Urgent call to ward medical team and specified staff who have core competencies in acute illness management to respond within 60 minutes. Consider sepsis.
4. **High** (NEWS 7 and above)

Response: Emergency call to the critical care team/outreach services who are skilled in advanced airway management and resuscitation to attend within 30 minutes. Consider sepsis. If there is no improvement within an hour of activity, for senior review. The senior comes to the patient.

The immediate ward response to any patient in the medium- and high-risk groups is the application of ABCDE, a measurement of the capillary blood glucose and a review of the urine output/fluid balance. The subsequent management plan from the on-call team will implement the necessary interventions and list the required observations, their frequency and the criteria for further review.

In many units an important development has been the availability of nurse-led critical care outreach teams, which can react rapidly to deteriorating warning scores by advising and initiating early interventions, assessing the response and liaising with the high-dependency unit and intensive care.

Once the staff have acted and a management plan is in place, NEWS is used to monitor improvement and ensures that patients who do not improve are identified and reassessed within an explicit time frame.

Urine output and the NEWS are equally important in acute illness. Although not scored in NEWS, the urine output contributes to the graded responses and must be considered whenever nursing observations are made, and the aggregate NEWS is calculated.

Thus NEWS 0–4 with a low urine output (catheterised: less than 100 mL over 4 h; not catheterised: has not passed urine for 8 h) should be acted on.

If NEWS 5–6 with a low urine output: treat as high risk. This may have to be modified in some situations where the risk of kidney damage is high – for example, in an unstable patient a urine output of less than 0.5 mL/kg for two consecutive hours would justify an immediate medical review.

Clinical concern: the NEWS does not replace clinical acumen and, regardless of the score, if there is concern about the patient's condition, there should be a clinical response and, if needed, escalation. *A clinical emergency is treated the same way as a patient who is in the high-risk group.*

SOFT SIGNS

NEWS does not replace or demote clinical intuition. The 'gut feeling' of an experienced team member can trump a low NEWS score. The following may be 'soft' signs of deterioration and are particularly important in certain patient groups – notably the frail elderly and those with learning difficulties.

- A patient who looks or feels awful
- A change in behaviour
- A desire to be 'left alone'
- Sudden fatigue
- Loss of interest in food or fluid
- Concerned relatives or usual carers

ADDITIONAL MONITORING

The NEWS does not look at every aspect of a patient's deranged physiology. In specific circumstances, additional monitoring will be required – for example, biochemistry (lactate – sepsis, glucose – diabetes), peak flow (asthma), Glasgow coma scale score (medical coma, meningitis), blood gases (chronic obstructive pulmonary disease [COPD]), pain (acute coronary syndrome) and hourly urine output (acute kidney injury).

NEWS2: OXYGEN TREATMENT AND TARGET OXYGEN SATURATION

Important new guidelines for acute oxygen therapy stress that except in emergencies, oxygen must, like any other drug, be prescribed, and the prescription must include a target oxygen saturation for each patient. For most patients who require urgent oxygen treatment, the target saturation will be between 94% and 98% – these patients are scored in accordance with the NEWS chart, noting that all patients on oxygen receive 2 points automatically before taking their saturations into account. However, in some patients, notably those with advanced COPD and high carbon dioxide levels (type II respiratory failure), because saturations that are too high would depress their drive to breathe and may further increase their carbon dioxide levels and worsen the clinical situation, the target saturation will be lower, at 88%–92%. For these patients only, NEWS2 introduces a Scale 2 for oxygen saturations.

These patients score 2 points for their oxygen treatment but should not score for achieving their target saturations of 88%–92% (patients without COPD, who are on Scale 1, would score 3 points for saturations of 91% or less – triggering an urgent review).

There is an important issue with patients who have COVID-19 and need oxygen to maintain their target saturations. They will score 2 because of the need for oxygen, but an increase in the oxygen flow rate to correct a sudden fall in saturation (as can typically happen in COVID-19 pneumonitis) may not be captured by the NEWS score, yet it is a very significant event and should lead to an alert.

NEWS2: ABCDE AND ACVPU

The introduction of NEWS2 (Figs. 1.2 and 1.3), the most recent version of the NEWS chart (2018), is of major importance to the early recognition of, and the timely and capable response to, the deteriorating medical patient. Its layout mirrors and reinforces the ABCDE approach to assessment and treatment; it emphasises that a *NEWS of 5 or more* is the key threshold for urgent review and action and, in particular, should trigger the clinical question: Is this patient septic? New-onset confusion has been added to the AVPU assessment (now called ACVPU) as it is acknowledged that even as an isolated observation, new confusion identifies patients at risk of deterioration – as such it is given a score of 3.

FIGURE 1.2 National Early Warning Score 2 (NEWS2) chart. Reproduced from the Royal College of Physicians, 2017. National Early Warning Score (NEWS) 2: Standardising the assessment of acute-illness severity in the NHS. Updated report of a working party. RCP, London. Before making any clinical use of the NEWS2 chart, please download the high-quality, full-colour version from the Royal College of Physicians website: www.rcplondon.ac.uk/projects/outputs/national-early-warning-score-news-2.

Physiological parameter	Score						
	3	2	1	0	1	2	3
Respiration rate (per minute)	≤8		9–11	12–20		21–24	≥25
SpO₂ Scale 1 (%)	≤91	92–93	94–95	≤96			
SpO₂ Scale 2 (%)	≤83	84–85	86–87	88–92 ≥93 on air	93–94 on oxygen	95–96 on oxygen	≥97 on oxygen
Air or oxygen?		Oxygen		Air			
Systolic blood pressure (mm Hg)	≤90	91–100	101–110	111–219			≥220
Pulse (per minute)	≤40		41–50	51–90	91–110	111–130	≥131
Consciousness				Alert			CVPU
Temperature (°C)	≤35.0		35.1–36.0	36.1–38.0	38.1–39.0	≥39.1	

FIGURE 1.3   National Early Warning Score 2 (NEWS2) scoring grid. Reproduced from the Royal College of Physicians, 2017. National Early Warning Score (NEWS) 2: Standardising the assessment of acute illness severity in the NHS. Updated report of a working party. RCP, London. Before making any clinical use of the NEWS2 chart, please download the high-quality, full-colour version from the Royal College of Physicians website: www.rcplondon.ac.uk/projects/outputs/national-early-warning-score-news-2.

COMMUNICATION: NEWS2 AND SBAR

NEWS2 ensures patients receive timely interventions but, importantly, also provides a concise and standardised way to communicate a patient's condition to another health professional – particularly when calling for assistance with a deteriorating patient. To ensure effectiveness and consistency, the NEWS2 is given within an overall communication framework known as SBAR.

- **S**ituation: The reason I am calling is …
- **B**ackground: Admission date and diagnosis. History and comorbidity. Treatment.
- **A**ssessment: NEWS. Fluid balance. Current medication. Do not attempt cardiopulmonary resuscitation status.
- **R**ecommendation: I need you to … (level of urgency). Meanwhile, what should I do?

Conclusion

The correct use of NEWS and the response to trigger scores (notably 5 and above) should identify a patient who is at risk and ensure that the staff who are giving the care have the appropriate skills in the management of the critically ill. NEWS is an aid to assessment; it does not replace common sense or intuition ('there is something not quite right here'), and it does not acknowledge the need to intervene when there are distressing symptoms or unrelieved suffering. It also does not recognise the critical role of history taking or that of relatives in recognising change. **One of the most telling signs of the at-risk patient (and importantly an opportunity to escalate treatment before it is too late) is the next of kin who wants to see a doctor because of their increasing concerns over the deterioration of their relative's condition.**

Further Reading

Care of Deteriorating Patients. SIGN Guideline 167, 2023. Available from: https://www.sign. ac.uk/our-guidelines/care-of-deteriorating-patients/
National Early Warning Score (NEWS) 2: Standardising the Assessment of Acute-illness Severity in the NHS. Updated Report of a Working Party, 2017. Royal College of Physicians, London.

Cardiology

11

Introduction

Heart disease is the most common single cause of emergency medical admission. The majority of these cases will be the result of ischaemic heart disease and present with a history of chest pain, symptoms of heart failure or non-specific ill health caused by decompensated heart disease. Acute medical wards are neither equipped nor staffed appropriately to deal with patients who have suffered an acute myocardial infarction, in whom the priority is for immediate angioplasty. Therefore a patient with an obvious myocardial infarction, unstable angina or a serious rhythm disturbance will be admitted straight to the cardiac care unit (CCU).

In many cases, however, the diagnosis will not be clear-cut. This is particularly true in the elderly, in whom the presentation of acute cardiac problems ranges from sudden confusion to abdominal pain and vomiting. Often, the clinical picture may overlap with non-cardiac conditions. In the classic situation, it is difficult to differentiate cardiac and respiratory breathlessness in patients with the common combination of chronic obstructive pulmonary disease (COPD) and ischaemic heart disease. Other examples include abdominal symptoms in congestive cardiac failure (CCF) and cachexia with weight loss in advanced decompensated valvular heart disease.

All these patients will be admitted to the acute medical unit (AMU), where the expectation is that they will be assessed, diagnosed and appropriately treated with the minimum of delay. The patients, particularly those who are older than 75 years, frequently have several medical conditions, and when admitted, are receiving complex treatment regimens. It is often the case that cardiac problems complicate other diseases that themselves were the reason for admission; the patient with anaemia from GI blood loss who develops angina after admission is a typical example.

The task for the clinician is to perform an accurate assessment that takes into account both cardiac and non-cardiac aspects of the patient's medical history. The patient's problems must be prioritised; for example, increasing angina will take priority over a recent change in bowel habit, and attacks of nocturnal breathlessness will be more urgent to address than newly diagnosed but stable type 2 (non-insulin-dependent) diabetes.

The management of heart disease must be based on an understanding of the underlying conditions, particularly *ischaemic heart disease* (coronary artery disease), *cardiac failure* and *atrial fibrillation*. There have been important advances in the diagnosis and management of these conditions that have altered our approach to patients:

- Active management of myocardial infarction
  - The use of high-sensitivity troponin-T measurements and other parameters for risk stratification
  - Urgent re-perfusion by primary percutaneous coronary intervention (PCI) or thrombolytic therapy in acute myocardial infarction
  - Prophylactic anti-platelet therapy (aspirin and ticagrelor or clopidogrel)
  - β-Blockers and intensive lipid-lowering therapy with statins to improve long-term outlook
  - Referral of unstable patients for coronary artery bypass grafting (CABG) or angioplasty
- New approaches to cardiac failure
  - The use of angiotensin-converting enzyme (ACE) inhibitors (e.g., enalapril)
  - The use of low-dose β-blockers
  - New pacing and electrophysiological techniques
  - Effective antiarrhythmic drugs: amiodarone and flecainide
  - Early involvement from an outreach specialist heart failure team
  - Ensuring all patients with heart failure are established on ACE inhibitors, spironolactone and β-blockers before discharge
- Recognition of the frequency and significance of atrial fibrillation
  - Increased use of anticoagulation in atrial fibrillation
  - The widespread introduction of new direct oral anticoagulants (DOACs) as safe alternatives to warfarin
  - Routine use of ablation to reverse atrial fibrillation

This chapter aims to provide the basis for this understanding by looking at disease mechanisms and by providing a logical approach to the patient with possible heart disease.

Common Clinical Problems

ACUTE SEVERE BREATHLESSNESS

Acute severe breathlessness is a common problem in the AMU, but there is often a diagnostic dilemma in deciding between pulmonary oedema and asthma or COPD (see in Chapter 3, The Breathless Patient: The General Approach). This chapter looks at the mechanisms and causes of cardiac failure, which will put into context both the clinical features and the management strategy of the patient with pulmonary oedema or congestive failure.

CHEST PAIN AND ATYPICAL MYOCARDIAL INFARCTION

Various clinical problems associated with ischaemic heart disease—infarction, angina and silent myocardial ischaemia—will be described. The chapter aims to clarify the management of chest pain, in particular, how to assess the urgency of the situation in a new patient.

ATRIAL FIBRILLATION

Atrial fibrillation is the most common arrhythmia encountered in the emergency ward. It causes cardiac failure, syncope and unexplained dizziness and can complicate any severe febrile illness, such as pneumonia or exacerbations of COPD. Atrial fibrillation is a common cause of stroke and is one of the major indications for anticoagulant therapy. The management of atrial fibrillation encompasses the use of a good assessment technique, a working knowledge of modern cardiac drugs and the ability to recognise and deal with complications such as cardiac failure and angina in an acutely distressed and anxious patient.

IMMEDIATE RELEVANCE OF HEART DISEASE TO OTHER ACUTE MEDICAL CONDITIONS

When assessing an unstable patient with any acute medical condition, it is important to consider the risk posed by any coexisting cardiac problem to the safety of the patient:

- High risk
  - Recent myocardial infarction
  - Unstable angina
  - Cardiac failure
  - Rapid atrial fibrillation
  - Significant aortic valve disease
- Medium risk
  - Stable angina
  - Previous myocardial infarction
  - Previous cardiac failure
- Low risk
  - Poorly controlled hypertension
  - Previous CABG, but now asymptomatic
  - Angina, but comfortable at a normal walking speed

Any patient within the first category needs to be assessed immediately and with particular care, and there should be no hesitation in involving senior medical staff if problems arise. In contrast, the cardiac conditions in patients in the medium- and low-risk categories are less likely to be immediately relevant to an acute admission, particularly during the first 24 h of admission. Box 2.1 lists some key questions that arise in the treatment of patients with cardiac disease.

Core Clinical Skills

Application of triage using ABCDE (covered in Chapter 1). The essential skill is to establish the safety of the patient. As with any acute illness, this is based on basic observations of the vital signs. The immediate priority is to establish adequate oxygenation and an effective circulation. In pulmonary oedema, for example, the patient can be so ill that other clinical considerations are overshadowed by the need to administer oxygen and intravenous (IV) furosemide to save the patient's life.

Reassurance of acutely distressed and anxious patients. The patient will be acutely unwell, with a combination of unpleasant and frightening symptoms: severe breathlessness, chest pain, rapid irregular palpitations and overwhelming fatigue. Not surprisingly, cardiac patients are among the most frightened and anxious, and this will not be helped by hearing staff talk of heart 'failure' and 'unstable' angina. Anxiety worsens breathlessness, can exacerbate angina, and will put an extra load on the heart. Reassurance is vital, and this is best provided by team members who understand exactly what is wrong and why and who can explain the details of their management. It is easy to forget, for example, that patients who are having intensive clinical observations and complex tests carried out may feel very anxious that they are not being told what all this information means and whether they are in fact going to recover.

Resuscitation skills. Acute cardiac illness is characterised by rapid changes in the patient's condition. The most difficult problems encountered on the AMU are

---

BOX 2.1 ■ Critical Questions in the Understanding and Treatment of Patients With Cardiac Diseases

- Is this chest pain cardiac in origin?
- What is the difference between cor pulmonale and CCF?
- How do I approach acute dyspnoea in a patient with asthma with known heart disease?
- The pulse is 135 beats/min; what is the next step?
- Why is this patient cold, clammy and shut down?
- Why are nitrates used to treat angina as well as pulmonary oedema?
- Why can morphine be used for acute left ventricular failure but not for treating asthma?
- Does this patient need urgent medical attention?
- How can I make sense of this patient's drug regimen?
- What can I say to the relatives of this patient with acute pulmonary oedema?

fulminating pulmonary oedema with hypoxia and hypotension, and the unexpected cardiac arrest. It is therefore important that all the staff are fully trained in CPR and are familiar with the resuscitation equipment.

Coordinated care within the clinical team. There is considerable overlap between nursing and medical responsibilities in the care of patients with acute heart disease. The initial clinical assessment will include important diagnostic information such as the nature of the predominant symptoms and the identification of ischaemic chest pain. Subsequently, documentation of the trends in the vital signs, urine output and symptomatic improvement is the main way to evaluate the patient's response to treatment. It is important that all this information is shared constructively within the team and that the duplication of tasks such as history taking and observations is kept to the absolute minimum, both to save time and reduce the burden on the patient.

ANTICIPATING PROBLEMS

With experience backed by a good understanding of the underlying disease mechanisms, some problems can be anticipated and often forestalled. Obvious examples include hypotension that can complicate the use of several cardiac drugs, and the development of ischaemic chest pain in a patient who develops rapid atrial fibrillation. It can be extremely helpful to assess how the patient has responded to similar situations in the past by examining the hospital records and noting what the patient and their relatives have to say about it.

Cardiac Failure

There are two components to heart failure: the primary problem, which damages the function of the heart, and the secondary mechanisms, which are activated to try and compensate for the impaired cardiac function. These are summarised in Fig. 2.1.

Primary Problems in the Heart
HEART MUSCLE DAMAGE

The most common cause of chronic heart failure is heart muscle damage from myocardial ischaemia due to coronary artery disease. Most patients have a history of long-standing angina and recurrent myocardial infarctions, but a significant proportion of cases, particularly patients with diabetes, have unrecognised silent ischaemia that presents for the first time as cardiac failure. Hypertension is also an important cause of cardiac failure. The response to long-standing, uncontrolled hypertension is an increase in the bulk and strength of the heart muscle to drive blood out of the heart against the increased pressure. In time, however, the muscle fatigues and weakens, leading to reduced cardiac reserve and eventual failure.

FIGURE 2.1 The mechanisms and management of cardiac failure: an overview. Numbers in the management box refer to numbers in the figure. *ACE*, Angiotensin-converting enzyme; *CABG*, coronary artery bypass grafting.

Other causes of heart muscle disease are listed in Fig. 2.1. Of these, alcoholic cardiomyopathy is probably the most important, as it is common and will respond to the combination of alcohol withdrawal and thiamine (vitamin B) replacement.

VALVULAR DISEASE

Although not as common as heart muscle damage, valvular disease can lead to chronic cardiac failure that, with correct management, can be alleviated or controlled. Heart valves normally act as one-way doors, which ensure that blood can pass in only one direction when the heart contracts (systole). To continue the analogy with a door— as a result of damage (e.g., past rheumatic fever or a congenital fault in the valve's structure) the valve can become permanently stuck half-open (stenosis), in which case the heart has difficulty expelling blood through it. This has two important consequences: the heart may become overworked and blood may dam up behind the stenosed valve.

Alternatively, a valve can lose its one-way facility so that instead of being normally closed in either systole or diastole (depending on which valve is being considered), blood can pass through it throughout the cardiac cycle: this is known as valve incompetence or valve regurgitation. In valve incompetence/regurgitation, the affected chamber not only has its normal quota of blood to expel each beat, but it also has the added amount that comes back to it as a result of the leaking valve. Thus in mitral incompetence, during left ventricular contraction, blood leaves by the usual route into the aorta, but some blood is also forced back into the left atrium through the incompetent mitral valve. This blood then returns, along with the normal quota of blood, during the subsequent relaxation (diastole). In aortic incompetence, blood leaks back into the left ventricle during diastole, when the aortic valve should normally be closed. The left ventricle has to deal with this backflow in addition to the normal amount coming to it from the left atrium. In time the heart muscle fatigues, either because of the extra pressure it has to generate (e.g., in aortic valve stenosis) or because of the additional volume of blood it has to cope with (e.g., in mitral valve incompetence). This fatigue, in turn, in time leads to clinical cardiac failure.

RHYTHM DISTURBANCE

Abnormally slow (bradyarrhythmias) or, more commonly, abnormally fast (tachyarrhythmias) cardiac rhythms can result in heart failure. A slow pulse leads to a fall-off in cardiac output, simply because the heart beats less often per minute. A healthy heart compensates for a slow pulse by having more time to fill before each contraction; the heart chamber responds to such stretching by producing a more forceful contraction, expelling an increased amount of blood. A diseased heart is unable to respond in this way, so a reduced heart rate causes a reduced cardiac output. Fast rhythms disrupt the events that occur during diastole—filling of the heart chambers and blood flow down the coronary arteries. Once again, a healthy heart can cope with a rapid rate, but a diseased heart can soon be compromised, particularly if the coronary arteries are narrowed. The most common rhythm disturbance to cause or contribute to cardiac failure is uncontrolled atrial fibrillation, in which the rate is both rapid and irregular. The onset of rapid atrial fibrillation can often trigger acute heart failure.

Secondary Compensatory Mechanisms in Cardiac Failure

In response to the basic problem of *reduced cardiac output*, two compensatory mechanisms are activated to try and maintain normal blood pressure:

1. Increased sympathetic nervous system activity (exaggerated stress reaction)
2. Activation of the renin–angiotensin–aldosterone hormone system (salt and water retention)

These two mechanisms, respectively, *increase the narrowing of the peripheral arterioles* and *increase thecirculating blood volume*—a strategy designed to keep the blood pressure up and maintain a good blood supply to the kidneys. Although this may work for a while, ultimately it leads to an increased load against which the heart must pump (in the case of the narrowed arterioles) and pulmonary congestion and ankle oedema (in the case of the increased circulating blood volume). Pumping against an abnormally high load eventually leads to heart muscle fatigue, the so-called pump failure or 'forward' heart failure (low blood pressure and poor organ perfusion). Conversely, the congestive component is known as 'backward' failure (pulmonary and peripheral oedema). These two components of cardiac failure are summarised in Fig. 2.2.

Modern management of cardiac failure aims to reverse these mechanisms by decreasing the resistance against which the heart must pump and unloading the congestion behind the failing heart. As shown in Fig. 2.3, this is achieved by:

- Dilating the arterioles (e.g., glyceryl trinitrate [GTN], isosorbide mononitrate, hydralazine),
- Reducing the salt and water retention (e.g., furosemide and bumetanide),
- Inhibiting the renin–angiotensin–aldosterone system (ACE inhibitors, angiotensin receptor blockers, aldosterone antagonists),
- Reducing sympathetic activity—the cautious use of sympathetic blockade (β-blockers), for example, bisoprolol

IMPORTANT BIOMARKERS OF CARDIAC FAILURE: B-NATRIURETIC PEPTIDE AND NT-PROBNP

When the ventricles are put under strain and begin to fail, the cardiac muscle cells release the hormone known as B-natriuretic peptide (BNP). BNP enters the circulation where it (or its close relative NT-proBNP) can be measured from a simple blood sample. BNP acts as an 'internal' anti-failure mechanism:

- It inhibits the increased sympathetic drive.
- It inhibits the renin–angiotensin–aldosterone system.
- It promotes the renal loss of water and salt.

There are two important clinical implications. First, the blood test can help diagnose cardiac failure and is particularly helpful in patients in whom the underlying cause

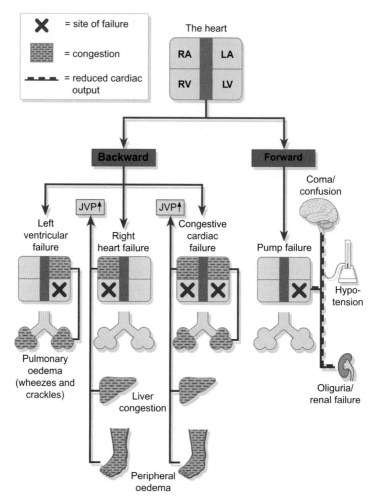

FIGURE 2.2 The two components (backward and forward) of cardiac failure. *JVP*, Jugular venous pressure; *LA*, left atrium; *LV*, left ventricle; *RA*, right atrium; *RV*, right ventricle.

of their acute breathlessness is unclear. Normal BNP levels (less than 100 pg/mL) or NT-proBNP levels (less than 300 pg/mL) in a patient with acute severe breathlessness rule out cardiac failure as the underlying cause. Second, drugs with the same chemical properties, such as BNP, are being developed to exploit their effects on reversing the underlying mechanisms of cardiac failure.

THE SPECIALIST HEART FAILURE TEAM

Hospitals should now provide an outreach team to optimise the management of heart failure:

- Based on the cardiology ward with a nurse-led outreach service

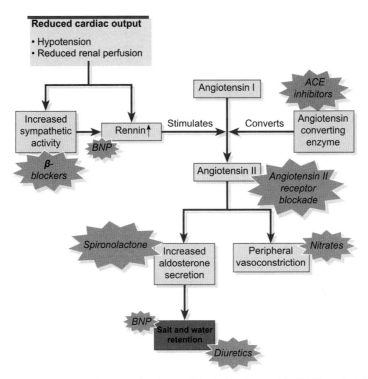

FIGURE 2.3 Further details of the mechanisms of B-natriuretic peptide (BNP) and of drug treatments in cardiac failure. *ACE*, Angiotensin-converting enzyme.

- Early and continuing involvement with patients with acute heart failure
- Advise on interventions, for example, when to introduce low-dose β-blockers/ ACE inhibitors
- Early outpatient assessment after discharge (2 weeks) with intensive up-titration of treatment over 6 weeks

Types of Heart Failure
LEFT-SIDED HEART FAILURE
In left-sided heart failure, the clinical problem is dominated by the buildup of fluid in the lungs because the failing left ventricle cannot cope with the increased circulating blood volume—blood dams up behind the left side of the heart, producing pulmonary congestion and pulmonary oedema. The symptoms of left-sided heart failure include:

- Breathlessness on lying flat (orthopnoea)
- Paroxysmal nocturnal dyspnoea (PND)
- Coughing frothy pink sputum (pulmonary oedema)

RIGHT-SIDED HEART FAILURE

In right-sided heart failure, the right ventricle cannot cope with the increased circulating blood volume and blood dams up in the veins, leading to liver congestion, ankle oedema and oedema over the sacrum. The symptoms of right-sided heart failure include:

- Swollen ankles
- Liver discomfort
- Abdominal swelling (ascites)

CONGESTIVE CARDIAC FAILURE

In CCF, there is a combination of left- and right-sided failure, giving a constellation of symptoms that include:

- Breathlessness
- Fatigue
- Pulmonary and ankle oedema

RIGHT HEART FAILURE AND CHRONIC OBSTRUCTIVE PULMONARY DISEASE

Many patients with acute exacerbations of COPD complain about the recent development of ankle oedema that coincided with the worsening of their chest symptoms. This is the result of the development of cor pulmonale—right-sided heart failure due to lung disease. The simplest explanation is that the right side of the heart has to do extra work to force blood through pulmonary arterioles that are abnormally narrow because of the low oxygen levels found in COPD (hence the benefit of long-term oxygen in selected patients with severe COPD).

DIASTOLIC HEART FAILURE

Diastolic heart failure is a newly recognised condition which may account for a fifth or more cases of cardiac failure. Typically seen in elderly, obese, hypertensive and diabetic females, diastolic failure results from an abnormally hypertrophied and stiffened ventricle, which contracts well enough but in diastole cannot relax sufficiently to accommodate returning blood. The symptoms—pulmonary and peripheral oedema—are the same as in other forms of failure; the diagnosis relies on the characteristic changes on an echocardiogram. The management is similar to the other forms of heart failure.

Echocardiography

Patients with suspected heart failure must have an echocardiogram within 48 h of admission—to assess heart muscle function and to look for valve disease.

Clinical Features and Management of Cardiac Failure

CHARACTERISTICS OF PATIENTS ADMITTED ACUTELY WITH CARDIAC FAILURE

In general, patients with heart failure comprise an elderly group of patients, with an average age of around 75 years and with a strong preponderance of ischaemic heart disease—half will have had a previous infarct. At least half of all these patients will be in atrial fibrillation, and for about a tenth the heart failure will have been triggered by their first attack of atrial fibrillation. One-third will also have COPD, and a fifth will be diabetic. In the majority, around 80%, the cause of the failure will be associated with poor heart muscle function; valve problems will only be seen in about 10% of the patients.

It can be helpful to characterise the patient's pre-existing level of disability. The New York Heart Association (NYHA) classification is the one most commonly used:

- **Class I**—no limitations (no fatigue, breathlessness or palpitations)
- **Class II**—slight limitations, fine at rest, but ordinary exertion leads to symptoms
- **Class III**—marked limitations, fine at rest, but symptoms on less than ordinary exertion
- **Class IV**—symptoms at rest

Patients in NYHA classes III and IV have a poor outlook, with 5-year mortality rates approaching 50%.

PRINCIPLES OF MANAGING CARDIAC FAILURE

- Management is based first on trying to correct the primary underlying problem:
  - Improving the coronary artery circulation (drugs, angioplasty, CABG)
  - Correcting any valve abnormality (valve repair and replacement)
  - Treating an abnormal heart rhythm (e.g., controlling atrial fibrillation with digoxin)
- In addition, or as an alternative, the compensatory mechanisms that are responsible for the clinical picture of chronic cardiac failure are addressed:
  - Reducing fluid retention (diuretics)
  - Reducing the load on the heart (vasodilators)
  - Counteracting excessive sodium retention (ACE inhibitors such as enalapril, angiotensin receptor blockers such as losartan)
  - Counteracting increased sympathetic activity (low-dose β-blockers)
    There is an obvious risk in correcting what are supposed to be compensatory mechanisms—in particular, over-diuresis and excessive use of vasodilators can produce hypotension, with a worsening of tissue perfusion (characterised by deteriorating kidney function).
- Using SGLT2 inhibitors to reduce the circulating fluid volume
- Device therapy

Cardiac resynchronisation therapy ('Device therapy'): In some patients with cardiac failure, delayed electrical activation of the left ventricle (recognised on an ECG by the pattern of left bundle branch block) produces a disjointed and inefficient cardiac contraction. If severely impaired, the contractile state can be resynchronised and improved using a novel permanent pacemaker which, unlike conventional pacemakers, paces the left as well as the right ventricle. This technique, termed dual-chamber pacing, will have an increasing role in selected cases of chronic cardiac failure, although the effects on quality of life surpass those on actual survival.

Implantable cardioverter-defibrillators (ICDs): Patients with heart failure are at least six times more likely to die suddenly than the general population. In carefully selected patients (e.g., severe failure and cardiac arrest survivors), ICDs are fitted to reduce mortality by treating any lethal ventricular arrhythmia.

Left ventricular assist devices: Introduced as a bridge to heart transplantation, this is a battery-powered pump fitted surgically between the left ventricle and aorta, which acts as a 'second heart'. With the advent of miniature devices which can be inserted percutaneously on a temporary basis, they will be used increasingly in very severe heart failure, even in patients ineligible for transplantation—a 'bridge to recovery'.

ACUTE LEFT VENTRICULAR FAILURE

Acute left ventricular failure (LVF) (Fig. 2.4) is a common cause of acute life-threatening breathlessness (the others being acute asthma, tension pneumothorax and pulmonary embolism). Case Study 2.1 illustrates the typical picture of heart failure due to ischaemic heart disease. Interestingly, the patient did not receive an ACE inhibitor after his infarct; these are now given routinely as post-infarct prophylaxis to lessen the risk of developing heart failure. The patient was given IV opiates and nitrates. Current guidelines stress that opiates and nitrates are no longer to be used routinely in acute heart failure. Opiates are now used only if there is chest pain or severe anxiety. Nitrates are reserved for diuretic-resistant congestion in the presence of normal or high blood pressure.

Critical Clinical Tasks in Acute Left Ventricular Failure

Ensure the patient is adequately oxygenated. Patients in acute LVF die of hypoxia due to pulmonary oedema. Therefore the safest practice is to start with high-flow oxygen or a non-rebreathing mask, aiming to give the patient at least 60% oxygen. This can be modified based on the oxygen saturation or blood gas measurements. The target oxygen saturation is between 94% and 98%. Patients must be propped upright—even if they are hypotensive. Their symptoms will improve because pulmonary oedema lessens in the sitting position.

Continuous positive airway pressure (CPAP) and high-flow nasal oxygen in acute LVF. Acute pulmonary oedema with resistant hypoxia, which is unresponsive to

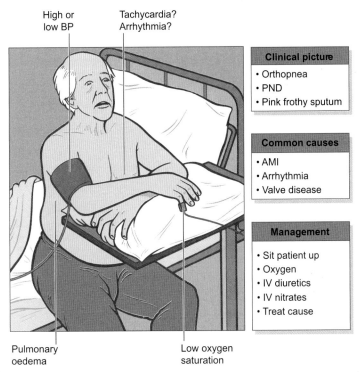

High or
low BP

Tachycardia?
Arrhythmia?

Clinical picture

- Orthopnea
- PND
- Pink frothy sputum

Common causes

- AMI
- Arrhythmia
- Valve disease

Management

- Sit patient up
- Oxygen
- IV diuretics
- IV nitrates
- Treat cause

Pulmonary
oedema

Low oxygen
saturation

FIGURE 2.4 Acute left ventricular failure. *AMI*, Acute myocardial infarction; *BP*, blood pressure; *PND*, paroxysmal nocturnal dyspnoea.

high-flow oxygen and diuretics, may respond to short-term (2-h) treatment with CPAP, often given with high-flow nasal oxygen.

Non-invasive ventilation with bilevel positive airway pressure (BiPAP) is only used if there is pulmonary oedema causing severe breathlessness and an acidosis on blood gases (denoting severe cardiorespiratory insufficiency). In extreme severity, full intensive therapy unit ventilation may be necessary.

Measure the Patient's Blood Pressure

Hypertension. Many patients with LVF become acutely hypertensive as a stress response; the blood pressure settles as their condition improves. Less commonly, hypertension is believed to be the cause, rather than the effect, of a patient's LVF. In such cases, it is usually severe (e.g., 210/140 mm Hg) and persistent and has to be lowered as part of the patient's immediate management. Fortunately, some of the drugs used to treat LVF, such as nitrates and diuretics, have a dual effect: they both eliminate pulmonary oedema and reduce the blood pressure.

Hypotension. Hypotension in the setting of LVF is an unfavourable sign, particularly if the blood pressure remains low after any abnormal cardiac rhythm has been corrected. It can indicate heart muscle damage; it limits the type and quantity of drugs that can

CASE STUDY 2.1	Left Ventricular Function due to Ischaemic Heart Disease

A 62-year-old male with a previous myocardial infarct was admitted with a 3-week history of increasing breathlessness. He had no other illnesses and was only taking low-dose aspirin. His blood pressure on admission was 180/120 mm Hg, the ECG showed heart strain and the chest film showed LVF. Urine testing showed proteinuria. His kidney function was normal.

The initial assessment was of a distressed and overweight male with a resting pulse of 120 beats/min which felt regular, a respiratory rate of 35 breaths/min with an audible wheeze, oxygen saturation on air of 85% and a blood pressure of 180/120 mm Hg. His peripheries were cold and clammy, and capillary refill time was prolonged. He complained of breathlessness but no chest pain.

The patient was propped upright and given high-flow oxygen with a reservoir mask; an intravenous cannula was inserted, and blood was taken, primarily to check the kidney function, cardiac enzymes, BNP, sugar and blood count. Arterial blood gases were checked. An ECG monitor to identify arrhythmias and an oximeter to confirm adequate oxygenation (target saturation 94%–98%) were attached to the patient. He was given:
- IV furosemide 80 mg
- IV diamorphine 2.5 mg
- Cyclizine as an antiemetic

Oxygen saturation increased to 94%, and the respiratory rate decreased to 25 breaths/min; his pulse remained high at 120 beats/min. The patient passed 1 L of urine in the first 1 h of admission but remained breathless. Bendroflumethiazide 2.5 mg was added orally.

An infusion of GTN was started, and plans were made for a trial of an ACE inhibitor. An urgent cardiac echocardiogram was requested. Thromboembolism prophylaxis with low-molecular-weight heparin (LMWH) was administered.

be used—because several cause hypotension themselves—and it can put kidney function at risk. Persistent hypotension is an indication of the need for inotropic support (drugs such as dopamine, which improve cardiac performance), particularly if the urine output is inadequate. Increasingly, ventricular assist devices (a 'second heart') are used as a bridge to transplantation or an anticipated recovery.

Evaluate the patient's pulse rate. The analysis of the patient's pulse rate is not easy from bedside observation, particularly if the patient is acutely ill, and a monitor and 12-lead ECG will be required. Nonetheless, atrial fibrillation (or its close relation, atrial flutter) is likely to be the cause of any rapid pulse of greater than 130 beats/min.

Occasionally, LVF can be accompanied by, and even caused by an abnormally slow pulse. Drug treatment, in particular with β-blockers, can be an important cause of this. The bradycardia resolves once the drug is withdrawn. Although low-dose β-blockers are now a mainstay of long-term treatment of heart failure, they are only introduced once the patient is stable and has a pulse rate of greater than 50 beats/min.

CRITICAL CLINICAL TASKS IN ACUTE LEFT VENTRICULAR FUNCTION
- Ensure adequate oxygenation
- Measure the blood pressure
- Evaluate the pulse

Important Clinical Tasks in Acute Left Ventricular Failure

Does the patient understand and comply with the oxygen therapy? Ensure that the patient understands the need for continuous (as opposed to symptomatic) oxygen administration. Is this reflected by appropriate improvements in the oxygen saturation?

Has the patient responded to the diuretic? An immediate diuresis is a good prognostic sign, whereas failure to establish a diuresis, especially if it is accompanied by hypotension, suggests a problem with maintaining blood flow through the kidneys. The aim in acute heart failure would be an initial daily diuresis of 3 L or more. In practical terms, this equates to a urine output of 100 to 150 mL/h during the first 6 h of treatment.

It is important to exclude retention as a cause of low output, particularly in older male patients. It is a common practice to obtain an exact assessment of the urine output in critically ill patients by using a urethral catheter. The patient's weight and kidney function must also be monitored during intensive diuretic therapy.

Is the patient less breathless and in a better clinical condition? As the treatment takes effect, the patient should become less breathless; they will be less distressed and their respiratory rate will decrease.

As the heart picks up, the peripheral circulation will also improve: extremities will be less clammy, and the feet and hands will warm up—the capillary filling should also improve.

IMPORTANT CLINICAL TASKS IN ACUTE LEFT VENTRICULAR FAILURE

- Ensure compliance with continuous oxygen
- Assess the response to diuretics
- Look for symptomatic improvement
- Demonstrate normalisation of the pulse and blood pressure
- Falling aggregate National Early Warning Score 2 (NEWS2)

Acute myocardial infarction can present as acute LVF, and chest pain may be ignored in the presence of severe breathlessness. It is therefore important to enquire specifically about pain and ensure that appropriate analgesia—morphine or diamorphine—is prescribed.

Have the blood pressure and pulse returned towards normal? Stress-induced hypertension should fall. Hypotension, unless it is the inevitable consequence of the drugs that are needed, should improve, either in response to inotropic support or spontaneously as the patient's general condition improves. Similarly, a rapid pulse should return towards normal, as a result of specific treatment (digoxin, cardioversion, etc.) or as a general response to overall improvement.

ACUTE ON CHRONIC CONGESTIVE CARDIAC FAILURE

The main clinical features of acute on chronic CCF are bilateral ankle oedema, debilitating tiredness and breathlessness on exertion (Fig. 2.5). The dominant problem is usually a progressive reduction in exercise tolerance, but in advanced failure, there is

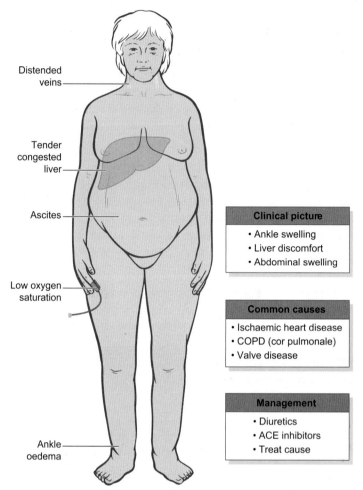

Distended veins

Tender congested liver

Ascites

Low oxygen saturation

Ankle oedema

Clinical picture
- Ankle swelling
- Liver discomfort
- Abdominal swelling

Common causes
- Ischaemic heart disease
- COPD (cor pulmonale)
- Valve disease

Management
- Diuretics
- ACE inhibitors
- Treat cause

FIGURE 2.5   Acute on chronic congestive cardiac failure. *ACE*, Angiotensin-converting enzyme; *COPD*, chronic obstructive pulmonary disease.

overwhelming fatigue: patients can be too tired to eat, they cannot cope with personal care and even mild constipation can prove a serious challenge. Patients are often increasingly dependent and depressed, sleep patterns are disturbed (frequent arousals are a consequence of Cheyne–Stokes respiration and paroxysmal nocturnal breathlessness) and the appetite is poor. Cardiac cachexia is a state of malnutrition caused by a combination of anorexia and impaired food absorption in advanced cardiac failure. Weight loss is often accompanied by abdominal pain and swelling due to liver congestion and ascites. Nausea and vomiting can have the same cause but are also seen in both hypovolaemia and diuretic-induced electrolyte disturbances, particularly hyponatraemia (low sodium).

IMPORTANT CLINICAL TASKS IN CONGESTIVE CARDIAC FAILURE

Identify Possible Causes of Cardiac Failure

Uncontrolled hypertension. Hypertension in the range of 160/110 mm Hg or higher can lead to cardiac failure but unfortunately may be ignored or inadequately treated. Contrary to earlier views, systolic and diastolic hypertension are equally damaging— treatment is started at sustained levels of 140–160 mm Hg systolic or 90–100 mm Hg diastolic. If hypertension is identified, the urine should be checked for protein (hypertensive kidney damage) and a family history should be taken to identify familial kidney diseases (especially polycystic kidneys) and unexplained hypertension. Is the patient's hypertension compounded by the presence of the other main cardiac risk factors: smoking, high cholesterol or diabetes? What is the HbA1c and the capillary glucose?

IMPORTANT CLINICAL TASKS IN CONGESTIVE CARDIAC FAILURE

- Identify possible causes of cardiac failure
- Establish the *exact* preadmission drug regimen
- Recognise significant hypotension
- Assess the lower limbs and pressure areas
- Assess the fluid balance

Ischaemic heart disease. A history of a previous infarct, angina or intermittent claudication makes it very likely that the basis for the cardiac failure is ischaemia.

Alcohol-induced cardiac failure. Chronic alcohol abuse often leads to heart muscle damage. The importance of recognising this lies in the good response that is seen with a change in lifestyle and treatment with vitamin replacements.

Chronic rheumatic valve disease. Forty years ago, rheumatic fever with cardiac involvement was common in adolescents in the United Kingdom. These patients are now in their 80s, with ageing valve replacements, chronic cardiac failure, complex drug regimens and extensive hospital notes. Hospital records make extremely interesting reading in these patients and are a useful starting point.

Often, the patient's current problems have been encountered and solved before and will have been documented fully. Examples may include:

- Previous episodes of cardiac failure with a documented cause (e.g., attempting to reduce diuretics).
- Previous episodes of renal insufficiency triggered by drug interactions (in particular the use of nonsteroidal anti-inflammatory drugs [NSAIDs]).
- The results of a previous ACE inhibitor trial (in general, the nursing notes give a more detailed account of individual problem episodes during a patient's stay than do the medical notes).

- Previous experience with recurrent arrhythmias and their management.
- Previous problems with anticoagulant control due to intercurrent illness, antibiotic administration or some other drug interactions.

Establish the exact preadmission drug regimen. Patients with chronic heart failure are usually receiving complicated drug regimens that have undergone serial changes as the clinical condition changes. The general practitioner and the hospital clinic may have been adjusting the drugs independently, so hospital letters and so forth may not reflect the actual situation. Even the instructions on the drug containers may not coincide with what the patient really takes. Important drug toxicity and interactions are common and often unrecognised. Examples include:

- Digoxin toxicity, especially in the elderly
- Warfarin overactivity due to antibiotic treatment or worsening CCF
- Electrolyte imbalance from diuretic therapy
- Worsening heart failure due to the use of NSAIDs
- Dangerous hyperkalaemia with spironolactone, particularly when combined with ACE inhibitors in patients with diabetes

Recognise significant hypotension. Hypotension is common and important in patients with acute on chronic CCF: a reduced blood flow to the brain and kidneys causes lethargy, near syncope and renal failure. The two most common causes of hypotension are *fluid depletion* and *drug therapy*. Fluid depletion may be caused by:

- Over-diuresis
- Vomiting and poor intake due to congestion of the GI tract and liver
- 'Concealed' GI bleeding (patients are usually receiving aspirin/warfarin)

Diuretics, nitrates, ACE inhibitors and virtually all antiarrhythmic drugs can induce postural hypotension, as can other classes of drugs that may have been 'added in', notably, any antidepressant.

In any cardiac patient with low blood pressure, it is also critical to exclude two other causes: *sepsis* and *acute myocardial infarction*. The most common sources of infection are cannulation sites, the respiratory tract (ask the patient to cough and inspect the sputum) and the urine. A rare but serious source of sepsis in these patients is infection of the heart valves (endocarditis). An unrecognised infarct may produce a combination of heart failure and hypotension, which will usually be diagnosed from the ECG and cardiac enzyme results.

Assess the lower limbs and pressure areas. Oedematous legs and poor cardiac output are potent causes of poor skin nutrition, soft tissue infection and damage to pressure areas, particularly in immobile elderly patients. In severe congestive failure, the legs may be blistered and weeping fluid, frequently on a background of chronically inflamed and eczematous ankles and calves. The feet should be examined with care because the poor blood supply and impaired nutrition can lead to fungal infections between the toes (soggy, inflamed-looking skin) and even areas of local gangrene. Early dermatological advice can be extremely useful in these situations. Patients who are immobile and oedematous develop oedema over the sacrum and are very susceptible to pressure sores. This area must be assessed with care so that appropriate pressure-relieving measures can be introduced.

Assess the fluid balance. This is a problematic area of management in patients with cardiac failure because it is difficult to maintain the balance between removing unwanted fluid from congested lungs while retaining enough fluid to support the circulation. The admission assessment will help to differentiate fluid overload from diuretic-induced fluid depletion.

- **Symptoms of congestion**—breathlessness, PND, orthopnoea, abdominal discomfort, weight gain
- **Signs of congestion**—increased respiratory rate, ankle oedema, abdominal distension (ascites)
- **Symptoms of fluid depletion**—thirst, nausea, lethargy, postural dizziness, weight loss
- **Signs of fluid depletion**—postural hypotension, poor capillary refill, poor urine output

The clinical decision of whether to increase or withhold diuretics and whether to restrict or push fluids depends on these basic observations in conjunction with the biochemistry results, particularly the levels of sodium, creatinine and urea. Low sodium is seen with both diuretic-induced fluid depletion and fluid overload, but only in fluid depletion will there be a progressive increase in urea and creatinine.

SPECIALIST INPUT

Advanced treatments may be required in difficult cases—those with diuretic resistance, particularly associated with congestion, worsening renal function and persistent hypotension. Techniques include emergency left ventricular assist devices (intra-aortic balloon counter-pulsation) and ultrafiltration—a portable and simplified version of dialysis used to remove salt and fluid from the patient's circulation without the need to compromise renal function by giving escalating doses of diuretics.

Answering Patients' and Relatives' Questions in Cardiac Failure

What does 'failure' mean? The heart has been put under temporary strain as a result of infection/angina/blockage of the heart's circulation. As a result it has become a less efficient pump. We are therefore trying to take the strain off the heart with a variety of drugs, bed rest and oxygen.

What will be the signs of improvement? Observations such as pulse rate and blood pressure will start to return towards normal. The patient will become less breathless. There will be an increase in urine output as we get rid of some of the excess fluid in the lungs and legs.

How can we help? The patient needs complete rest—keep visitors to a minimum to start with. Encourage the patient to keep the oxygen on at all times and to stay propped up in bed. Fluids are likely to be rationed for a time.

What about the diet and fluid intake once the patient is discharged? Salt-rich foods should be avoided, and salt should not be on the table or in the cooking. The main salt-rich foods are cheese, crisps, bacon, sausages and processed meat foods such as pies. Fluid intake is not usually restricted unless persistent fluid retention becomes a particular problem.

What about weight? If there is obesity, aim for a reduction of around 2 lb (1 kg) or so per week towards a realistic target. Weight gain can be the first sign of fluid retention (worsening heart failure), and regular weighing can be very helpful as part of the patient's follow-up care.

Provide small frequent meals (perhaps with calorie supplements if there is cachexia) and consider water-soluble vitamin supplements (B complex and C). Alcohol may be taken in moderation unless there is an alcoholic cardiomyopathy.

What about smoking? Smoking must be stopped immediately.

What about exercise? Regular non-tiring exercise should be encouraged. 'Reconditioning' with regular graded exercise will help to improve endurance in some patients with cardiac failure. This probably needs to be supervised in some form of hospital-based programme.

Addressing compliance problems. Lack of compliance is a major factor in triggering readmissions in cardiac disease, especially in the elderly who are often on complex regimens. Side effects, notably constipation, anorexia and confusion, make the drugs unpopular with the patients, and this may be compounded by forgetfulness. It is therefore vital to discuss details of the patient's regimen with the relatives and carers.

Ischaemic Heart Disease

More patients present to the AMU with the consequences of ischaemic heart disease than with any other single condition. Atheromatous narrowing of the coronary arteries leads to cardiac failure, angina, myocardial infarction and cardiac arrhythmias (Fig. 2.6). Fortunately, the combination of improved treatment for established disease and the widespread introduction of preventative measures has reduced mortality from coronary artery disease by 10% in the past decade. However, cardiac ischaemia continues to present major issues for the AMU: recognising its various manifestations (heart failure, chest pain, arrhythmias), dealing with atypical clinical features in the elderly and identifying those patients who need urgent coronary care.

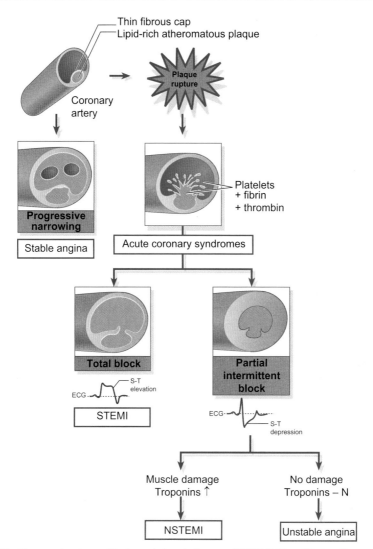

FIGURE 2.6 The mechanisms of ischaemic heart disease. *NSTEMI*, Non-ST-elevation myocardial infarction; *STEMI*, ST-elevation myocardial infarction.

Chest Pain

APPROACH TO THE PATIENT WHO HAS CHEST PAIN ON THE ACUTE MEDICAL UNIT

Context

Chest pain in a patient with a history of angina, previous myocardial infarction or any serious cardiovascular disease should be assumed to come from the heart until proven otherwise. Whereas pain in a young male with a recent chest infection and no risk factors is

CASE STUDY 2.2	Myocardial Infarction in the Acute Medical Unit

CASE 1

A 75-year-old female presented with acute sweating, malaise and mild heartburn. She denied chest pain. The ECG was done on admission but not seen for several hours: it showed an acute inferior myocardial infarction. Patients with an atypical history slip through the net. On a CCU, the emphasis is on urgent re-vascularisation for the true infarcts. In the AMU, there will be delays because, by their nature, these patients are atypical. A system of triage is needed.

CASE 2

A 90-year-old female awoke with a left-sided stroke. She was alert and denied any chest pain. Her ECG showed a recent inferior infarction and her cardiac enzymes were elevated.

likely to be pleurisy, in the case of an elderly female with a recent fall and vertebral collapse, chest pain is as likely to be referred from the back as it is to be angina. The situation in which the pain arises is as important as the nature of the pain in establishing the diagnosis.

Chest pain can be so difficult to describe that it is preferable to be overcautious in your management. After all, if the history was crystal clear, the patient would not be in the AMU in the first place (Case Study 2.2), but in the CCU. This seems to be a particular issue in female patients and in patients from ethnic minorities in whom, for some reason, cardiac symptoms are all too often dismissed as insignificant, leading to diagnostic delays.

Onset

Classically, angina builds up over a few minutes into a dull, heavy, central chest ache and spreads into the jaw, upper arm, or wrists. It is *not* usually localised to a single spot on the chest or associated with local tenderness; however, the so-called 'atypical angina' can be positional, worsened by breathing and may even radiate through into the back and to the upper abdomen.

Commonly used descriptions of angina include pressure, weight, chest tightness and constriction. Patients often also describe a feeling of breathlessness. Triggers on the ward include showering, temperature changes and strong emotions.

Common reasons for worsening angina on the AMU are as follows:

- Anaemia (e.g., recent upper GI bleed, anaemia due to cancer or chemotherapy)
- Sudden onset of atrial fibrillation
- Stress of acute illness (especially exacerbations of COPD)

Other Important Symptoms and Signs

Serious anginal episodes are accompanied by pallor, sweating and hypotension. Prolonged pain, lasting for more than 15 min, especially if it is accompanied by nausea and vomiting, is more in keeping with an infarction than with angina, although the distinction can be difficult, particularly in the elderly.

In the elderly, the symptoms of acute ischaemic heart disease are often atypical and include:
- Breathlessness without pain
- Acute confusion
- Dizziness
- Abdominal pain
- Syncope

It should be remembered that around one in four acute myocardial infarcts are painless or unrecognised by the patient. This is a particularly common situation in patients with diabetes.

Why Obtain an ECG While the Patient Is in Pain?

A resting ECG should be recorded during any episode of acute chest pain or discomfort. There will usually be changes during an attack of angina, indicating a temporary reduction in the blood supply to the heart muscle. Persistence of ischaemic changes after the pain has resolved suggests either unstable angina or an actual infarction. An ECG with 'dynamic changes'—fluctuating changes synchronous with episodes of chest pain—requires urgent intervention.

Acute Coronary Syndromes, ST-Elevation Myocardial Infarctions, Non-ST-Elevation Myocardial Infarctions and Unstable Angina

Ischaemic heart disease occurs when the enlargement of cholesterol-rich plaques within the coronary artery walls leads to arterial narrowing, which is sufficient to starve the heart muscle of oxygen. Slow progressive narrowing results in stable angina. However, if a plaque becomes unstable and ruptures, a sudden combination of platelet clumping and thrombosis clots off a coronary artery. The resulting clinical conditions are termed acute coronary syndromes (ACS) (see Fig. 2.6). There are three types of ACS, depending on the extent of the blockage and the degree of resulting heart muscle damage: ST-elevation myocardial infarction (STEMI), non-ST-elevation myocardial infarction (NSTEMI) and unstable angina.

A complete block results in severe damage and then, within 45 min, irreversible death of the cardiac muscle. Troponin levels are markedly increased, and the ECG reflects damage to the full thickness of the heart muscle wall with *elevation* of the ST-segments (STEMI). A partial or intermittent block results in *depression* of the ST-segments accompanied by evidence of heart muscle damage and elevated troponin levels (NSTEMI) or the same ECG changes with no heart muscle damage and normal troponin levels (unstable angina).

The clinical picture in a STEMI is most commonly that of the classic 'heart attack': severe crushing pain, sweating and nausea; in NSTEMI and unstable angina, it is usually one of intermittent pain or increasing exertional pain culminating in episodes of pro-longed pain at rest.

The sooner the coronary artery can be reopened (re-perfusion), the lesser the damage and the lower the mortality risk. STEMIs were previously treated with urgent throm-bolytics but should now receive immediate PCI (per-cutaneous intervention) in the form of balloon angioplasty and stent to unblock the coronary artery and salvage any damaged heart muscle. Thrombolytics are now only used when it is not possible to get a PCI within 2 h of the ECG diagnosis of a STEMI. NSTEMIs and unstable angina need timely diagnosis and urgent risk assessment to identify the level of intervention required to prevent progression from partial to complete coronary artery blockage. This will range from immediate treatment combining antiplatelet drugs (aspirin with either ticagrelor or clopidogrel) with anti-thrombin agents (subcutaneous fondaparinux or enoxaparin) escalating, in the high-risk patient, to intravenous glycoprotein IIb/IIIb inhibitors (tirofiban and eptifibatide) and urgent re-vascularisation with angioplasty or coronary artery bypass.

The current organisation of care for a classic STEMI (severe pain at home—ambu-lance—diagnostic ECG—PCI unit) means that they are seen with increasing rarity outside the specialist centres. Unstable angina and NSTEMIs, however, can have a less straightforward presentation (often initially labelled as 'atypical chest pain'), and both can present to the AMU, where early recognition and treatment are vital to lessen the risk of further life-threatening cardiac damage.

TROPONIN T AND TROPONIN I IN THE ASSESSMENT OF CHEST PAIN

The diagnosis of myocardial infarction is based on three elements: the history, the ECG (which is all that is needed to immediately diagnose a STEMI) and the measurement of biomarkers in the blood, troponin T and troponin I, which are released from the heart muscle when it is damaged. Troponins are highly specific for cardiac muscle and are sensitive to even minor degrees of damage. Troponin levels rise 3–6 h after the onset of damage, peak at 24 h, and remain elevated for up to 10 days. As a general rule, a normal troponin T level (less than 0.01 mcg/L) 6 h after the onset of suspicious chest pain rules out myocardial infarction (but not unstable angina). Levels in the intermediate range (0.01–0.03 mcg/L) need follow-up blood tests to identify rising values as even small increases can indicate damage, while cases where the levels are above 0.03 mcg/L have definite damage and, depending on other risk factors, need urgent damage limitation with anti-platelet drugs, anti-thrombins and possible angioplasty. Recent improvements in the measurement of troponin ('high-sensitivity troponin testing') have reduced the timing of the second blood test in suspected ACS from 6 h after presentation to 3 h. Usual practice, therefore, to rule out ischaemic heart muscle damage, would be to check high-sensitivity troponin levels at presentation and after 3 h.

RISK STRATIFICATION IN THE MANAGEMENT OF CHEST PAIN

Chest pain is a very common medical emergency—accounting for around a quarter of all emergency medical admissions. It is vital to recognise those patients, many of whom will not have 'classic' cardiac pain, who are at particular risk of progressing to acute myocardial infarction or who may need emergency re-vascularisation or who may even suffer sudden death. It is now recognised that reliance on the history of the ECG changes or even troponin levels is insufficient to accurately identify those at risk—patients will be missed and either falsely reassured or managed inappropriately. Reliable scoring techniques are now available which stratify patients with acute chest pain by their risk of a subsequent myocardial infarction or sudden death and therefore determine the degree and urgency of preventative action required. Most reliable is the GRACE system of risk stratification, which is used to grade patients with acute chest pain according to age, ECG ST segment changes, troponin levels, admission heart rate, admission systolic blood pressure, degree of heart failure, renal function and whether or not the patient suffered a cardiac arrest on admission. As an example, an NSTEMI or unstable angina with a GRACE score in the intermediate or high-risk category (a predicted 6-month mortality risk of more than 3%) should have cardiac catheterisation with or without PCI within 72 h of admission. If the patient is clinically unstable (low blood pressure, LVF, fluctuating ECG changes), the time frame is reduced to 24 h.

COCAINE AND THE HEART

Cocaine is a potent cause of cardiac damage—the catecholamine surge, which is seen within an hour of ingestion, can trigger acute hypertension and spasms of the coronary arteries, leading to an ACS or myocardial infarction. It is important to recognise cocaine use as a cause of acute heart damage as it requires specific management. Treatment is aimed at sedating the patient with diazepam and reducing the spasm with IV nitrates and diltiazem—β-blockers worsen the situation, and drugs conventionally used for ACS, aimed at 'plaque stabilisation', such as aspirin and clopidogrel are of no value.

WHAT ARE THE OTHER CAUSES OF ACUTE CHEST PAIN?

Pleurisy is severe and stops the patient from moving around the bed or taking a full breath. Acute pericarditis occurs in the setting of a viral infection with pleuritic-type, left-sided chest pain.

In the frail elderly, rib fractures and vertebral collapse are common causes of acute, severe, intractable pain. This situation is seen after falls, after bouts of severe coughing and particularly in patients with osteoporosis. Oesophageal pain and biliary colic can both easily be confused with heart pain. Musculoskeletal pain is positional and is not usually severe. The pain from shingles, however, can be extreme and often appears a day or so before the rash is recognised.

When to Call Senior Medical Staff

At-risk patients have cardiac-sounding pain, may be in the convalescent period from a recent infarct, or may have a definite history of cardiovascular disease. If these patients have rest pain, there should be a liaison with the medical staff, particularly if the pain is associated with ECG changes or a decrease in blood pressure. Unstable angina needs active and immediate intervention, probably in a CCU. Such patients, if left in a general ward, do worse in terms of time to angioplasty, treatment of serious arrhythmias, management of acute haemodynamic changes and their chances of survival from a cardiac arrest.

Prior to transfer, if an ACS has been diagnosed, the immediate treatment is likely to be loading doses of aspirin, ticagrelor (or clopidogrel) and an intravenous β-blocker, usually metoprolol. If there is a STEMI, prepare the patient for probable urgent intervention (PCI). If it is an NSTEMI the patient will be given LMWH (or its close relative, fondaparinux) and then risk stratified to assess whether and with what urgency angiography (and possible PCI) is needed. If there is persistent, uncontrolled chest pain, the more potent anti-platelet drugs, intravenous eptifibatide and tirofiban may have to be added. It is important to site IV lines in the left arm, as access for PCI will usually involve the right radial artery.

WHEN TO TRY GLYCERYL TRINITRATE?

A patient with known angina will be familiar with their pain and can advise you whether any particular episode is unusually severe or prolonged. Their 'usual' angina can be treated with simple sublingual GTN, but the patient must first be assessed for the severity and frequency of their attacks.

WHAT TO SAY TO THE PATIENT?

'We may have to "nip this problem in the bud" using anticoagulants, IV nitrates and perhaps a procedure to unblock the coronary artery. You must report any further chest pain to the nursing staff immediately'.

Case Study 2.3 illustrates the management of a patient with breathlessness and chest pain.

CRITICAL CLINICAL TASKS IN THE PATIENT WITH CHEST PAIN

ABCDE triage. Chest pain with hypotension and arterial desaturation needs urgent/immediate medical attention. The possible causes in a collapsed patient include a myocardial infarct and a pulmonary embolus; a less common cause is acute aortic dissection.

Monitor oxygen saturation. Only give oxygen if the saturation is less than 94%, aiming for a target saturation of 94%–98%.

CASE STUDY 2.3   Breathlessness and Chest Pain

An 83-year-old male, an independent retired widower, was admitted at 6 p.m. with a 4-h history of increasing breathlessness. There had been no response to nebulised salbutamol, which he had tried at home. He had COPD and, because of an exacerbation, he had been receiving antibiotics and oral steroids for 3 weeks prior to admission.

INITIAL ASSESSMENT

On admission, he was distressed, dyspnoeic and frightened. His oxygen saturation was 87% on high-flow oxygen. Respiratory rate was 36 breaths/min. His pulse was 120 beats/min and regular. His blood pressure was 170/120 mm Hg. There was a severe wheeze and mild ankle oedema. He had been given sublingual GTN and high-flow oxygen by the paramedics. His current medication was:

- Uniphyllin (dose unknown)
- Inhalers of salbutamol, Becotide and salmeterol
- Nebulised ipratropium (Atrovent) and salbutamol (Ventolin)

His ECG showed a tachycardia and mild left heart strain. His blood gases on 28% oxygen via a Ventimask showed an acceptable pO$_2$ (of 9.4 kPa) and normal pCO$_2$. Chest film showed mild congestion.

INITIAL DIAGNOSIS

- Exacerbation of COPD
- Possible LVF

Correctly, the paramedics had considered a cardiac cause for his symptoms and tried GTN. A painless myocardial infarction would have to be excluded with ECGs and cardiac enzymes.

It can be difficult to decide in an emergency what is the relative contribution from COPD, and the initial management may have to target both conditions. The priority at this stage is:

- To maintain oxygenation
- To correct any reversible underlying cause (LVF, arrhythmia, bronchoconstriction)

MANAGEMENT

The patient was propped upright and reassured; 28% oxygen was administered and a cardiac monitor was put in place. He was given:

- IV *furosemide* 80 mg
- Nebulised *salbutamol* 5 mg (caution is needed if acute cardiac ischaemia is a suspected possible diagnosis as salbutamol can overstimulate the heart — this dose may have been too large)
- IV *hydrocortisone* (for presumed bronchoconstriction)
- oral *amoxicillin* (if there had been pneumonia on the chest film, this would have been given intravenously to a patient as ill as this)

Theophylline levels were checked urgently:

- To guide further aminophylline doses if they are needed
- To exclude theophylline toxicity as the cause for his marked tachycardia

The patient had an immediate diuresis; this was charted and a strict fluid balance chart was started.

Progress. At 2 a.m. the patient became more breathless and cyanosed. He was sweating profusely and looked extremely unwell. He complained of anterior chest pain that had started 30 min before.

Assessment. The patient was severely distressed. His saturation was 75% on 28% oxygen, respiratory rate of 40 breaths/min, pulse rate of 140 beats/min and regular and blood pressure of 170/75 mm Hg. His abdomen was soft and non-tender, and there was no sign of acute urinary retention. (Intra-abdominal catastrophes such as a ruptured aortic aneurysm can present in the elderly with acute sudden cardiovascular deterioration. Acute retention is common in males of this age after IV diuretics.)

(Continued)

CASE STUDY 2.3   Breathlessness and Chest Pain—cont'd

The ECG had not changed, and neither had the chest film. The possibilities at this stage were:

- Worsening respiratory failure
- Increasing LVF
- Possible acute myocardial infarction

The oxygen delivered was changed to 60% using a reservoir mask (in an acutely deteriorating patient, correcting hypoxia takes precedence over all other considerations). The patient was given:

- IV *furosemide* 120 mg.
- IV *diamorphine* 2.5 mg for chest pain and LVF (this must be used with extreme caution in patients with a possible respiratory component to their illness as it will depress ventilation).
- An *aminophylline* infusion was started (the initial theophylline level was in the normal range so a loading dose was not given). Aminophylline has the advantage of working in both pulmonary oedema and bronchoconstriction, although it is not generally used as a first-line treatment in either situation.

A decision was made to consider ventilation if the patient did not improve (using information about his previous level of independence and health from the admission assessment). His relatives were contacted and brought in.

The patient's arterial blood gases at this stage showed an acceptable oxygen level but, possibly as a result of the diamorphine, an increasing pCO_2. His oxygen mask was changed again to 28%, and the patient was given two further 120 mg doses of IV furosemide. By 7 a.m. after a significant diuresis, there was notable and continued improvement. He was eventually well enough to be discharged back to his home.

Subsequent cardiac enzymes (Table 2.1) showed that he had suffered an acute myocardial infarction, which had presumably caused the sudden deterioration in the early hours of the first morning after his admission.

TABLE 2.1 ■ Cardiac Enzymes From Case Study 2.3

Enzyme Level	Day 1	Day 2	Day 3
Troponin T (mcg/L)	<0.01	0.40	0.30
Creatine kinase (IU/L)	114	559	354

Obtain a 12-lead ECG. This is useful to confirm a myocardial infarction or unstable angina. A normal ECG is not particularly helpful in ruling out other conditions. The way to gain the most information from an ECG is to compare it with others from the case record.

Take an overall look at the patient. If the patient is stable, a more measured approach can be used. However, this is not the case if:

1. The pain sounds anginal and has lasted more than 20 min.
2. The patient is also breathless, that is, pulmonary oedema or pulmonary embolus.
3. The blood pressure has dropped.
4. The pain is taking place soon after an infarct.

Severe angina, myocardial infarction, or pulmonary embolus produces a pale, sweaty and clammy patient. A patient who cannot take a full breath because of pain probably has pleurisy. Biliary colic makes the patient roll around the bed in pain.

Ask Key Questions

- Where is the pain, and where does it radiate?
- What makes it worse (deep inspiration, minor exertion such as showering)?
- What relieves it (e.g., GTN, breathing shallowly)?
- Has it occurred before? Is it like your usual angina/previous heart attack?

CRITICAL CLINICAL TASKS IN THE PATIENT WITH CHEST PAIN

- ABCDE triage
- Monitor oxygen saturation
- Obtain a 12-lead ECG
- Take an overall look at the patient, including the NEWS2
- Ask key questions

Sudden Cardiac Death

Sudden cardiac death (SCD) describes a sudden collapse, usually in ventricular fibrillation, ventricular tachycardia or asystole. There are few warning symptoms, perhaps a few seconds of chest tightness, palpitations or weakness. The outlook is variable, with the best survival rates seen in patients experiencing witnessed in-hospital arrests in which the rhythm is ventricular fibrillation or ventricular tachycardia—of whom 20% will leave the hospital alive.

Ischaemic heart disease is responsible for 70% of SCDs, and although it may be the first symptom, more commonly it occurs during the first 12 months after an acute myocardial infarction. The use of preventative measures post-infarct, particularly in patients with poor left ventricular function, has a significant impact on reducing the incidence of SCD. A typical regimen in a high-risk case would consist of:

- An ACE inhibitor or an angiotensin II receptor antagonist
- A β-blocker
- Spironolactone
- Intensive statin therapy
- Aspirin with ticagrelor or clopidogrel

Patients who survive a cardiac arrest after a STEMI, **even if they remain unconscious**, require urgent coronary angiography with a view to PCI to stabilise the heart and improve the outlook.

There is increasing interest in preventing SCDs with ICDs. These would be considered, for example, in high-risk survivors of cardiac arrest such as those with poor left ventricular function and in whom electrophysiological testing demonstrates instability of their cardiac rhythm.

Atrial Fibrillation and Arterial Emboli

Normally, the heart beats in an orderly fashion and is led by the rhythmic activity of the sinoatrial (SA) node. Each atrial contraction is followed immediately by that of the ventricles. The SA node establishes the heart rate through the rhythmic discharge of a small electrical impulse that spreads, wavelike, through each atrium, producing atrial contraction. The impulse then passes through the atrioventricular (AV) node and onward continues onward to initiate ventricular contraction. Thus if the SA node is firing regularly 75 times per minute, the AV node will, in turn, be activated at the same rate, leading to a regular ventricular response (and, of course, pulse rate) of 75 contractions per minute.

In atrial fibrillation (Fig. 2.7), organised atrial activity is replaced by random electrical impulses which spread chaotically through the atrium. The atrium responds by muscular activity that can be described as a shivering motion (fibrillation) rather than a coordinated contraction. There are two important consequences:

- The atrial 'squeeze', which expels the final 10% of the blood into the ventricle at the end of diastole, is lost. This loss can be important, particularly if the ventricle relies on atrial contraction to ensure it is properly filled, for example, when the valve between the atrium and ventricle is already narrowed (as in mitral stenosis).
- The AV node is activated at random by the chaotic atrial electrical activity at rates of anything between 60 and 140 times per minute. The ventricles respond to this random activation accordingly and produce irregular pulse rates within this wide range. Clearly, an irregular heart rate of 140 beats/min will not be tolerated by the heart for long.

Thus atrial fibrillation reduces cardiac output (Box 2.2).

Causes of Atrial Fibrillation

Cardiac failure from whatever cause can be associated with atrial fibrillation. The most common situations in which atrial fibrillation is seen on the AMU are as follows:

- The ageing heart (8% of all those older than 80 years old are in atrial fibrillation)
- Ischaemic and hypertensive heart disease
- Chronic heart valve disease
- Binge alcohol drinking
- Atrial fibrillation triggered by hypoxia or infection in COPD

Atrial fibrillation can also be triggered by an acute myocardial infarction and by a pulmonary embolus.

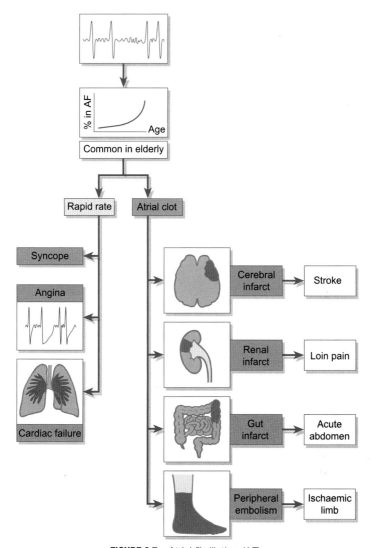

FIGURE 2.7   Atrial fibrillation (AF).

BOX 2.2 ▮ Why Atrial Fibrillation Reduces Cardiac Output

■ Loss of atrial contraction
■ Too-rapid ventricular response
■ Irregular ventricular rate

Atrial fibrillation can occur in a normal heart; indeed, this is the case in around 50% of all patients with recurrent attacks of atrial fibrillation (paroxysmal atrial fibrillation). In these patients, such short-lived episodes are extremely unpleasant and, particularly, when prolonged, pose a risk of embolic complications.

Importance of Atrial Fibrillation
UNCONTROLLED ATRIAL FIBRILLATION
Cardiac Failure

Atrial fibrillation itself can cause right and left heart failure if the ventricular rate is excessive. This is particularly the case in elderly patients. More commonly, the onset of atrial fibrillation in someone with pre-existing valvular or heart muscle disease will tip the patient into cardiac failure (Case Study 2.4).

Angina

Uncontrolled atrial fibrillation can reduce the blood supply to the heart muscle and trigger angina simply because there is not enough time for adequate coronary artery blood flow to occur. The reverse may also occur—an attack of ischaemia can trigger atrial fibrillation—so it is important to take a good history to see which came first, the pain or the palpitations.

Syncope and Near Syncope

The cardiac output may suddenly decrease in acute atrial fibrillation, sufficiently to reduce cerebral blood flow, leading to syncope or presyncope. This is a particular risk if there are existing problems with blood flow because of either aortic valve stenosis or disease in the carotid arteries (Case Study 2.5).

There are several important issues in Case Study 2.5. The patient's old hospital records showed he had previously been investigated for unexplained blackouts. Some had been associated with transient atrial fibrillation, but his heavy alcohol intake had been blamed for this. The murmur had been heard but not investigated. Aortic stenosis is a common valve problem and usually results from degenerative calcification of a congenitally abnormal valve. Rheumatic valve disease is a much less common cause of aortic stenosis. The stenosis leads to three symptoms: increasing angina, recurrent syncope and sudden death. All are a manifestation of obstruction to blood flow out of the left side of the heart. If undiagnosed, it can eventually lead to LVF. Critical stenosis is potentially

CASE STUDY 2.4	Sudden Atrial Fibrillation in Unrecognised Mitral Stenosis

A 68-year-old female was admitted severely breathless, coughing up copious frothy pink sputum, characteristic of pulmonary oedema. Her pulse rate was 145 beats/min and irregular, and her blood pressure was 70/40 mm Hg. Her oxygen saturation was 70%.

The patient was treated with high-flow oxygen and IV diuretics. Her atrial fibrillation was controlled with IV amiodarone (electrical cardioversion was considered but she improved rapidly with initial treatment and it was unclear from the history how long the atrial fibrillation had been present). Subsequent examination and investigation demonstrated tight mitral stenosis. There was no history of cardiac disease, but she had had rheumatic fever as a teenager.

CASE STUDY 2.5   Aortic Stenosis and Paroxysmal Atrial Fibrillation

A 68-year-old male was admitted as an emergency with a 4-month history of feeling unwell and collapsing to the floor. Some of the episodes were accompanied by fast palpitations. On the day of admission, he had a rushing feeling in his head and collapsed to the floor. His wife said that he was grey and clammy and stayed unconscious for around 10 min. There were no convulsive movements. When he came round he was slightly confused and had been incontinent of urine.

The only finding on admission was a murmur coming from what was thought to be a stenosed aortic valve. The patient's pulse was normal at 86 beats/min.

Three hours after admission, he suddenly went into rapid atrial fibrillation and felt very faint. His atrial fibrillation stopped without treatment after 2 min, but it was followed by a long pause on the ECG during which time the patient felt worse.

He was referred to the cardiologists and urgently transferred to the CCU. A cardiac echo showed severe aortic stenosis. Syncope due to a structural heart defect needs urgent attention.

CASE STUDY 2.6   Sudden Atrial Fibrillation

A patient was admitted with severe diabetic ketoacidosis: blood sugar 55 mmol/L, pH 6.85 and an unrecordable blood pressure. His pulse rate was 140 beats/min and was initially misinterpreted as a normal rhythm. He was given aggressive fluid replacement with no improvement in his blood pressure. After 4 h, his heart rhythm suddenly reverted from what was now clearly rapid atrial fibrillation to sinus rhythm. His blood pressure immediately increased to 110/70 mm Hg.

lethal yet easily managed with valve replacement—a diagnosis not to be missed. In this patient, the atrial fibrillation combined with the stenosis led to syncope and the excess alcohol intake may well not have been of immediate relevance, except for obscuring the true nature of the problem.

Sudden Atrial Fibrillation Causing Hypotension During Severe Illness

Acute atrial fibrillation can cause a sudden decrease in blood pressure and, if this decrease occurs in the setting of a severe illness, it can be misinterpreted as hypovolaemia or sepsis (Case Study 2.6).

In a sick patient, it can be difficult to tell whether severe tachycardia is the primary cause of low blood pressure or whether, along with the hypotension, it is one of the effects of the acute illness.

COMPLICATIONS OF ATRIAL FIBRILLATION

Atrial Fibrillation and the Formation of Left Atrial Clots

Unfortunately, blood stagnates in a fibrillating atrium and is liable to clot. A clot that breaks loose (*embolus*) can, in the case of those originating in the left atrium, have disastrous consequences: *stroke* as a result of cerebral embolus, *kidney damage* as a result of renal emboli and *acutely ischaemic limbs* as a result of peripheral vessel emboli. Transthoracic or transoesophageal echocardiography can help to assess the risk of embolisation by examining overall cardiac function, looking for enlargement of the left atrium and identifying left atrial clots.

Of these complications, the risk of embolic stroke is much the most important and is quite common—approaching 5% of patients in atrial fibrillation per year. The risk of stroke is particularly high in those older than 65 years, especially if there are other risk factors present such as diabetes, cardiac failure, hypertension and previous cerebrovascular disease. This group of patients will be considered for anticoagulation as soon as atrial fibrillation has been diagnosed.

Diagnosis of Atrial Fibrillation

Atrial fibrillation causes a chaotically irregular pulse, which can be fast or slow. If the ventricle contracts quickly and irregularly, the amount of blood expelled with each beat will vary, and the very weak beats will not be palpable at the wrist. This produces a deficit between the apical rate (measured with a stethoscope at the apex) and the rate measured by palpation at the wrist.

This is a common pitfall in uncontrolled atrial fibrillation—the pulse can be 80 beats/min at the wrist and 130 beats/min at the apex. *If the pulse feels irregular, measure both the apical and the radial rates. Confirm atrial fibrillation with a 12-lead ECG.*

Management of Atrial Fibrillation

Unless there is a contraindication, most patients with atrial fibrillation will be started immediately on anticoagulation using LMWH. The choice then lies between:
- Observation
- Converting the atrial fibrillation to a normal rhythm (cardioversion)
- Controlling the atrial fibrillation by slowing the ventricular rate

Management options are summarised in Box 2.3.

Observation. This would be appropriate for the first 24 h in a patient with slow atrial fibrillation in which the rhythm was not compromising cardiac function. If the patient

---

BOX 2.3 ▉ Management Options in Atrial Fibrillation

- Immediate anticoagulation and observation
- Immediate anticoagulation and rate control with digoxin/β-blocker/diltiazem
- Immediate anticoagulation and cardioversion
- Immediate anticoagulation and planned cardioversion in 3 weeks

is acutely unwell due to atrial fibrillation, urgent action is required to restore a normal heart rhythm or control the heart rate.

Cardioversion. It is possible to convert atrial fibrillation to a normal rhythm by using drugs (chemical cardioversion) or by a synchronised shock (electrical cardioversion). In general, in rapid atrial fibrillation of recent onset (less than 48 h), cardioversion is the treatment of choice, particularly if the abnormal rhythm is having an adverse effect on the patient. The sooner that cardioversion is tried, the better the chances of success. Unless the situation is critical, drugs are tried before a synchronised shock is attempted—intravenous amiodarone is the most commonly used drug.

If atrial fibrillation has been present for longer than 48 h, it is essential to anticoagulate the patient for at least 3 weeks before attempting cardioversion because of the risk of dislodging a clot from the left atrium. Rather surprisingly, the evidence suggests that patients with well-established atrial fibrillation fare just as well from control of the ventricular rate as they do from re-establishing normal rhythm with cardioversion.

Controlling atrial fibrillation. In many acute situations, the duration of the atrial fibrillation will be unclear, and urgent cardioversion could put the patient at risk of an embolus. As untreated, rapid atrial fibrillation compromises the heart, in an unstable patient, it is important to use a drug such as metoprolol or digoxin which acts quickly (and may need to be given intravenously). Where there is severe heart failure (hypotension, pulmonary/peripheral oedema), intravenous amiodarone is used—but only after specialist advice.

STROKE PREVENTION VERSUS BLEEDING RISK: $CHAD_2DS_2$-VASC AND HAS-BLED

Anticoagulation significantly reduces the chances of stroke in atrial fibrillation, but this benefit must be balanced against the risk of bleeding. $CHAD_2DS_2$-VASc is used to score stroke risk factors that are present in a patient in addition to their atrial fibrillation. These factors are heart failure, hypertension, diabetes, previous stroke/transient ischaemic attack (TIA)/embolus, vascular disease (previous MI, peripheral vascular disease) and an age of at least 65 years. Any one of these additional risk factors is sufficient to make anticoagulation worthwhile (aspirin confers no benefit in reducing stroke risk in these patients or those with no additional risk factors). Conversely, a patient younger than 65 years with atrial fibrillation but no other risk factors does not benefit from anticoagulation.

HAS-BLED estimates the risk of a major bleed while on anticoagulants. A high HAS-BLED score does not preclude the use of anticoagulants; it signals the need for targeted follow-up with attention to anticoagulant control, alcohol intake, use of NSAIDs and the treatment of any potential upper GI bleeding sources. In the United Kingdom, the ORBIT score is replacing HAS-BLED as it is easier to use and can be applied to DOACs, which, in most situations, are now the anticoagulants of choice.

ORBIT takes into account age, history of previous bleeding, blood count, kidney function and current use of blood thinners.

Atrial fibrillation in the elderly. Atrial fibrillation is present in 8% of the population over 80 years of age and is associated with a high risk of complications—there is a sixfold increased risk of emboli and atrial fibrillation is implicated in one-third of all strokes in this age group. Although long-term anticoagulant therapy has dangers in the elderly, particularly in those experiencing confusion, it also has major benefits, with large reductions in the risk of stroke, provided that there is careful selection of the patient and monitoring of the anticoagulant control. Importantly, a perceived increased risk of falls is NOT a contraindication to anticoagulation.

The risk of warfarin-induced haemorrhage (in particular, intracerebral haemorrhage) can be reduced by maintaining an international normalised ratio (INR) between 2.0 and 3.0, avoiding the combined use of aspirin, fall reduction strategies and careful blood pressure control.

Atrial fibrillation induced by alcohol. Case Study 2.7 describes the management of a patient whose atrial fibrillation was caused by excess alcohol intake. The important points from this case study include:

- Alcohol itself can directly trigger atrial fibrillation and is the precipitating factor in up to a quarter of cases of acute atrial fibrillation (it can also eventually damage the heart muscle by causing thiamine deficiency).
- Up to half of all cases of first-time atrial fibrillation will return to a normal rhythm without treatment.

CASE STUDY 2.7   Atrial Fibrillation Induced by Alcohol

A 43-year-old male was admitted to hospital as an emergency at 3 a.m. on a Sunday, complaining of palpitations and chest tightness. He had consumed two bottles of red wine and three pints of beer during the course of a dinner party the evening before. He was awoken at 2 a.m. with rapid palpitations and chest tightness. The history was negative, but he drank on average 30 units of alcohol per week and smoked 20 cigarettes per day.

On admission, the patient was anxious with an irregular pulse of 110 at the wrist and 140 beats/min at the apex. Blood pressure was 160/90 mm Hg, and the full examination was negative. The chest film was clear and the 12-lead ECG confirmed atrial fibrillation with no evidence of a myocardial infarction.

He and his wife were reassured that this was probably not a heart attack, he was monitored and blood was taken for cardiac enzymes and biochemistry. He was started on a treatment dose of subcutaneous LMWH and a decision was made that, as this was a short-lived arrhythmia (and hence there had not been time for a clot to form in the left atrium), it would be safe to try cardioversion, initially with an IV infusion of amiodarone. Fortunately, while waiting for the results of his blood tests his monitor showed a sudden return to sinus rhythm with immediate relief of his symptoms. Electrical cardioversion was not needed.

A cardiac echogram was arranged to look at the heart valves and heart muscle function, and he was discharged home with an appointment for the cardiology clinic. He was strongly advised to moderate his alcohol consumption to prevent any recurrence.

- If the atrial fibrillation is new (less than 48-h old), there is little risk of a clot having formed in the left atrium and cardioversion can be tried without first giving prolonged anticoagulation.
- The alternative to cardioversion would have been to control the rate of atrial fibrillation initially with digoxin, if necessary, adding a β-blocker or verapamil.

WARFARIN AND NEW DIRECT ACTING ORAL ANTICOAGULANTS (DOACS)—EDOXABAN, DABIGATRAN, APIXABAN AND RIVAROXABAN

- A new class of anticoagulants—DOACs—has been introduced which are at least as effective as, and are largely replacing, warfarin in reducing the risk of stroke. They have superior safety profiles in terms of the risk of major bleeding events—in particular, except for dabigatran, with regard to intracranial bleeding. Their major advantage is that INR monitoring is not necessary, so more patients will have effective treatment (a high proportion of patients on warfarin spend a significant proportion of their time under-anticoagulated) and compliance will be improved. Their drawbacks are that they should not be used in patients with renal failure or patients with mechanical heart valves and that, unlike warfarin, their effects on clotting cannot as easily be reversed.
- If anticoagulation is contraindicated because of the bleeding risk, intolerance or poor compliance, the left atrial appendage (where most clots arise) can be sealed off using a specialised percutaneous technique.

CRITICAL CLINICAL TASKS IN ATRIAL FIBRILLATION

The aim of the clinical assessment is to document the effect that the atrial fibrillation is having on the patient and hence to determine the urgency of the situation. If atrial fibrillation is causing angina, hypotension or heart failure, then corrective action is necessary as soon as possible. Slow atrial fibrillation with no acute complication may simply require a period of observation.

Assess the rate of atrial fibrillation. Atrial fibrillation at a pulse rate of 80–100 beats/min is unlikely to cause acute cardiac decompensation, whereas at 130–140 beats/min, problems will arise. It is important to document both the apical and the radial rate. In uncontrolled atrial fibrillation, not all the apical impulses are conducted to the radial pulse, which leads to a difference between the rates (pulse deficit); this gap narrows as the heart rate comes under control with treatment.

Identify chest pain. A history of chest pain may mean that the atrial fibrillation has been triggered by an ischaemic episode or even by a myocardial infarction. More commonly, however, rapid atrial fibrillation can cause rate-related anginal pain.

CRITICAL CLINICAL TASKS IN ATRIAL FIBRILLATION
- Assess the rate of fibrillation
- Identify chest pain
- Look for heart failure
- Document hypotension

Look for heart failure. Symptoms of breathlessness, particularly on lying flat, and associated with signs of an increase in respiratory rate and bilateral ankle oedema, suggest that the atrial fibrillation is causing, or contributing to, cardiac failure.

Document hypotension. Sudden rapid atrial fibrillation can decrease blood pressure acutely. This can have a critical impact, especially if the atrial fibrillation is further complicating major acute illnesse such as pneumonia or diabetic ketoacidosis.

IMPORTANT CLINICAL TASKS IN ATRIAL FIBRILLATION

Watch for emboli caused by atrial fibrillation. The three areas particularly prone to emboli are the brain, limbs and intestine—presenting as stroke-like illness or sudden confusion, acutely painful, pale and pulseless limbs and, particularly in the elderly, an acute abdomen.

Identify factors that could have triggered the atrial fibrillation. Common non-cardiac causes of acute atrial fibrillation are pneumonia, exacerbations of COPD and any source of sepsis, particularly if there is pyrexia.

Obtain an accurate drug history. The names and doses of all cardiovascular drugs need to be recorded. This is especially important for digoxin (under- or overtreatment can cause problems with uncontrolled atrial fibrillation), oral theophyllines (overtreatment is a potent cause of any arrhythmia) and anticoagulants. Some patients on DOACs, particularly the elderly, may not be aware that these drugs are the equivalent of warfarin.

Regimens will often need to be cross-referenced with information from relatives and the GP's surgery.

IMPORTANT CLINICAL TASKS IN ATRIAL FIBRILLATION
- Observe for emboli (brain, limbs, gut)
- Look for non-cardiac triggers
- Obtain an accurate drug history

Answering Relatives' Questions in Atrial Fibrillation

What is it, and why is it important? Atrial fibrillation is a prolonged, irregular heart rhythm. It makes the heart pump less efficiently and can cause the blood to stagnate and form potentially dangerous clots. It is often temporary, especially if it has been triggered by some other acute illness.

How will it be treated? If it is troublesome, we can slow the pulse down to normal with drugs or try and jolt the heart back into a normal rhythm using either an injectable drug (flecainide/amiodarone) or a small electrical impulse delivered under an anaesthetic ('synchronised DC shock'). While the pulse is irregular, we will keep the blood watered down with heparin/warfarin to prevent it from clotting.

Infective Endocarditis

Infective endocarditis is a serious condition in which there is an infection of the heart valves, usually the mitral or aortic valve. In the past, only damaged or mechanical valves have been involved, but the increasing incidence of IV drug abuse has put even normal heart valves at risk. Other major risk factors are advanced age, diabetes and recent dental, operative and endoscopic procedures, which can result in bacteria entering the bloodstream.

Infective endocarditis is a serious acute medical problem. The affected valve may fail suddenly as it is destroyed by infection. Pieces of infected material can break off and spread via the blood to vital organs, resulting in:

- Foci of sepsis, especially in the kidneys
- Septic cerebral emboli (stroke-like illness)

How Infective Endocarditis Presents
PYREXIA OF UNKNOWN ORIGIN

The picture is of severe malaise associated with night sweats and generalised aches and pains. Usually, there will be a known valve lesion, valve replacement or previously diagnosed congenital heart defect.

CATASTROPHIC VALVE FAILURE

Infection can destroy a cardiac valve and even form an abscess within the heart muscle or in the conducting system. This can lead to devastating cardiac failure, particularly in the case of the aortic valve, and the patient can deteriorate acutely with sudden pulmonary oedema and hypotensive shock.

INFECTED EMBOLI

The history here is of a recent feverish illness complicated by the acute onset of a stroke (cerebral embolus), ischaemic limb (large vessel embolus) or, in the case of right-sided endocarditis, infected pulmonary emboli as described in Case Study 2.8.

CASE STUDY 2.8	Endocarditis and Intravenous Drug Use

A 45-year-old male with a history of previous IV drug use (which was only obtained 2 days after admission) was admitted with severe pleurisy, haemoptysis and widespread shadowing on his chest film. The provisional diagnosis was multiple pulmonary emboli, and treatment was started with heparin.

The patient's condition deteriorated suddenly and, on the basis that this could be pneumonia, IV amoxicillin and clarithromycin were started. He remained severely hypoxic, deteriorated further and died.

The autopsy finding was a staphylococcal endocarditis involving the tricuspid valve—a typical finding in bacterial endocarditis caused by the use of infected intravenous needles (the infection passes through the veins to the right side of the heart, and when infected particles break off the tricuspid valve, they embolise to the lungs).

Role of the Acute Medical Unit in Suspected Endocarditis

Prompt investigation of any illness accompanied by fever. Infected heart valves shed bacteria into the bloodstream, resulting in positive blood cultures. If endocarditis is suspected, then three sets of blood cultures are taken at 30-min intervals; each sample of 10 mL is taken from a peripheral vein using an obsessively aseptic technique and is divided between aerobic and anaerobic blood culture bottles. The urine should also be cultured.

Recognition of high-risk patients. These include patients with valve disease or congenital heart disease admitted to the hospital with fever or unexplained deterioration and illicit drug users with breathlessness and fever.

Appropriate action on finding proteinuria and haematuria. In endocarditis, microemboli of infected material lodge in the kidneys and set up an inflammatory response. As a result, blood and protein appear in the urine. Clearly, in patients with fever, haematuria and proteinuria are more likely to indicate a simple urinary infection; nonetheless, if other risk factors are present, this finding can be critical in guiding the medical staff towards the correct diagnosis.

PRINCIPLES OF MANAGEMENT IN THE FIRST 24 H

Ensure the Safety of the Patient

- Treat cardiac failure
- Treat any arrhythmia
- Involve the cardiologists and the microbiologists

Secure the Diagnosis

- Identify at-risk patients
- Take several blood cultures (avoid the casual use of antibiotics on the ward)
- Conduct urine testing and culture
- Examine the valves (cardiac echo)

Initiate Antibiotic Therapy

- Insert IV lines
- Repeat blood cultures at 72 h to check the effectiveness of the treatment
- Monitor antibiotic levels

Prepare the Patient for a 'Long Haul' of Antibiotic Therapy (Several Weeks)

- Take particular care with IV cannulation sites

Observe for Complications

- Look for antibiotic allergy
- Look for left heart failure (breathlessness, respiratory rate, oxygen saturation, pulse, blood pressure)
- Monitor temperature
- Measure urine output
- Look for septic emboli (any sudden event, e.g., confusion, stroke, cold limb)

Drugs in the Management of Acute Heart Disease
INTRAVENOUS FUROSEMIDE
Indications
Acute pulmonary oedema
  Severe congestive cardiac failure
- Furosemide is a well-tolerated and powerful diuretic with a very wide dose range—from 20 to 250 mg or more. Low doses are used in patients not previously exposed to the drug; higher doses are needed with patients taking oral furosemide, patients with renal failure and patients with severe heart failure.
- Diuresis starts within 10 min of the IV dose, although it is also a vasodilator and may act even more quickly on pulmonary oedema by causing blood to pool in the peripheries.
- As well as advantages, there are also dangers of a sudden diuresis: this may precipitate acute retention, causing hypovolaemic hypotension and sudden electrolyte changes (predominantly urinary potassium loss).
- For doses greater than 50 mg, the rate of IV administration should not exceed 4 mg/min to avoid the risk of acute hearing disturbance.
- Increasingly, the furosemide is given as a bolus followed by a continuous infusion.

ANTIPLATELET AGENTS

Aspirin, ticagrelor, clopidogrel

Indications

Acute coronary syndromes

- The dual combination of aspirin with either ticagrelor or clopidogrel started immediately in ACS and STEMIs reduces cardiovascular mortality, recurrent infarction and stroke.
- The combination also reduces the risk of stent blockage in patients who require PCI.
- The immediate loading doses are aspirin 300 mg, ticagrelor 180 mg, clopidogrel 300 mg. Aspirin is continued long term, ticagrelor and clopidogrel are stopped after 12 months.

INTRAVENOUS NITRATES

Isosorbide dinitrate (Isoket), glyceryl trinitrate (Nitrocine)

Indications

Unstable angina
  Acute LVF

- Nitrates have three important actions: dilate the coronary arteries, unload the heart by reducing the load against which it pumps (peripheral arterial dilatation) and increase the pooling of blood in the veins (which unloads the right side of the heart). They are therefore useful in both angina and cardiac failures, particularly when present together.
- Patients rapidly develop tolerance to nitrates, so the initial dose may have to be increased repeatedly to overcome this (Table 2.2).
- There is a risk of hypotension with IV nitrates, particularly when the heart is already in a parlous state.

TABLE 2.2 ■ **Characteristics of Intravenous Nitrates**

Drug Parameters	Nitrocine	Isoket
Infusion strength[a]	100 μg/mL	100 μg/mL
Starting rate angina	10 μg/min	15 μg/min
Starting rate left ventricular function	20 μg/min	30 μg/min
Step up rate every 30 min	10–20 μg/min	15–30 μg/min
Maximum dose	100–200 μg/min	300 μg/min

[a]Data sheets must be used with care when preparing the admixture of the drugs and the saline or dextrose vehicle. For example, Isoket is provided in 0.05% and 0.1% strength ampoules, and the examples used in the preparation instructions express the doses in *milligrams per hour* (2–20 mg/h). In contrast, the doses of Nitrocine are expressed in *micrograms per minute*. Local protocols are invaluable in these situations.

- Nitrates are no longer recommended as first-line treatment for acute heart failure unless there is continuing ischaemia or severe hypertension, and their use is now probably confined to a high-dependency unit setting where the blood pressure response can be carefully monitored.
- The advantage of the IV infusion of nitrates is that the onset of action is immediate, and the dose can be titrated continuously to balance haemodynamics (the blood pressure and pulse) with the beneficial clinical response.
- As IV nitrates are incompatible with PVC infusion sets (Viaflex, Steriflex) they must be administered through polyethylene or glass containers.

DIGOXIN
Indications
Atrial fibrillation
Cardiac failure
- The major beneficial effect of digoxin is to slow down the ventricular response to atrial fibrillation and atrial flutter. It does this by slowing the conduction of electrical impulses through the AV node.
- Digoxin increases, albeit to a modest degree, the strength of the heartbeat.
- Rapid control of atrial fibrillation requires IV loading:
  - 0.75–1 mg of digoxin in 50 mL of fluid over 2 h
- Lower doses are needed in the elderly, those with renal failure and those who have received digoxin within the past 2 weeks.
- Oral digitalisation can be achieved over 24 h using divided doses of the total loading dose of 1.0–1.25 mg.
- The symptoms of digoxin toxicity (drug levels more than 3 mg/L) are anorexia, nausea, vomiting and an abnormally slow pulse (less than 50 beats/min). Toxicity is more likely if there is potassium deficiency from diuretic therapy.

INTRAVENOUS DILTIAZEM
Indications
Rapid control of atrial fibrillation
- Intravenous 0.25 mg/kg up to three doses and 120–300 mg orally daily in three doses.
- Diltiazem can depress cardiac function and worsen heart failure.

ANGIOTENSIN-CONVERTING ENZYME INHIBITORS
Captopril, enalapril, lisinopril, ramipril

Indications

Cardiac failure
  Hypertension
  Post-myocardial infarct
  Diabetic renal disease

- ACE inhibitors have proved an important advance in the treatment of heart failure and hypertension. They improve survival and symptoms in heart failure and after myocardial infarction, and they have a beneficial effect on diabetic renal disease.
- Their use requires close supervision—particularly in the elderly, those with inter-current illness and those in cardiac failure—because they can adversely affect kidney function through their mode of action, which is to inhibit mechanisms that are normally in place to protect renal blood flow (the renin–angiotensin system).
- First-dose hypotension is a recognised problem but is usually relieved by lying the patient down. The hypotensive response can be exaggerated in a patient who has severe cardiac failure and is already receiving high-dose diuretics. A small test dose should be given and the blood pressure monitored for 2 h.

INTRAVENOUS AMIODARONE

Indications

Rapid termination of serious arrhythmias (rapid atrial fibrillation/flutter, ventricular tachycardia)

- Amiodarone is unusual in that it is an effective antiarrhythmic drug that does not depress the function of the heart. It is therefore relatively safe to use in heart failure, when it is the drug of preference in a critically ill patient with life-threatening arrhythmias.
- The drug causes local phlebitis. Although the loading dose can be given through a peripheral vein, the follow-up, 24-h continuous infusion needs a central line.
- The loading dose is 5 mg/kg (usually 300 mg) in 250 mL 5% dextrose over 20 min.
- The infusion dose is 15 mg/kg (usually 1.2 g) in 500 mL 5% dextrose over 24 h.
- Once there is a response, the infusion is replaced, if indicated, by oral amiodarone.
- There are several important drug interactions, notably, with warfarin and digoxin, and some potentially serious side effects on the thyroid gland, lungs and liver. Most of these are associated with long-term rather than acute therapy.

SPIRONOLACTONE AND EPLERENONE

Indications

Post-infarct
  Cardiac failure

Spironolactone is used in cardiac failure. Its close relative, eplerenone, is used in combination therapy with an ACE inhibitor and a β-blocker to minimise left ventricular damage in high-risk patients after a myocardial infarct.

Further Reading

Heart Failure

Morton, G., Masters, J., Cowburn, P.J., 2017. Multidisciplinary team approach to heart failure management. Heart. https://doi.org/10.1136/heartjnl-2016-310598.
NICE guidelines, 2014. Acute Heart Failure: Diagnosis and Management. Updated 2021. https://www.nice.org.uk/guidance/cg187.

Ischaemic Heart Disease

Edmondstone, W.M., 1995. Cardiac chest pain: does body language help the diagnosis? British Medical Journal 311, 1660–1661.
NICE Guideline (NG196), 2021. Atrial Fibrillation. https://www.nice.org.uk/guidance/NG196.
NICE guidelines, 2010 updated 2016. Chest pain of suspected cardiac origin: assessment and diagnosis. https://guidance.nice.org.uk/CG95.
Chest pain. https://cks.nice.org.uk/topics chest pain.

Respiratory Medicine

Introduction

Respiratory emergencies are a major source of work in the acute medical unit (AMU). Their management is based on two fundamental clinical issues:

- The assessment and relief of breathlessness
- The prevention and treatment of respiratory failure

This chapter explains the basic principles underlying these two areas and applies them to the assessment and management of the types of respiratory cases that you will encounter on a day-to-day basis: asthma, chronic obstructive pulmonary disease (COPD) and pneumonia.

The Breathless Patient: The General Approach

IS THIS PATIENT'S BREATHLESSNESS DUE TO HIS HEART OR LUNGS?

The two most important and most difficult questions in a breathless patient are always:

- Is this cardiac or respiratory breathlessness?
- Is this a pulmonary embolus?

Differentiating the causes of breathlessness can be very difficult, and the history and examination will not always provide an answer. Symptoms and signs are shared by many of the common respiratory and cardiac conditions. Thus a patient with left ventricle failure (LVF) and a patient with acute asthma will both have nocturnal breathlessness and severe wheezing. Ankle swelling is characteristic of congestive heart failure, but it can also be a complication of severe COPD. The difficulties are often age related. If a young person presents with a history of intermittent wheezing, breathlessness and cough, the diagnosis is almost certain to be asthma; but what about the obese, wheezy, 70-year-old smoker with previous myocardial infarcts and chronic venous disease in both legs? Why is the patient short of breath? COPD? Pulmonary oedema? Pulmonary embolus?

WHAT TESTS WILL BE NEEDED TO MAKE THE RIGHT DIAGNOSIS?

It can be helpful to remember a few ground rules about the investigation of patients with unexplained breathlessness.

- In breathlessness caused by COPD and asthma:
  - The chest x-ray may be normal; it may show overinflation, but it will not show pulmonary oedema.
  - The peak flow rate (PFR) and spirometry will always be very abnormal.
- Breathlessness caused by LVF:
  - The chest x-ray will show pulmonary oedema.
  - The electrocardiogram (ECG) is abnormal, showing ischaemia, strain or arrhythmia.
  - An echo-cardiogram will usually confirm poor left ventricular function.

- In breathlessness caused by pulmonary emboli:
  - The diagnosis is often missed, usually because it is not considered.
  - Risk factors are usually present (recent surgery, phlebitic legs, etc.).
  - When in doubt, start oral anticoagulation within an hour of your suspicion and scan the lungs later to confirm the diagnosis.

PRINCIPLES OF EMERGENCY TREATMENT

The principles of emergency treatment are set out in Box 3.1. It must be recognised, however, that on occasions, in a critically ill patient with unexplained breathlessness, it may be appropriate to cover a number of diagnostic options until the picture becomes clearer, and the results of further tests become available.

Respiratory Failure

Normal ventilation is a process in which fresh air is brought through the airways to the alveoli, where it is in intimate contact with blood in the pulmonary capillaries. Gas exchange occurs across the alveolar–capillary interface: oxygen passes from the alveoli into the blood, and carbon dioxide passes from the blood into the alveoli. We measure blood gas partial pressures to assess the efficiency of this two-way traffic: the arterial pO_2 tells us about oxygenation; the arterial pCO_2 indicates how well the lungs are venting carbon dioxide.

BOX 3.1 ■ Principles of Emergency Treatment

1. Correct the immediate and life-threatening problems (ABC)
   - Hypoxia   Oxygen
                              Ventilation
   - Acidosis   Correct high arterial carbon dioxide
   - Hypotension   Fluids ± inotropic support
2. Treat the cause
   - Pulmonary oedema   Diuretics
                                Vasodilators
   - Bronchoconstriction   Bronchodilators
                                Steroids
   - Pulmonary embolism   Anticoagulants
   - Pneumonia   Antibiotics
   - Tension pneumothorax   Intercostal drain
   - COVID-19   Dexamethasone
                                Antivirals
                                Immunomodulators
3. Prevent further attacks
   - Asthma   Education (assess–adjust–review)
   - Pulmonary oedema   Review previous cardiac therapy
   - Pulmonary embolism   DOACS/warfarin

ABC, Airway, breathing, circulation; *DOAC*, direct acting oral anti-coagulant.

Respiratory failure describes a state in which the lungs can no longer oxygenate the blood and is diagnosed by measuring the arterial blood gases (ABGs). Conditions that interfere with any part of the process of normal ventilation may cause respiratory failure. Examples from the AMU include patients who depress their respiratory drive with drug overdosage; patients with progressive paralysis (the most common example is the Guillain-Barré syndrome), in whom respiratory muscles become increasingly weak and ineffective and, by far the most common causes, acute asthma and COPD, in which there is direct impairment of gas exchange as a result of lung damage.

Type I and Type II Respiratory Failure

The lungs are more efficient at venting carbon dioxide than they are at oxygenating blood. As a result, during the development of respiratory failure, problems with oxygenation occur well before carbon dioxide starts to build up. When things start to go wrong, the patient compensates for lesser degrees of carbon dioxide retention by increasing ventilation and blowing off the build-up of carbon dioxide. Thus if you look at the blood gases in a case of acute asthma, you will find that, in the early stage of an attack, carbon dioxide levels in the blood are often lower than normal.

Unfortunately, this compensatory mechanism does not work at all well for problems with oxygenation. You will find, for example, that arterial oxygen levels decrease early on in an asthma attack. Several conditions have a similar pattern of *hypoxia without carbon dioxide retention*: this pattern is termed 'type I' respiratory failure (Fig. 3.1 and Box 3.2). (Look at ward blood gas results in some of the conditions mentioned in Box 3.2—in type I respiratory failure, the arterial pO_2 is less than 8 kPa, with a normal or low carbon dioxide at 4 kPa or less. You need to remember that these figures apply to patients whose gases are measured while they are breathing room air; once oxygen is given to patients with type I respiratory failure, the pO_2 increases.)

With more advanced diseases in which the compensatory mechanism of trying to blow off carbon dioxide has 'worn out', *carbon dioxide retention occurs in addition to hypoxia*. This is type II respiratory failure (pO_2 < 8 kPa, pCO_2 > 6 kPa while not receiving oxygen; see Fig. 3.1). Examples are listed in Box 3.3; the patient in Case study 3.1 has type II respiratory failure.

Hypoxia and hypercapnia: the blood gases. Carbon dioxide is a central nervous system depressant, and its build-up (termed hypercapnia) leads to a cycle of confusion, lack of cooperation, increasing drowsiness and hence further carbon dioxide retention. Hypoxia impairs the function of the heart, brain and kidneys. The combination of excessive carbon dioxide and tissue hypoxia causes an *acidosis* that produces its own damaging effects on major organ functions. (The pH in the blood gas results reflects the degree of tissue acidosis. A pH of less than 7.3 in respiratory failure indicates a major problem and a pH of less than 7.25 requires urgent and aggressive intervention to improve gas exchange.)

FIGURE 3.1 Type I and type II respiratory failure: an overview. *COPD*, Chronic obstructive pulmonary disease.

BOX 3.2 ■ Examples of Type I Respiratory Failure

- The early part of an attack of asthma
- The thin, breathless patient with emphysema
- Pneumonia
- Pulmonary oedema (left ventricle failure)
- Pulmonary embolism

BOX 3.3 ■ Examples of Type II Respiratory Failure

- Severe life-threatening asthma (type I failure progresses to type II failure)
- The obese oedematous patient with severe chronic obstructive pulmonary disease
- Respiratory centre depression in a severe drug overdose
- Obesity/hypoventilation syndrome

CASE STUDY 3.1   Confusion and Falls Due to Respiratory Failure

A 68-year-old non-smoking female was admitted because of increasing drowsiness following a fall at home. The emergency doctor thought she had probably had a stroke.

She and her husband led 'separate lives' at home but he said that she had become increasingly immobile and had taken to sleeping in an armchair over the previous 3 years. Her only medication was a mild diuretic. After a fall in her bedroom, she had not been able to get up and became increasingly difficult to rouse.

On admission, she was drowsy and uncooperative; she was morbidly obese and deeply cyanosed. Her respiratory rate was 5 breaths/min; she was wheezy and her legs, thighs and abdomen were grossly oedematous. There was no evidence of a head injury or any focal neurological signs. Her chest film was normal. Her arterial gases showed a pO_2 of 4.5 kPa, a pCO_2 of 16 kPa and a pH of 7.1. A diagnosis of severe type II respiratory failure due to a combination of obesity/hypoventilation syndrome and asthma was made.

The anaesthetists declined to ventilate her and attempts at non-invasive ventilation (NIV) (see page 81, non-invasive ventilation in COPD) were only partially successful. Intravenous doxapram infusion, 24% oxygen and a combination of twice-daily high-dose furosemide and aminophylline were started. With considerable difficulty, she was nursed in a sitting position. On this regimen, she had marked diuresis with a reduction of her oedema; although with a negative deficit of 10 L, she still weighed 150 kg. She became increasingly alert and started to cough up purulent sputum. She slowly mobilised and lost weight over several weeks in the continuing care ward. NIV was reintroduced successfully and continued overnight after discharge.

NIV is always the preferred option to doxapram (a largely out-dated respiratory stimulant), which is now only considered as a very last resort.

PRINCIPLES OF TREATMENT

For the treatment of respiratory failure to be effective, it must reverse the process by correcting the cause, which, depending on the disease, may include any combination of the following:

- Airway narrowing
- Respiratory muscle weakness

- Alveolar damage
- Respiratory infection
- Impaired respiratory effort

Before vital organ function is compromised, the blood gases must be corrected at the simplest level by giving additional oxygen and, in more complex cases, by assisting or even replacing normal respiratory efforts. The introduction of new forms of 'non-invasive' respiratory support (i.e., the patient does not need endotracheal intubation) now means that selected patients with quite severe respiratory failure can be managed on the AMU with a 'half-way house' type of ventilation. Ideally, these patients should have an early transfer to a respiratory support unit (RSU), run by the respiratory team, where expertise in continuous positive airway pressure (CPAP), NIV, HFNO and proning (see later) is concentrated.

This approach does not have the implications of full intensive therapy unit (ITU) treatment with the problems of endotracheal tubes, weaning, hospital-acquired infections and so forth.

Pulse oximetry. The oximeter measures the oxygen saturation in the arterial blood. The range of values for a normal saturation is small; thus a saturation of 97% is seen in the healthy population, whereas a saturation of 90% can indicate impending respiratory failure. The pulse oximeter is invaluable in recognising early respiratory failure, particularly when readings are taken on admission before the patient has been given oxygen. You must remember, however, that the oximeter only measures oxygen saturation—it will tell you nothing about the level of carbon dioxide or the degree of acidosis.

Why and when do we do blood gases? Oxygen saturations will be low in all cases of respiratory failure. Only the blood gases will tell you whether this is type I or type II respiratory failure. In acute asthma, for example, there is a world of difference between the patient with hypoxia and a normal pCO_2 and the patient who is similarly hypoxic but, having passed from acute asthma to near exhaustion, the patient is now retaining carbon dioxide. If you are in doubt about the severity of the patient's condition, examine the blood gases. As a general rule, in AMU patients, ABGs must be checked when the oxygen saturations are less than 92% with the patient breathing room air (you will see patients with severe type II respiratory failure who have been given unlimited oxygen on their way into the hospital: the oxygen saturations look wonderful at 97%, but the gases reveal grossly increased levels of carbon dioxide).

Acute Severe Asthma

Acute severe asthma continues to be a major challenge to the team at the AMU. The assessment must be quick and accurate, and the treatment has to be tailored to the severity of the attack. The patient's condition can change dramatically and, unfortunately, there is still a significant mortality rate.

Mechanisms

WHO GETS ACUTE SEVERE ASTHMA AND WHY?

Any patient with asthma may have an acute attack, but those who are at particular risk of dying from acute asthma include:

- Chronic severe asthma sufferers
- Patients who are non-compliant with therapy and follow-up
- Overusers of reliever inhalers (more than a canister per month)
- Patients with no written self-management plan (personalised asthma action plan [PAAP])
- Patients with previous acute/near-fatal attacks
- Patients who were admitted for asthma in the past year
- Patients who are poor at recognising the severity of their asthma
- Patients exposed to a high allergic load with a strong history of allergy
- Patients who normally require regular oral steroids
- Patients with a history of brittle asthma/frequent Accidents and Emergency Department (AED) attendance
- Patients with serious psychosocial problems
- Patients with learning difficulties, a history of psychosis or major tranquiliser use
- Patients who have a history of childhood abuse
- Patients who were inappropriately prescribed β-blockers and non-steroidal anti-inflammatory drugs
- Patients with obesity

The number of acute exacerbations per year in which asthma treatment has to be intensified is a useful marker of the severity and control of the underlying asthma. The patient in Case Study 3.2 had been getting attacks of nocturnal breathlessness for months but had not appreciated their significance.

Three major factors narrow the airways in acute asthma:

- Airway muscle contraction
- Thickening of the airway wall with inflammatory cells
- Airway clogging by thickened secretions

Without inhaled steroid treatment, the patient's airways will have been chronically inflamed (see Case Study 3.2). Uncontrolled airway inflammation in asthma is a potent cause of persistent symptoms and repeated severe attacks.

WHAT GOES WRONG DURING AN ATTACK?

As an attack develops, breathing becomes progressively more difficult because the patient has to drag and push air through increasingly narrow tubes. Air becomes trapped behind the blocked tubes so that the lungs overinflate, making the work of breathing even harder. There are two consequences as the asthma attack progresses:

- Gas exchange worsens
- The muscles used for breathing start to fatigue

CASE STUDY 3.2	Acute Severe Asthma

A 38-year-old male had asthma for 30 years. Contrary to medical advice, his only treatment was occasionalinhaled salbutamol. He described chronic sleep disturbance from early morning wheezing, but even the presence of frequent symptoms did not dissuade him from the view that 'normal people like him' should not need to rely on inhalers. His asthma worsened over 2 weeks despite using oral steroids. After a day of exposure to building dust and grass cuttings, he became severely breathless and collapsed. He was admitted after his wife dialled 999.

The patient was too breathless to speak and unable to tolerate a mask. The peak flow could not be recorded. He was clammy with quiet breath sounds and a pulse rate of 160 beats/min. He was given high-flow oxygen via a reservoir mask, nebulised bronchodilators and IV steroids. Emergency blood gases with the patient breathing oxygen showed a pO_2 of 5.6 kPa, a pCO_2 of 16 kPa and a pH of 6.9. A portable chest film showed no sign of a pneumothorax.

The patient was transferred immediately from the AMU to ITU and ventilated for 48h. His peak flows thereafter slowly improved on 40mg of prednisolone and nebulised salbutamol. He continued to have early morning wheezing for the next four mornings, which required extra nebulisers before his symptoms slowly improved. He was transferred to the chest unit. He was discharged with a written personalised asthma management plan and an early out patient review with a respiratory consultant.

The abnormal gas exchange, if uncorrected, goes through two phases:

1. Early in an attack of asthma, a combination of necessity and fear drives breathing sufficiently hard to blow off carbon dioxide. At this point, the levels of carbon dioxide in the blood are normal or low. In contrast, oxygen uptake is impaired and there is hypoxia, even at this early stage. The patient in Case Study 3.2 had already passed this stage by the time he was admitted to hospital.

2. Later, *as breathing tires*, carbon dioxide builds up, oxygen levels continue to decrease and the patient's condition becomes critical. The increase in carbon dioxide, which can be rapid and dramatic, now causes a sudden and dangerous decrease in the blood pH. If this is unchecked, a respiratory arrest will follow.

The implications for emergency management are to identify the patients who are at risk:

- Those who are tiring (history, observation and blood gases)
- Those with severe airway narrowing (peak expiratory flow rate)
- Those with hypoxaemia (oxygen saturation) and a build up of carbon dioxide (blood gases)

Assessment of Acute Severe Asthma

History. By its nature, acute asthma must be assessed quickly. You must find out from the history whether the patient is in a high-risk group. Four features will warn you of the likely difficulties:

- Previous severe attacks, AED attendance and hospital admissions with asthma
- Patients who are taking, or who have previously needed, steroid tablets
- Recent nocturnal attacks (a major sign that asthma is out of control)
- A history of psychosocial problems, non-compliance, self-discharge or substance use disorder

It is unusual for the patient to overestimate the severity of their attack. Patients like that in Case Study 3.2 who are panicking and uncooperative are far more likely to be doing so because of impending asphyxia than because of overanxiety.

Examination. The signs of severe asthma must be recognised:

- A pulse rate of more than 110 beats/min
- A respiratory rate of more than 25 breaths/min
- The patient is too breathless to complete a sentence in 1 breath
- A PFR between a third and a half of their best or their predicted peak flow

A common sequence leading to respiratory arrest is of a desperately breathless patient who becomes ashen, clammy and quietly 'cooperative'. The chest becomes quiet, the pulse slows and respiratory efforts become increasingly feeble. You may have seen patients who are poor at perceiving the severity of their own attacks and noted how they can pass from the severe to the life-threatening stage with little apparent fuss.

The signs of *life-threatening asthma* are any one of the following:

- Oxygen saturations of less than 92%
- Cyanosis
- A silent chest with feeble respiratory effort and exhaustion
- Increasing confusion or a reduction in conscious level/sudden collapse
- Bradycardia or arrhythmia
- Hypotension
- PFR less than one-third of their best or their predicted peak flow
- PaO_2 < 8.0 kPa (if the $PaCO_2$ is also >6.0 kPa, the asthma is *very* severe)

Peak flow rate. The PFR is the simplest and most important objective way to assess acute asthma and monitor the effectiveness of treatment (Fig. 3.2). It must be measured in every case; most patients can produce a reading. However, even the observation that the patient is 'too breathless to do a peak flow' is a clear indication of the severity of the asthma.

It is important to try and find out how the patient is when at their best. There is a world of difference between an admission peak flow of 250 L/min in a steroid-dependent asthmatic patient who never blows better than 275 L/min and a peak flow of 250 L/min in a previously 'mild' asthmatic individual who is used to peak flows of 550 L/min. This information may be available in their hospital case notes, GP records and in-home peak flow diaries. *The best-ever peak flow* is not necessarily the same as the *predicted peak flow*, but both values are useful to decide the current state of the patient's asthma. To know the predicted PFR, you will need a table giving the normal value for a person of the same height, age and sex. These tables should be freely available on the AMU.

- An initial PFR of less than 50% of the predicted value or, if available, 50% of their best-ever PFR reading indicates severe asthma. Peak flows down to one-third of these values indicate life-threatening asthma. As a rough guide, acute severe asthma is associated with PFR readings of less than 300 L/min for most males and less than 200 L/min for most females.

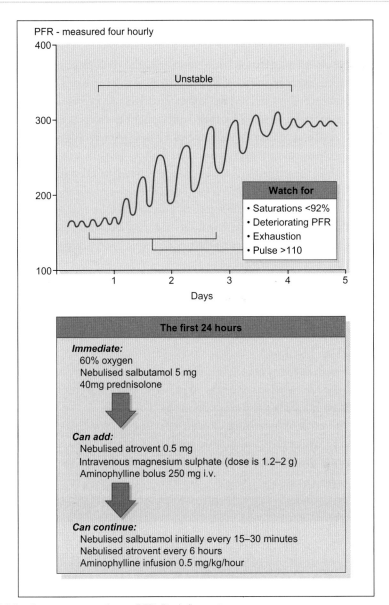

FIGURE 3.2 Acute severe asthma. *PFR,* Peak flow rate.

- The change in PFR with emergency treatment predicts the likely course of events. Unless in a high-risk group, which includes pregnancy, a patient whose PFR rises an hour after treatment to 75% of their best/predicted value can usually be discharged.
- The subsequent PFR chart shows the level of asthma control and stability. Peak flows seesaw as an attack resolves (see Fig. 3.2). Patients are particularly vulnerable during the morning dips in PFR, which occur during the first 2 to 3 days after an acute attack.

Caring for the Patient With Acute Severe Asthma

The balance between resuscitation and communication will depend on your initial assessment. Patients with an unrecordable peak flow, a pulse rate of 140 beats/min and an oxygen saturation of 75% will not welcome a discussion on preventative inhalers. The patients will, however, be terrified by their suffocating breathlessness and will be desperate for your reassurance that they are not going to stop breathing and die (Box 3.4). There will be excellent educational opportunities before the patient is discharged, while the attack is fresh in the patient's mind. Your approach will be tailored to the individual patient. There will be an obvious difference between the communication issues in a case of chronic asthma with repeated admissions to hospital and the case of a new asthmatic presenting with their first attack. There will also be sometimes surprising similarities, not least in the most basic of requirements: the understanding and practical use of inhalers.

CRITICAL CLINICAL TASKS DURING THE ACUTE ATTACK

Give reassurance and support. Take patients through the ways in which each aspect of their treatment acts to bring the attack to an end and enables them to regain control of their breathing (see Box 3.4).

Explain. Explain the importance of effective, continuous oxygen therapy. Show the patient how to use the nebuliser and how to perform a peak flow reading. Explain how the patient can get immediate assistance from the staff.

Minimise the work of breathing. Provide effective and timely asthma medication. Sit patients up in their most comfortable position (this will often involve the patient wanting to sit up, either leaning over a bed table or on the edge of the bed).

BOX 3.4 ■ Reassurance for Patients With Acute Severe Asthma

- I will measure your peak flow rate; we will treat you and we will see how it improves.
- The hard work of breathing will lessen with treatment.
- You will regain control of your breathlessness soon.
- We will stay with you until the treatment works.
- We will sort things out for you—try and relax if possible.
- Find your most comfortable position.
- Slow your breathing rate.
- Take deep, slow breaths through the mask.
- Allow the nebuliser to do its work.
- If the mask is too claustrophobic, we can use oxygen tubing to your nostrils.
- The ward team will be here near you at all times.
- Call us if your breathing seems to be getting more difficult.
- Do not worry about all the noises from the monitors and drips.
- The oximeter shows that you are getting enough oxygen into your lungs.
- Steroid side effects will be minimised by the short course that you need.

CRITICAL CLINICAL OBSERVATIONS IN ACUTE SEVERE ASTHMA

- Pulse rate
- Respiratory rate
- PFR before and after each nebuliser
- Oxygen saturation (preferably before oxygen is started)
- Ability to complete a sentence

IMPORTANT CLINICAL OBSERVATIONS IN ACUTE SEVERE ASTHMA

- Blood pressure (which may be increased by anxiety)
- Urine dipsticks (for steroid-induced diabetes)
- Sputum colour (wallpaper glue-like sputum is common in asthma)
- Temperature (a sign of respiratory infection)
- Inhaler technique (critical for future management)

CRITICAL CARING TASKS DURING THE ACUTE ATTACK

- Give reassurance and support
- Provide explanations
- Minimise the work of breathing
- Monitor the patient's progress (National Early Warning Score 2 [NEWS2])
- Plan to prevent this from happening again

Monitor the patient's progress. This may need to be continuous for the critical first hour or so. Beware of an increasing pulse rate, decreasing peak flow and a tiring patient. Do not be falsely reassured by a normal oxygen saturation if the patient looks awful. Just before a respiratory arrest, many asthmatic patients become quiet, clammy and cooperative.

Plan to prevent this from happening again. Identify why this attack occurred. Start a re-evaluation of the patient's long-term management that must then be taken over by appropriate follow-up arrangements.

Management of Acute Severe Asthma

INITIAL EMERGENCY TREATMENT

- **Oxygen** (to correct gas exchange): High-flow oxygen at 40% to 60% and oxygen-driven nebulisers (at 6 L/min). The target oxygen saturations are 94% to 98%
- **Bronchodilators** (to increase airway calibre): Nebulised (with oxygen at 6 L/min) salbutamol 5 mg combined, if there are life-threatening features, with nebulised ipratropium (Atrovent) 0.5 mg
- **Corticosteroids** (to reduce airway inflammation): IV hydrocortisone 100 mg and/or 40 to 50 mg oral prednisolone

SUBSEQUENT TREATMENT

If there is no improvement by 15 minutes:

- Repeat the salbutamol and ipratropium.
- Consider a single dose of IV magnesium sulphate, 1.2 to 2 g, over 20 min.
- Continue to give nebulised salbutamol every 15 (in a poorly responding severe attack, consider using a special nebuliser to give continuous salbutamol at 10 mg/h). Continue ipratropium from 4 to 6 h a day.
- Consider IV aminophylline (5 mg/kg) over 20 minutes. Particular care is needed in choosing the doses, especially if patients have been taking theophylline as their usual asthma therapy, in which case theophylline levels should have been checked on admission. Start an infusion of aminophylline 0.5 to 0.7 mg/kg/h over 24 h. Check theophylline levels (aim for 10–20 mg/L) daily.

ASSESSING RESPONSE

Following the PFR and oximetry. The key to assessment lies in the measurement of PFR. This is done on admission and, while the patient is in the unstable phase, at 15-min intervals. Thereafter, measure the PFR before and after bronchodilator treatment at least four times per day. The oximetry is monitored continuously with the aim of keeping the oxygen saturations in the range of 94% to 98%.

Repeating the blood gases. During the first few critical hours, you may need to use the ABGs if there is any doubt about the patient's progress. The purpose of the blood gas measurement is to identify an increase in $PaCO_2$ (and a fall in pH). Thus the blood gases should be repeated 1 h after the start of treatment (or earlier) if:

- Poor blood gases on admission (pO_2 < 8.0 kPa, with a normal or high pCO_2)
- Saturations cannot be kept above 92%
- The patient's condition deteriorates

Patients ought to have improved by 4 to 6 h, but if not, the blood gases should be repeated.

Transfer to intensive therapy unit? If the patient is tired, confused or drowsy, if the PFR is deteriorating or unchanged and the patient feels worse and particularly if the pCO_2 is increasing and the pH is decreasing, you should prepare to move the patient to the ITU (see Case Study 3.2). The ITU outreach team should have already been made aware of the patient. Respiratory arrest, when it complicates acute asthma, occurs with alarming speed and always poses a major challenge to the resuscitation team. With proper assessment and by monitoring the response to treatment, you can avoid this complication.

Non-invasive ventilation (NIV)? CPAP/BiPAP (two levels [Bi] of positive airway pressure) are of unproven value in acute severe asthma and should only be considered in an ITU setting.

A good response to treatment. In most cases, you will see a rapid response to treatment. Salbutamol and ipratropium can be reduced to 4 or 6 hourly. The PFRs increase and the patient will feel better. However, if you examine the PFR charts of patients who are recovering from acute asthma, you will often see that, despite a trend of improvement, the readings continue to fluctuate for several days. These patients remain at risk, particularly in the early morning when their peak flows are at their lowest. You will find that some asthma guidelines use the degree of variation in PFR between the morning and evening as an indication that the patient is fit to be discharged from the hospital. As a minimum, a patient should not be discharged if their PFR is less than 75% of their predicted or best-ever value. Ensure a trained asthma liaison nurse is involved in providing a written PAAP based on symptoms and a PFR diary. Robust follow-up arrangements are critical—inform the patient's primary care practice within 24 h of discharge.

In a 'difficult-to-each' asthmatic patient, the aftermath of an acute asthma attack provides a golden opportunity to reassess their asthma. There are now several 'biologics'—monoclonal antibody therapies such as benralizumab which can be life changing for patients with chronic severe asthma (only 20% of whom are currently offered this treatment).

Acute Severe Asthma in Pregnancy

Control deteriorates in about a third of asthmatics during pregnancy, particularly in the second and third trimesters. Acute severe asthma will threaten the life of both the mother and the foetus. Fortunately, the drug treatment for severe asthma is the same as for the non-pregnant. Oxygenation is a priority with urgent measures to keep saturations between 94% and 98%. Foetal monitoring is required from the onset, and if there is any doubt about foetal well-being the patient will need to be transferred to ITU.

Excellent Asthma Care

- Use of British Thoracic Society guidelines for the treatment of acute asthma
- Admission peak flow rates recorded
- Blood gases measured if saturation was under 92% and appropriate action was taken
- Serial PFRs documented
- The documentation of 'best-ever' lung function (PFR or spirometry)
- Referral for follow-up to a respiratory nurse or chest team
- Review of educational needs, inhaler technique, compliance and PAAPs for each patient

Answering Relatives' Questions in Severe Asthma

The patient's relatives will have found this as frightening as the patient and will also need reassurance. You may need to address several issues with them.

Should we have acted sooner? Examine their understanding of asthma. Establish if they were aware of a self-management plan. Consider referral to the asthma service or recommend up-to-date written information (e.g., National Asthma Campaign leaflets).

Was there anything else that we could have done? Had the patients been underestimating the severity of their asthma? Had there been overreliance on the reliever medication? What were the methods used to assess the severity of the attack? What about the use of rescue steroid medication?

The patient has been under stress—is it all nerves? Provide reassurance about the physical nature of asthma. Any 'nervous' component is almost certainly an effect rather than a cause of asthma. Ensure that the patient's visitors do not have an adverse effect on the patient's management, particularly in the early stage when cooperation with oxygen therapy, nebuliser treatment and so forth is critical.

Could any of the patient's other medications upset the asthma? Examine and list all of the patient's medication. Some drugs, such as aspirin, non-steroidal anti-inflammatories and β-blockers (tablets or β-blocker-containing eye drops), can worsen asthma. Assess the patient's compliance with their asthma medication. Involve close relatives with the management plans.

Upper Airway Obstruction: Not to Be Confused With Asthma

Upper airway obstruction also produces severe airway noise and breathlessness. Although it can be difficult, a distinction in these cases must be made from acute severe asthma (Case Studies 3.3 and 3.4).

CASE STUDY 3.3 Acute Epiglottitis

A 35-year-old male had flu-like symptoms for 5 days, culminating in a severe sore throat. For 24 h, he could not swallow fluids and had a hoarse voice. On admission, he was flushed, pyrexial and breathless. He had a harsh superficial inspiratory and expiratory upper airway noise (*stridor*), which was easily heard at the mouth. He could open his mouth but could not swallow his saliva. His tonsils were inflamed but not particularly enlarged. His PFR was 250. Based on the characteristic history and examination a diagnosis of acute adult epiglottitis with impending respiratory obstruction was made. Intravenous antibiotics were started, and he was transferred, accompanied by a competent anaesthetist, to the ENT (Ears, Nose and Throat) unit for close observation and upper airway management.

CASE STUDY 3.4 Stridor and Haemoptysis Due to Tracheal Cancer

A 55-year-old male smoker was admitted with increasing breathlessness, panic attacks and noisy breathing. On direct questioning, he was admitted to occasional haemoptysis. He had a virtually unrecordable peak flow. Bronchodilators were ineffective and it became clear his wheeze was in fact stridor. At bronchoscopy, his trachea was narrowed to a pinhole at its midpoint by a carcinoma. Urgent laser treatment and chemotherapy produced an excellent symptomatic response.

Chronic Obstructive Pulmonary Disease

MECHANISMS

What Is COPD?

The term COPD describes patients who suffer from long-standing progressive airflow obstruction but in whom the response to bronchodilator therapy, no matter how intensive, is either absent or incomplete. The airflow obstruction is predominantly fixed, so most of the patients have symptoms that, unlike in asthma, vary little from day to day or from week to week. Acute exacerbations occur when infection temporarily worsens the airflow obstruction with an increase in breathlessness, cough and/or sputum.

COPD embraces a spectrum of cases that range from the patient who is steroid-dependent with chronic asthma to the individual with heavy-smoking chronic bronchitis with advanced emphysema. The 'mix' in any one patient with COPD depends on how much is asthma (reversible) and how much is irreversible smoking-related damage to both the alveoli (emphysema) and the small airways (Case Study 3.5).

CASE STUDY 3.5   **Acute Exacerbation of COPD**

A 67-year-old male was admitted with breathlessness, general weakness and a productive cough. He had smoked 20 cigarettes a day since his late teens but had given up 3 months previously. He had been 'chesty' for more than 10 years with wheeziness and chest tightness. Colds always went to his chest, leaving him with a prolonged cough with green sputum. He eventually retired in his late 50s because of respiratory problems: a chronic cough, frequent chest infections and increasing breathlessness on exertion. For 2 weeks his cough and wheeze had worsened, he had become weaker and his ankles had started to swell. He had suffered a myocardial infarction 2 years previously and had occasional attacks of angina. He had also been troubled by chronic varicose veins, complicated by a venous ulcer. Being a widower, he lived alone.

On admission, the patient was pink, overweight, tremulous and mildly confused. He was receiving oxygen at 15 L/min via a reservoir mask, which had been started by the paramedics. He had a weak, productive-sounding cough but could not bring sputum up. He was wheezy, tachypneic at 28 breaths/min and had quite marked ankle oedema.

The patient's temperature was 37.6°C, and he had an irregular pulse, with an apical rate of 125 beats/min. His oxygen supply was changed to 24% by Ventimask, but his saturations on pulse oximetry decreased to 75%. Immediate physiotherapy helped him to cough up moderate amounts of green sputum and, after an air-driven nebuliser of ipratropium (Atrovent) 0.5 mg, he appeared less drowsy. His ABGs on admission, breathing room air were pO_2 4.5 kPa, pCO_2 10 kPa, pH 7.25. An ECG confirmed atrial fibrillation and a chest film showed overinflation but no evidence of pneumonia.

The inspired oxygen was increased by changing to a 28% mask. This improved the patient's oxygen saturation to 85% but gases repeated after an hour showed a rising CO_2 level, and the patient had become more drowsy. At that stage, NIV (non-invasive ventilation) was successfully introduced.

The clearest indication for NIV is type II respiratory failure with a pCO_2 >6.0 kPa and an arterial pH less than 7.35 despite 1 h of maximum medical treatment and controlled oxygen administration.

There are four elements to COPD, all of which are seen in Case Study 3.5.

1. **Asthma.** This provides the responsive component to the airflow obstruction, which will improve with aggressive bronchodilator treatment. The patient will exhibit wheeze and chest tightness. There will be features of airway irritability: tightness on exposure to cold air and fumes and an early morning wheeze.

2. **Chronic bronchitis.** A smoking-related condition in which there is a long-standing productive cough as a result of the formation of excessive mucus (phlegm) in the lungs. This is usually worse in the winter months. When the mucus becomes infected, the airflow obstruction temporarily worsens.

3. **Emphysema and small airway damage.** These are fixed changes in the structure of the lungs. In emphysema, the alveoli are destroyed and the lung's elastic supporting tissue is lost. Airways collapse through loss of support and the lungs overinflate to try and hold them open. Patients with overinflated lungs appear barrel chested and, to prevent airway collapse, breathe out through pursed lips: a common sign in severe emphysema that becomes particularly obvious during acute exacerbations. Some emphysematous patients maintain normal blood gases at the expense of severe chronic breathless ness (fighting for breath) - generating the term "pink puffer".

4. **Acute exacerbations.** These are episodes of increased breathlessness, cough and sputum which develop over 1 to 2 weeks. They have a major impact on the patient's health, recovery is slow—taking up to 8 weeks. Each exacerbation speeds up the loss of lung function. Exacerbations become more frequent as the COPD worsens. Importantly, the new combination inhalers (e.g., Trimbow, Trelegy and Spiolto Respimat) improve the quality of life in patients with COPD but also reduce the frequency of exacerbations.

The combination of airway damage and alveolar destruction disrupts the primary function of the lungs: the exchange of oxygen and carbon dioxide between the air and the blood. Too much disruption and the patient becomes hypoxic (blue) and loses the battle to blow off carbon dioxide; a combination described previously and termed type II respiratory failure.

COPD Complicated by Cor Pulmonale

Why did the patient in Case Study 3.5 develop ankle oedema, and why is it of such importance to his future management? Patients who are chronically hypoxic eventually develop fluid retention. A major reason for this is the increased strain on the right side of the heart that occurs because the heart has to force blood through abnormal lungs. The first sign of fluid retention, the development of ankle oedema, often occurs (as in the case study) during an acute exacerbation of COPD. The presence of ankle oedema should act as a warning to take a more aggressive approach to the treatment of the underlying lung disease. Right-sided heart failure that occurs as a result of lung disease is known as cor pulmonale. The most common cause of cor pulmonale is COPD (the combination of cyanosis and oedematous limbs generated the term "blue bloater" for this clinical combination), but it can occur in the setting of any chronic severe lung disease.

Long-Term Oxygen Therapy

Patients with COPD who develop cor pulmonale can be helped by long-term oxygen therapy, which is administered for 15 h/day or more. By correcting the underlying problem, hypoxia, the length and quality of the patient's life can be improved. Once the patient in Case Study 3.5 has recovered from the exacerbation, he should be referred to the respiratory team for possible long-term oxygen therapy.

Assessment of Acute Exacerbations of COPD

Patients with COPD who are ill enough to be admitted to hospital during an exacerbation do not fare particularly well. The in-hospital mortality is around 10%, and only 50% of the patients will still be alive 5 years after the exacerbation. One in three patients will be readmitted within 3 months—a risk strongly associated with frailty, severity of COPD and the presence of comorbidities. Information from the initial assessment will help discussions on possible ventilation should the need arise, but such decisions are fraught with difficulty. The patients most in need of ventilation are least able to give a good history. Relatives' information is vital, but may not be objective. There has to be particular caution when a patient as in Case Study 3.5 comes in, who is not previously known to the hospital service. Quite often, the patient has been on suboptimal treatment and may do well once the crisis has passed. The prognosis in patients with COPD does not seem to depend on whether they require emergency ventilation but more on the severity of their pre-existing lung disease and their overall frailty.

History in COPD

Important points in the history include:
- Baseline breathlessness and overall frailty using the extended Medical Research Council dyspnoea score (Table 3.1).

TABLE 3.1 ■ eMRCD Scale

Grade	'In the past 3 months when you were feeling at your best which of the following statements best describes your level of breathlessness?'
1	Only breathlessness on strenuous exercise
2	Short of breath when hurrying on the level or walking up a slight hill
3	Walks slower than contemporaries or stops on the level after 15 min
4	Stops for breath after walking about 100 m or after a few minutes on level ground
5a	Too breathless to leave the house unassisted but independent of washing and/or dressing
5b	Too breathless to leave the house unassisted and requires help with dressing and washing (includes help with putting on socks and shoes)

eMRCD, Extended Medical Research Council dyspnoea.

- The number of exacerbations per year.
- Previous hospital admissions and their outcomes.
- Does the patient have an 'oxygen alert' card indicating they are at risk from oxygen-induced CO_2 retention?
- Any history of ankle oedema suggesting episodes of cor pulmonale?
- Comorbidity, especially heart disease, diabetes, depression/anxiety, obesity and sleep apnoea
- Is the patient using nebulisers?
- Is the patient on long-term oxygen therapy?
- Is the patient still smoking?
- Is there evidence of an advanced directive or of the wishes of the patient concerning resuscitation and escalation to ITU with a view to ventilation?
- Has the patient been in contact with COVID-19?

The initial assessment must take note of:

- Is the patient being given oxygen inappropriately? (The patient in Case Study 3.5 was receiving a potentially disastrous quantity of oxygen.)
- Is the patient confused? (Confusion suggests CO_2 retention.)
- Is the respiratory rate at or above 25 breaths/min? (The patient is already at their limits of reserve.)
- Is the pulse more than 110 beats/min?
- Does oximetry indicate saturations on room air (or their usual oxygen prescription) of less than 88%?
- Is the temperature above 38.5°C? (It indicates severe infection, particularly pneumonia.)
- How long has this attack lasted? (Is the patient likely to be tired?)
- Is the cough effective and are there retained secretions?
- Is the sputum purulent?
- Is breathing hard work? (Pursed lips, overuse of accessory muscles, patient sitting forward with arms fixed.)
- Breathlessness can be quantified from 0 (not at all breathless) to 10 (worst breathlessness I have ever experienced). A score over 5 suggests a serious exacerbation.
- How much wheezing is there? (Bronchodilators and steroids should help.)
- Is there ankle oedema (cor pulmonale)?
- Results of immediate testing for COVID-19 and influenza.

CRITICAL CLINICAL OBSERVATIONS

- Respiratory rate
- Oxygen saturation (preferably before oxygen is started)
- Is the patient at all confused? (possible CO_2 retention)
- Is there an effective cough?
- Is there ankle oedema?

IMPORTANT CLINICAL OBSERVATIONS

- Peak flow rate
- Pulse rate
- Sputum colour
- Temperature (a sign of respiratory infection)
- Will the patient cooperate with the oxygen mask?

Analysis of the blood gases of the patient in Case Study 3.5 indicates that he needs urgent and aggressive intervention. Any of these results needs to be acted on quickly.

- pO_2 less than 6.7 kPa
- pCO2 is more than 9.3 kPa
- pH is less than 7.3

Management of Acute Exacerbations of COPD

In an unfamiliar patient, it can be hard to differentiate a case of end-stage COPD from a case of moderately severe COPD made worse by a reversible factor such as pulmonary embolus, infection or heart failure. If there is any doubt, it is safer to assume there is a treatable component and to manage the patient aggressively. If all else fails, this may have to include ITU ventilation.

Controlled oxygen therapy. Many patients with severe COPD and type II respiratory failure are in a parlous state with regard to their oxygen needs. During periods of instability, there is a fine balance between:

1. The deleterious effects of hypoxia (low oxygen levels) on cardiac, cerebral and kidney function
2. The stimulant effects of hypoxia on respiratory drive

If too little oxygen is given, hypoxia damages the function of vital organs. If too much oxygen is given, the respiratory drive is switched off, carbon dioxide builds up, and as a result, the patient becomes acidotic (pH falls), which in itself causes organ damage.

How much oxygen is safe? The aim of controlled oxygen treatment is to maintain oxygen saturations between 88% and 92% without triggering worsening hypercapnia and a decrease in pH (increasing acidosis). Venturi masks giving 24% or 28% oxygen are safe as an initial step until the arterial gas results are known. Pending blood gas results, the target saturation for all patients with COPD should be 88% to 92% and no higher.

It should be noted that patients with COPD with very high respiratory rates (>30 breaths/min) may not receive sufficient gas flow with a 24% Venturi mask at the specified 2 L/min and in these cases, the flow rate should be increased to 3 L/min. Nasal cannulae may give more than 28% and are probably not safe as first-line treatment in unstable patients, although occasionally patients will not tolerate a mask. Gases should be rechecked 1 h after controlled oxygen is started. A good response sees the pO_2 increasing above 7.5 kPa, with no fall in pH or increase in CO_2. A poor response sees a falling pH and difficulty in keeping oxygen levels above 6.6 kPa.

If the pO_2 can only be corrected at the expense of a decreasing respiratory effort (as indicated by the falling pH and increasing pCO_2), then an additional stimulus or aid to respiratory drive may be needed to drive off CO_2. Intervention must not be delayed, and if, despite controlled oxygen, the pH decreases to 7.35 or less and the pCO_2 is more than 6, assisted ventilation should be considered. There are two ways to provide respiratory support:

- NIV, also known as BiPAP
- Formal ventilation on the ITU

Why measure gases when we have an oximeter? Pulse oximetry measures oxygen saturation, and as such, it can be a useful guide to oxygen requirements. It must be clearly understood, however, that oximetry does not measure pCO_2 or pH, both of which are critical factors in type II (hypercapnic) respiratory failure, particularly during the first 12 h of treatment. It is dangerous to rely entirely on pulse oximetry in unstable patients, in whom blood gases must be measured regularly to evaluate the effect of any change in treatment.

Bronchodilators in COPD. The response to bronchodilators is modest in COPD. Nebulised salbutamol 2.5 to 5 mg 4 hourly should be tried until the patient is well enough to revert to lower-dose treatment. Some patients with COPD probably respond as well or better to nebulised ipratropium (Atrovent) 0.5 mg 6 hourly. For severe exacerbations, the combination of nebulised salbutamol (Ventolin) and ipratropium (Atrovent) is usually given. *If the patient is hypercapnic, the nebuliser must be driven with compressed air and not oxygen. If the patient needs constant oxygen, this can be continued with nasal cannulae during nebulization.* The driving gas should be stated on the prescription. Intravenous theophyllines can be tried if nebulisers are ineffective, but the response is unpredictable and toxicity may occur. These drugs may have a role with high-dose furosemide when there is resistant oedema in severe cor pulmonale.

Antibiotics in exacerbations of COPD. Most exacerbations of COPD are primarily viral in origin. Nonetheless, antibiotics are generally given to patients with COPD who exhibit increasing breathlessness if the quantity and colour of the sputum are changing. Amoxicillin is the first choice unless it has been given unsuccessfully at home. A 5-day course is usually sufficient. The emergence of the organisms *Moraxella catarrhalis* and *Chlamydia pneumoniae* as pathogens in some exacerbations of COPD means that other antibiotics such as co-amoxiclav (Augmentin) and erythromycin may need to be considered. Although the choice of antibiotics should be determined by the result of sputum cultures, in most cases, these are not available until the patient has been in the hospital for several days. If the patient remains unwell with persistent breathlessness, a productive cough and sputum that will not clear, it is justified to try a potent IV antibiotic such as a third-generation cephalosporin. Severe and frequent exacerbations may be associated with the colonisation of damaged lungs with pseudomonas, a notoriously resistant bacteria.

If pneumonia is diagnosed from the chest film, the patient is treated in accordance with the appropriate guidelines.

Oral steroids in exacerbations of COPD. Steroids are used in COPD in much the same way that they are given in acute asthma: 40 mg of oral prednisolone daily for 5 days. There is some evidence that steroids will shorten the duration of an acute exacerbation. The response will be less marked than in asthma; peak flows will show only modest increases as the patient's symptoms improve. Typical values would be peak flows of around 120 L/min on admission and perhaps 150 L/min before discharge. The question of whether oral steroids should be followed by inhaled steroids will have to be considered at a later stage. In selected, severely affected cases, inhaled steroids reduce the frequency of exacerbations and slow the decline in quality of life. Overall, about 10% of patients with COPD will benefit from long-term inhaled steroids (combined in a triple inhaler with long-acting relatives of salbutamol and ipratropium), although they can be difficult to identify during an acute illness. Inappropriate maintenance of oral steroids, a common problem in COPD, causes more harm than benefit but can only be withdrawn under careful supervision.

Non-invasive Ventilation. NVI is the best way to treat patients with acute exacerbations of COPD who remain in type II (hypercapnic) respiratory failure despite 1 h of maximum medical treatment and controlled oxygen therapy (see Case Study 3.5). A delay in initiating NIV reduces the chance of recovery, so it should be started within 2 h of arriving in hospital. When done properly, it is successful in 8 out of 10 cases.

Patients receiving NIV are less likely to need tracheal intubation, stay in the hospital for less time and are more likely to survive than patients treated conventionally. Success is not guaranteed, however, and before embarking on NIV, there must be an explicit decision as to whether or not the patient should be intubated and ventilated if NIV fails—a decision that will be critically dependent on the patient's pre-existing level of dependency, which must be documented in the notes.

There must be an explicit record of whether NIV is the ceiling in any management plan or whether the patient can go on to intubation if NIV fails.

Ventilator. The simplest and most popular machine is a BiPAP ventilator, which provides two levels (Bi) of **p**ositive **a**irway **p**ressure (PAP): a higher pressure in inspiration (IPAP) to drive air into the lungs and blow off carbon dioxide and a lower pressure during expiration (EPAP) to keep the bases of the lungs expanded, thus helping oxygenation. The machine senses the onset of an inspiratory effort and is triggered to assist the patient by pushing in a bigger breath than would otherwise have been taken. If the machine is not triggered, either because the effort is too feeble or because the patient's respiratory rate is too low, the machine takes over and supplies the whole of the breath.

Masks. The full-face mask is easier to fit than the nasal mask, and it ventilates more effectively, as many patients can only breathe through their mouths. There are established techniques for sizing and fitting the masks, ensuring that leaks are minimised and that the patient is reassured and comfortable. Masks are usually 'vented'—there is an intentional leak to allow carbon dioxide to be expelled.

Setting IPAP and EPAP levels. The starting level for IPAP is 10 cm H_2O, increasing by 2 cm H_2O every 10 to a maximum, if tolerated, of 20 cm H_2O. EPAP is set at 4 to 5 cm H_2O and is not usually changed.

Oxygen. This is fed into the circuit (through a T connector and not directly into the mask) to keep the saturations in the range of 88% to 92%; a typical initial flow rate would be 4 L/min.

The first 24 h on NIV. Patients who do well settle on the NIV and synchronise with the machine, struggle less to breathe, use their accessory (neck) muscles less, their respiratory rate falls, and, within 1 to 2 h, their blood gases start to improve. Patients who do less well show lots of air leaks, they are confused or restles, their chest does not expand well in time with the machine ('asynchrony'), their vital signs are unstable and blood gases at 4 h are unchanged or worse. The aim of NIV is to allow oxygenation to take place without an increase in CO_2. If it is successful, the CO_2 will slowly fall and the pH will rise (Fig. 3.3).

Typical signs of success would include:

- Respiratory rate falling below 24 breaths/min
- Heart rate below 110 beats/min
- Saturations more than 90% on oxygen 4 L/min
- pH greater than 7.35 (blood gases are checked at 0, 1, 4 and 12 h)

Failure of NIV is usually due to:

- Mask intolerance
- Persistent mask leaks
- Asynchrony
- Excessive airway secretions
- Nasal bridge erosions
- Patient choice
- The need to escalate treatment (intubation)

The first 24 h of NIV. Success is determined by improvement in ABGs after NIV has been started. These are taken after 1 h (to optimise the NIV settings and oxygen administration), after 4 h (a critical result that often determines the escalation of care to ITU and ventilation if improvement is not apparent by then) and after 12 h. Failure to improve after 4 h of NIV requires specialist respiratory input within 30 minutes of identifying the issue.

Frequent clinical observations (accompanied by intensive reassurance) are critical during the first 4 h: every 15 minutes during the first hour, and every 30 minutes for the next three hours. Thereafter, hourly observations are continued until 12 h and then reduced further as appropriate.

Observations include:

- Mask comfort and compliance
- Oxygen saturations (continuous oximetry)
- Respiratory rate
- Pulse and blood pressure

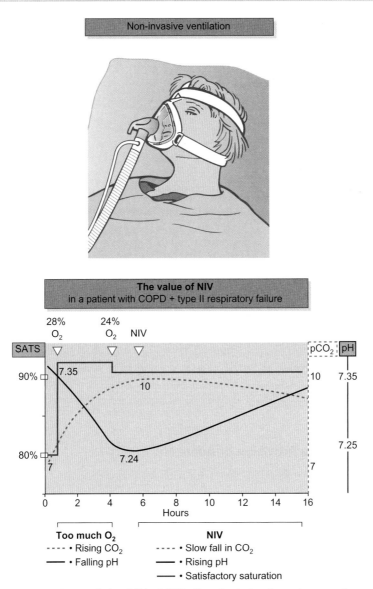

Figure 3.3 Non-invasive ventilation (NIV). *COPD,* Chronic obstructive pulmonary disease; *SATS,* saturations.

- Extent of chest movement, use of accessory muscles and asynchrony
- Conscious level and degree of confusion (AVPU plus new-onset confusion)
- The times when NIV starts and finishes
- Head and neck position: excessive neck flexion, particularly when the patient is not fully awake, can cause upper airway obstruction and is a common source of NIV failure. Prop the patient up and seek physiotherapy advice

A typical 5-day NIV regimen

0–24 h

As long as possible but a minimum of 6 h. One 10-min break/h for nebulisers, oral intake and personal care.

24–48 h (day 2)

NIV for 16 h, including 6 to 8 h overnight.

48–72 h (day 3)

NIV for 12 h, including 6 to 8 h overnight.

72–96 h (day 4)

NIV for 2 h in the morning and afternoon and 6 h overnight.

96–120 h (day 5)

NIV overnight only.

Clearly, some patients will recover with only 2 to 3 days of NIV and will not require weaning; remaining stable for 4 h off NIV suggests it can be taken off. Others will decide for themselves when to discontinue based, often, on intolerance of the whole process. Some patients need longer than 5 days; indeed, some may require long-term overnight NIV. Late failure of NIV (after using it for 48 h) has a poor outlook, unless the patient is suitable for treatment escalation with ITU care, intubation and ventilation.

The outlook after ITU ventilation for COPD is surprisingly good: mean survival times are around 3 years. The patients who do well have usually been on suboptimal treatment before their admission to hospital. There is a general view that, in the United Kingdom, too few patients with COPD and respiratory failure are given the chance of ITU ventilation.

Excellence in the Provision of Acute NIV?

A cohort of appropriately skilled staff with defined competencies
1. Administering NIV in designated areas (preferably an RSU
2. Minimum nurse: patient ratios of 1:2 during the first 24 h of NIV
3. Structured training: induction and annual updates
4. Written protocols and patient/relative information leaflets
5. Individualised NIV 'prescriptions' and documentation of compliance and hours of use
6. Appropriate use of the NEWS2 and the supplementary scale for patients with COPD at risk from too much oxygen
7. Explicit documentation concerning ceilings of care and plans for escalation
8. Annual audit/NIV register or database

Caring for the Patient With COPD

Patients who are admitted with COPD often have complex nursing and medical needs. Most will have several major health problems besides COPD, and there is invariably a background of increasing disability and dependence. For a number, however, their usual treatment will have been less than optimal, and there may be some treatable condition that has tipped the balance and brought them into hospital. As a general rule, therefore, your safest course is to assume that there is a major reversible component in all of your patients with COPD. Remember, most of your patients will respond to treatment; they will be discharged with a new and better management plan and will have an improved quality of life. For those who do not improve or for those who deteriorate despite maximum treatment, your role becomes one of symptom palliation, but this will not be clear to you in the first 24 h of the patient's admission. Your priorities are therefore to address airflow obstruction, improve gas exchange and prevent respiratory failure. The skill for you as a clinician is to combine this with an understanding of the psychological burden that this condition carries and which colours the patient's physical response to it (Box 3.5).

CRITICAL CARING TASKS DURING THE ACUTE ATTACK

Give reassurance and support. Take a positive approach. Most patients with COPD will have experienced very negative attitudes toward their condition. Some patients will be very fearful that they have reached the terminal phase of their illness. Reassure them about the new techniques and approaches to treatment that we are now using.

CRITICAL CARING TASKS DURING THE ACUTE ATTACK

- Give reassurance and support
- Provide explanations
- Minimise the work of breathing
- Monitor the patient's progress
- Prepare the patient for possible active intervention

BOX 3.5 ▪ Reassurance for Patients With Exacerbations of Chronic Obstructive Pulmonary Disease

- Your breathlessness and tightness will improve as our therapies start to work.
- You will start to cough up sputum and clear your chest as the treatment takes effect.
- The more you cough up, the better you will feel.
- You can have the nebuliser on frequent occasions during the first few days.
- Because you are getting oxygen through the mask, you do not have to fight for breath.
- Try not to panic about the mask; it needs to stay on to boost your oxygen levels.
- The oximeter reading is more than 80%, so you are getting plenty of oxygen into your lungs.
- Your ankle swelling is due to fluid retention; it will improve slowly with treatment. It is not a sign of heart weakness.
- Find your most comfortable position, even if it means sitting out in the chair.
- You will start to eat again as the infection clears and your oxygen levels improve.
- We will work hard on your chest for the next 24 h, and you can rest after that.
- You will get some sleep once things improve; a sleeping tablet would be dangerous.
- We will give you your other medications just as you were taking them at home.

Explain. Despite its inconvenience, the mask *must* be kept on because it is not there simply to relieve breathlessness; it is part of the continuing treatment. Take some time to familiarise the patient with the mask and to ensure it fits comfortably. Prepare the oedematous patient for the effects of the diuretics. For a severely breathless patient, asking for and using a bottle or bedpan will be a major undertaking.

Minimise the work of breathing. Many of your patients with COPD will be bordering on panic. Prop the patient up with pillows or allow them to rest on pillows across a bed table. Excessive neck flexion with the head flopping forward while on NIV must be corrected. Patients with obesity and oedema will be nursed best sitting out or resting with their legs over the side of the bed. One close relative can be very helpful in ensuring cooperation with masks and so forth; any more than this is counterproductive.

Monitor the patient's progress. The first 12 h are critical. Keep oxygen saturation in the target range of 88% to 92%. Patients who are becoming drowsy or confused need a detailed reassessment, including blood gases. Fluid balance becomes critical if diuretics are being used. Monitor the pulse: your patients are at risk from arrhythmias, particularly if they are hypoxic, are receiving aminophylline or have a cardiac history.

The new NEWS2 Scoring Scale 2. The new oxygen saturation scoring scale is used for patients with hypercapnia and COPD with a prescribed oxygen target range of 88% to 92%. These patients now score 0 points when in the target range, reducing the risk of unnecessary escalation.

Prepare the patient for more active intervention if there is no improvement. Explain about the possible need for invasive ventilation. Many patients will feel relieved that the work of breathing is going to be taken from them. It is helpful to give some warning about the need for ITU ventilation if this looks like becoming an option.

Excellent Care for COPD

- Documentation of existing exercise tolerance and quality of life
- The use of validated scoring systems (DECAF and PEARL) to identify high-risk patients and calculate the immediate and long-term prognosis
- Attempts to identify the patient's wishes regarding active treatment and resuscitation
- Documentation of discussions with the patient's family
- Chest film report is in the notes
- Evidence that old hospital notes have been reviewed
- Due regard to comorbidities (especially anxiety, heart disease, diabetes and upper GI problems)
- Appropriate use of blood gases
- Safe oxygen prescribing
- Documentation of inspired oxygen at the time arterial gases were measured
- Appropriate use of the oxygen saturation section 2 on the NEWS2 charts in patients with target saturation of 88% to 92%
- Statement of treatment aims (e.g., 'to maintain saturations in the range 88%–92%')
- Availability of NIV
- PFR chart or regular spirometry
- Close liaison with early discharge COPD teams and urgent referral for pulmonary rehabilitation

Answering Relatives' Questions in COPD

The patient's relatives are likely to have witnessed the effects of the progressive loss of lung function first hand. They will be anxious about the immediate outcome and will often express strong views about the patient's existing quality of life. While these are important, they are subjective and will not necessarily mirror those of the patient. When discussing prognosis, you can emphasise the positive benefits of re-examining aspects of the patient's long-term management, particularly when combined with cessation of smoking. Bear in mind, however, that the hospital mortality in COPD with respiratory failure is as high as 10%, so reassurance must be tempered with caution. There are two important prognostic scores based on routine data collection which predict the immediate ('DECAF') and longer-term ('PEARL') risks of death and readmission. Their use will inform any discussion with the patient and their relatives and make a major contribution to the management plans.

Is this asthma or emphysema? The lay view is that emphysema is untreatable and often fatal. Explain that, in most cases of COPD, there is a mixture of asthma and emphysema and that our aim is to correct the asthmatic component. Emphasise the role of smoking cessation in preventing further deterioration.

Why is the patient so depressed and lacking in energy? This may be caused by a chronic lack of oxygen, and we can look into this after this episode is over. There may also be a true depressive element or an anxiety state. If you suspect this, note it down for future action.

Why does the patient keep coming back in so quickly? You may have to accept that your patient has reached a stage where there is no further respiratory reserve. However, readmissions can also be due to social factors such as loss of confidence, fear and isolation. These issues should be noted and tackled later. Social work and occupational therapy input is likely to be helpful here.

Relatives should be involved in encouraging smoking cessation and attendance at pulmonary rehabilitation sessions. Frequent hand-washing, mask wearing and appropriate social distancing have reduced COPD exacerbation rates during COVID-19, so are probably applicable as a general rule in troublesome COPD. However, this should not be at the expense of full physical activity and social interaction.

Is the heart affected? Patients with COPD often have coexisting heart disease, simply because they share the main risk factors: age and smoking. More often than not, however, ankle swelling is due to cor pulmonale rather than to congestive cardiac failure. Reassure the relatives that, as the lungs improve, the ankle oedema should resolve.

Can we get a nebuliser or oxygen for the patient? There are guidelines for nebulisers and home oxygen in COPD. These are best applied after specialist assessment by the respiratory team.

What can we do when the patient panics at home? Stay with the patient and provide a nebuliser, followed, if it is available, by oxygen. Wait to see the effect. If the patient deteriorates, particularly if the patient appears to be drowsy, more blue than normal or confused, ask for help.

Respiratory Infections and Pneumonia

Respiratory infections are a common cause of admission to the AMU (Case Study 3.6). Prior to COVID-19 (see later), most occur in a setting of pre-existing lung disease, usually COPD, or some other debilitating condition. An infective exacerbation of COPD is characterised by an increase in cough, an increase in the volume and stickiness of the sputum and a change in sputum colour to green. There may be a fever and the infection may precipitate respiratory failure or cor pulmonale. In a frail, debilitated patient, a respiratory infection may simply cause a general deterioration with nothing more in the chest than a fruity-sounding cough and an increase in the respiratory rate. Major risk factors for the development of respiratory infection are mouth sepsis, a weak and ineffective cough and associated conditions such as stroke or coma that increase the risk of aspiration.

Pneumonia

Pneumonia is a type of respiratory infection that leads to consolidation of part of the lung. Consolidation impairs gas exchange and is visible on the chest x-ray. Even in a previously fit person who acquires pneumonia outside hospital, it can be a clinical challenge, and there are still a substantial number of deaths. The mortality rate in cases of pneumonia admitted to hospital is 10%, but this increases to 50% in patients who are ill enough to need ITU care. The term 'community-acquired pneumonia' is used to differentiate it from cases occurring after the patient has been admitted (e.g., while on a ventilator in ITU).

SIGNS AND SYMPTOMS OF PNEUMONIA

The clinical features of pneumonia are due to a combination of lung involvement and sepsis:

- Breathlessness
- Cough and sputum
- Cyanosis

CASE STUDY 3.6 | **A Bad Case of Flu or Severe Pneumonia?**

A 54-year-old fit male had been unwell for 8 days. His symptoms progressed from generalised flu-like symptoms to severe malaise and confusion. On admission, he was pyrexial and unwell, with a respiratory rate of 30 breaths/min and a blood pressure of 80/40 mm Hg. His chest x-ray showed a solid upper lobe in the right lung. His blood count showed a very low white cell count (polymorphs 0.2×10^9), a raised urea of 25 mmol/L and a low albumin of 19 g/L. The bacterium *Streptococcus pneumoniae* was grown in both sputum and blood. The pneumococcal antigen was positive in the urine. The CURB-65 score was 4, indicating severe pneumonia.

The patient was treated with IV co-amoxiclav and clarithromycin, oxygen and aggressive fluid replacement, combined with careful monitoring of the urine output. His temperature settled over 4 days, and he slowly improved.

- Chest pain (usually pleurisy)
- Marked tachypnea
- Fever
- Systemic illness

In severe pneumonia, there are signs of systemic upset, including myalgia (muscle pains), diarrhoea and, in extreme cases, restlessness and shock. Even without pre-existing lung disease, pneumonia can cause severe type I respiratory failure. Any two of the following key features are associated with a mortality rate of 20%:

- Respiratory rate more than 30 breaths/min
- Diastolic pressure less than 60 mm Hg
- Blood urea greater than 7 mmol/L

ASSESSMENT OF PNEUMONIA

The history will identify patients who are particularly vulnerable to the development of pneumonia:

- Over 65 years of age
- Chronic lung disease, especially in heavy smokers
- Underlying ill health or alcohol use disorder
- Patients who are immunosuppressed (recent chemotherapy, AIDS, myeloma, etc.)

THE SEVERITY SCORE IN PNEUMONIA: CURB-65

CURB-65 (Table 3.2) is a simple 5-point scoring system based on clinical observations and a blood test. It is used to assess the severity of pneumonia by stratifying patients by their risk of death and is a fundamental part of the initial assessment. A CURB-65 score of 0 to 1 is associated with a low risk of death (less than 5%). A score of 2 is associated with an intermediate risk of 3% to 15%. A CURB-65 score of 3 to 5 carries a

TABLE 3.2 ■ **CURB-65**

Confusion	New-onset disorientation for time, place or person(AMTS 8 or less)	Score 1
Urea	Greater than 7.0 mmol/L (as a new finding)	Score 1
Respiratory rate	30 breaths/min or more	Score 1
Blood pressure	Systolic of less than 90 mm Hg or diastolic 60 mm or less	Score 1
65	65 years of age or older	Score 1

Score 0–2 = mild; Score 3–5 = severe; Score 4–5 = move to HDU/ITU.
AMTS, Abbreviated Mental Test Score; HDU, high-dependency unit; ITU, intensive therapy unit.

high mortality risk of more than 15%, and these patients should be considered for early transfer to a high-dependency unit (HDU) or ITU bed.

FINDING THE CAUSE OF PNEUMONIA

To identify the likely cause of pneumonia (which is critical in severe cases) and therefore to choose the most appropriate treatment:

- Note the history (AIDS, recent travel, contact with COVID-19, etc.).
- Culture blood, sputum, urine and pleural fluid (if an effusion is present).
- Send the blood and urine for immunology (legionnaires, *Pneumococcus*, atypical pneumonia) and arrange for convalescent samples to be sent for comparison at 10 days. There should be an urgent testing and reporting service for Legionnaires' urinary antigen that should be used for patients with severe pneumonia. If the urinary antigen is positive, respiratory secretions must be sent for *Legionella* culture. Nasal and throat swabs are tested for COVID-19.
- The polymerase chain reaction (PCR), a molecular diagnostic technique, can accurately type viral and bacterial infections and can be applied to blood, throat swabs and respiratory secretions. During the winter months, early identification of influenza is particularly important. PCR will also confirm a diagnosis of COVID-19.

CRITICAL CLINICAL OBSERVATIONS

- Respiratory rate
- Blood pressure
- Conscious level (particularly new confusion)
- Oxygen saturation
- Pulse (rate *and* rhythm)

IMPORTANT CLINICAL OBSERVATIONS

- Temperature
- Sputum colour
- Presence of pleuritic pain
- Evidence of mouth sepsis (including oral *Candida*)
- Evidence of existing airway disease

ASSESSING THE EFFECT OF PNEUMONIA ON THE PATIENT

A few simple tests will give you an accurate measure of the impact that the pneumonia is having on the patient:

- The extent of shadowing on the chest film
- An ECG, particularly to look for atrial fibrillation, a common complication in severe cases
- The degree of hypoxia (pO_2 less than 8 kPa)

- The degree of acidosis (pH less than 7.3)
- White cell count is either less than 4 (marrow depression in severe sepsis) or more than 20×10^9/L
- Blood urea greater than 7 mmol/L (indirect evidence of hypovolemia and potential kidney damage)
- Low serum albumin (albumin less than 35 g/L) as a result of the toxic effect of severe infection on protein manufacture

MANAGEMENT OF PNEUMONIA

If the assessment indicates features associated with a high risk of death (respiratory failure, shock, acidosis, disseminated intravascular coagulopathy) and particularly if the CURB-65 score is 4 or more, the patient should be managed where ventilation is available at short notice. The key to treatment lies in the following:

- Oxygenation
- Fluid balance
- Appropriate antibiotics given within 4 h of admission
- Early mobilisation and deep venous thrombosis prophylaxis

BASIC AIMS OF TREATMENT

Fluids. Suitable fluids are administered:

- To maintain a blood pressure of more than 90/60 mm Hg
- To maintain a urine output of more than 0.5 mL/kg/h, crystalloids such as normal saline are preferable to colloids such as polygeline (Haemaccel). Fluids may need to include inotropic support

Oxygen. Sufficient oxygen is administered to maintain saturations of between 94% and 98%. In the absence of COPD (where the target saturations would be 88%–92%), patients with pneumonia are not at risk from a worsening of CO_2 retention by receiving too much oxygen. A high-concentration reservoir mask should be used. NIV or CPAP should be used in pneumonia only in an HDU/ITU setting, as at least half the patients who reach this stage will need tracheal intubation and ventilation of the lungs. The management of COVID-19 pneumoniais covered separately later in the chapter.

Antibiotics. Appropriate antibiotics are administered to cover the likely causative organisms. These are based on the 'best guess' for the likely organism within the context of local antibiotic guidelines. The choice of antibiotics may have to be modified once the results of cultures and blood tests become available.

Which antibiotic is for which patient? Examples of suitable initial regimens pending microbiological results include:

- CURB-65 = 0 to 1 Mild pneumonia
  - Amoxicillin 500 mg tds orally
    if allergic to penicillin:

- Doxycycline 200 mg, then 100 mg daily orally
  or clarithromycin 500 mg bid orally
  or if pregnant, erythromycin 500 mg qds
- CURB-65 = 2 Moderate pneumonia
  - Amoxicillin 500 mg tds orally
    plus
  - Clarithromycin 500 mg bid orally
    if allergic to penicillin:
  - Doxycycline 200 mg, then 100 mg daily orally
    or clarithromycin 500 mg bid orally
    or if pregnant, erythromycin 500 mg qds
- CURB-65 = 3 to 5 Severe pneumonia
  - Co-amoxiclav 500/125 mg tds or 1.2 g tds IV
    plus
  - Clarithromycin 500 mg bid orally or IV
    or if pregnant, erythromycin 500 mg qds
    if allergic to penicillin:
  - Levofloxacin 500 mg bid, orally or IV

Regimens must be reviewed within 24 h when the initial microbiology results are available. Intravenous antibiotics are a major burden for the AMU in terms of both time and expense, so patients should be transferred to oral antibiotics at the earliest opportunity. Antibiotics should be stopped after 5 days, provided the temperature has been normal for 48 h.

PLEURAL EFFUSION AND PLEURAL EMPYEMA

One of the most common complications of pneumonia is the development of a pleural effusion. If the fluid in an effusion becomes infected, an empyema (pus in the pleural cavity) will develop.

Empyemas are seen in the elderly and debilitated, particularly when the treatment of pneumonia has been delayed (Case Study 3.7). An empyema should be suspected if there is persistent fever associated with weight loss, pleuritic pain and weakness despite

---

CASE STUDY 3.7   **Delayed Treatment of Pneumonia**

A 17-year-old youth was admitted with severe chest pain and malaise. Three weeks before admission, he had become acutely unwell with a cough, shivering and breathlessness. He treated himself with aspirin. On examination, he was pyrexial, pale and looked unwell. He had a productive cough, severe right-sided chest pain on inspiration and signs of a right-sided pleural effusion. His chest film showed a solid right lower lobe and fluid in the pleural space.

A diagnosis of unresolved pneumonia with possible empyema was made. His effusion was aspirated to dryness and sent for examination. He was started on ampicillin and erythromycin.

appropriate antibiotics. The treatment of an empyema involves clearing the infected fluid from the pleural cavity by intercostal drainage.

ASPIRATION PNEUMONIA

Frail patients, especially those with swallowing difficulties due to neurological disorders, are at risk of pneumonia through aspirating food or nasopharyngeal secretions into the lungs. The usual antibiotic regime for aspiration pneumonia is IV co-amoxiclav 1.2 g tds. Metronidazole is given with IV cefuroxime if the patient is allergic to penicillin. Aspiration pneumonia due to methicillin-resistant *Staphylococcus aureus* (MRSA) should be considered if:

- The patient has had previous MRSA.
- The patient has come from a nursing or residential home and there are chronic breaks in the skin.
- There is a long-term catheter.
- The patient has been in the hospital within the past 6 months.

Caring for the Patient With Pneumonia

The patient with pneumonia combines the challenges of uncontrolled sepsis with the management of threatened or actual respiratory failure (see Case Study 3.7). For many patients, the pneumonia will complicate pre-existing medical conditions, so your assessment will need to be comprehensive and searching. For example, has your patient with a cerebral vascular accident developed pneumonia because he cannot swallow and has aspirated? Your most important immediate task is to grade the severity of the pneumonia. This is simple to do and is based on the combination of vital signs (notably respiratory rate and blood pressure) and basic laboratory investigations. As a general rule, the more 'multisystem' the symptoms appear (e.g., diarrhoea, muscle pains, headache), the worse the pneumonia. Some organisms attack several systems at once. Has your patient with pneumonia, a splitting headache and photophobia also gotten meningitis? If you are lucky, the history may help you establish the cause of the pneumonia (e.g., in a recent case, a failure to seek out appropriate risk factors led to a lengthy delay in recognising an AIDS-related pneumonia). The history is more likely, however, to highlight other relevant medical conditions that will influence the speed of recovery.

Patients with pneumonia will be in need of reassurance (Box 3.6).

 CRITICAL CLINICAL TASKS DURING THE ACUTE EPISODE
- Provide timely therapy
- Provide explanations
- Monitor the patient's progress
- Assess the need for analgesia
- Watch for complications

BOX 3.6 ■ Reassurance for the Patient With Pneumonia

- Pneumonia is a treatable infection in the lungs. We are trying to trace its source.
- It would be very unusual for other members of your family to be at risk.
- The drip is to give you fluid and antibiotics.
- For the first few days, you will be helped by continuous oxygen through the mask.
- The chest pain is due to inflammation in the lining of the lung; it is not from your heart.
- Your fever and sweats will take several days to subside.
- Your breathlessness is due to temporary lung damage, which is starting to heal. Although you will feel better in a few days, we would not expect your x-ray to clear completely for 3 or 4 weeks.
- It is quite normal to have no appetite at all and feel very weak at first.
- You will probably be able to cough up sputum more effectively as you start to improve.

FIVE CRITICAL CARING TASKS DURING THE ACUTE PHASE

Provide timely therapy. Once the diagnosis is suspected, your patient must receive their antibiotics. Hypotension needs urgent attention with fluids. Hypoxia is treated with high concentrations of oxygen.

Explain. Explain the importance of continuous oxygen. Reassure the patient that the IV antibiotics are given for the first few doses only.

Monitor the patient's progress. The hypotensive and ill patient will need a urinary catheter to ensure an adequate urine output (20+ mL/h). Oxygen saturations should be maintained between 94% and 98%. The pulse and temperature should start to decrease within 24 to 48 h of the start of treatment. Persistent confusion in your patient is a worrying sign.

Assess the need for analgesia. Opiates are not advisable because of respiratory depression, but you must try to relieve any pleuritic pain. The pain of pleurisy prevents an adequate cough and impairs deep inspiration.

WATCH FOR COMPLICATIONS

- Persistent fever and anorexia: pus in the pleural cavity or an abscess
- Ankle oedema and extreme lethargy: either cardiac failure or low albumin due to systemic illness (lung abscess?)
- Low urine output and nausea: renal failure complicating sepsis

Answering Relatives' Questions in Pneumonia

Pneumonia has a bad reputation with the lay public, who still associate it with death, especially in the elderly. This reputation is not undeserved, particularly when pneumonia complicates other serious diseases such as cancer, diabetes and stroke. Many patients with pneumonia will have passed through a flu-like stage at home and will have seen their family doctor on two or three occasions, with or without the prescription of antibiotics. Many of you will recognise the words, 'Why wasn't something done sooner', and you may have had to deal with combinations of resentment and anger. You must remember that it is easy to diagnose pneumonia in hindsight, particularly with the aid of on-site chest films. It is probably best to explain to the relatives how the disease can progress rather than imply any criticism of their initial management. Common questions that you will have to deal with are listed below.

Is this bronchopneumonia, lobar pneumonia or double pneumonia? The term 'bronchopneumonia' is commonly used to describe the terminal respiratory distress in a frail and usually elderly patient. In practice, it means infection, usually in the lung bases, as a result of retained secretions and an ineffective cough.

'Bronchopneumonia' is often stated on the death certificate as the immediate cause of death in patients in whom it was simply the terminal event after, say, a severe stroke, advanced malignant disease or dementia. 'Lobar pneumonia' is a more exact term, indicating the extent (a lobe) of the consolidation. 'Double pneumonia' is an entirely lay expression, presumably indicating the involvement of both lungs.

Can the rest of us catch it? There can be a common source of infection (such as a faulty water-cooling system in an outbreak of legionnaires disease), but, with the exceptions of COVID, person-to-person spread is rare.

Will the confusion be clear? If the oxygen mask is kept on and the antibiotics work, the confusion will clear. It is, however, an indication of the severity of the case that you are dealing with.

Will there be any permanent lung damage? There should be a complete recovery, but this should be seen as an opportunity to ensure that the patient stops smoking.

What if the patient gets worse? If your patient has poor prognostic signs, introduce the relatives to the possibility of ITU care and possible ventilation. One way to discuss this is as a "stop-gap" measure to allow the lungs to rest while the antibiotics get to work'.

Can you feed the patient? The patient has not eaten for days. To start with, the priority is fluids, antibiotics and oxygen. As the patient improves, appetite will return.

Why don't you x-ray the patient again to look for progress? We will if we suspect complications, the chest x-ray will not improve for at least 2 weeks. The best sign of recovery is when the patient starts to feel better. Special tests, such as CT scans, are helpful to sort out any complications.

How soon will the patient be back to normal? Pneumonia is a serious illness, and symptoms can take a while to clear—typically a week for the fever, 4 weeks for chest discomfort and excessive sputum, 6 weeks for breathlessness and cough and 12 weeks or more for generalised tiredness.

Spontaneous Pneumothorax

A spontaneous pneumothorax occurs when a defect on the surface of the lung 'pops', letting air out under positive pressure into the pleural space. This pressurised air prevents expansion of the lung and can push the mediastinal structures to the opposite side of the chest (a tension pneumothorax implies a large, high-pressure pneumothorax with a major effect on lung function). The symptoms are pain, breathlessness and, in severe cases where there is a tension pneumothorax, cardiorespiratory collapse.

The diagnosis of a tension pneumothorax needs a high degree of clinical suspicion. The features are low blood pressure, low oxygen saturation and severe breathlessness. It may occur on the AMU:

- With blocked, kinked or displaced chest drains
- After cardiopulmonary resuscitation (rib fractures causing a pneumothorax)
- During NIV (which can be confused with a lack of NIV progress)

As you can see, a pneumothorax can be confused with three major medical conditions:

- Pulmonary embolus
- Myocardial infarction
- Pleurisy

Small pneumothoraces (a rim of air less than 2 cm wide on the chest x-ray) produce few symptoms and improve without treatment. A rim of more than 2 cm is a 'large' pneumothorax; the patient is usually breathless and intervention is necessary. Active treatment of a pneumothorax involves removing the air from the pleural cavity by simple aspiration or, in more difficult cases, by placement of an intercostal drain. Tube drainage is best performed with a small bore (9–14 F) catheter inserted very easily using a Seldinger technique and attached to either an underwater seal or a flutter valve.

Whether a patient is admitted for observation and possible intervention depends primarily on:

- The degree of lung collapse
- The amount of breathlessness
- The presence of pre-existing lung disease. Patients with emphysema and asthma are prone to pneumothoraces. (Even a small pneumothorax in a patient with severe lung disease or occurring during an asthma attack can be the last straw.)

A *primary* pneumothorax occurs in otherwise normal lungs; a *secondary* pneumothorax is caused by underlying lung disease (usually emphysema) or trauma.

Simple aspiration is preferable to tube drainage for any primary pneumothorax and should be tried first. Aspiration is successful in 60% of cases, with re-expansion of the lung. These patients can be discharged rapidly but, as with *all* cases of pneumothorax, they must be told to return to hospital if they suddenly become short of breath and they should be given an early (1–2 weeks) appointment for the chest clinic.

If aspiration does not lead to re-expansion of the lung, or if there is expansion followed by further collapse within 72 h, then an intercostal drain will be needed (Fig. 3.4). Except

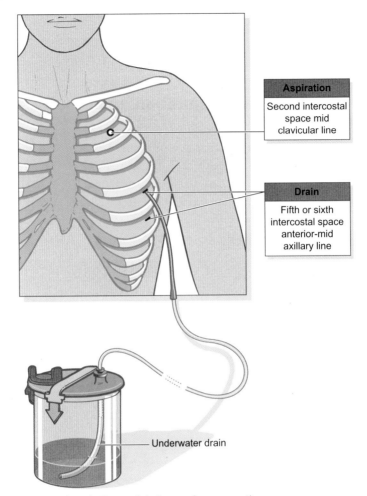

FIGURE 3.4   Intercostal aspiration and drainage of a pneumothorax.

when they are very small and asymptomatic, all *secondary* pneumothoraces require tube drainage. Once a drain is in place,

- It should be clamped only under exceptional circumstances (*not* because the patient is going for a chest film).
- Chest drains that are still bubbling should not be removed unless they are to be replaced.
- If the drain is in place for more than 24 h, the patient should be referred at that time to the respiratory team.

The management of a pneumothorax can be troublesome, particularly if there is also chronic lung disease present. A safe course of action is to refer all cases of pneumothorax to the respiratory team within 24 h of admission. Interestingly, there is a strong move towards outpatient management of spontaneous primary pneumothoraces (i.e., no underlying lung disease). An ambulatory device such as the Pleural Vent (Rocket Medical, United Kingdom) allows the drainage of the pneumothorax to occur at home, provided there is a system in place for close outpatient supervision.

Safety Issues: Pleural Aspiration and Pleural Drainage

There are increasing concerns about the safety of pleural aspiration and drainage when it is carried out on non-specialist wards, including the AMU, particularly when performed 'out of hours'. Inexpertly placed drains can penetrate the liver, lung, spleen and heart; inattention to sterile techniques can lead to infection; inadequate pain relief and a clumsy technique can leave the patient (and the staff) traumatised. Current guidelines provide clear advice to minimise the risk and reduce the stress and discomfort to the patient:

- Except where urgent clinical need dictates, pleural procedures should not be done 'out of hours'.
- Unless there is an absolute emergency, there must be documented patient consent.
- These are sterile procedures (clean space, adequate skin cleansing, gowns, gloves and drapes).
- Commercial chest drain packs should be used, which contain almost everything that is needed: gowns, drapes, skin preparations, syringes, needles, scalpels, appropriate dilators, guide wires, drains, three-way taps and a variety of connections.
- The positioning of the patient and the choice of aspiration/drainage sites are critical to success.
- For pleural effusions, bedside ultrasound is mandatory for identifying safe aspiration and drain insertion sites.
- Intravenous midazolam (1–2 mg) or morphine (2.5 mg) as premedication reduces the patient's pain and anxiety.
- Oxygen saturation must be monitored throughout the procedure.
- The staff who are responsible for the patient must be familiar with the management of chest drains.
- Patients should be encouraged, when appropriate, to take some responsibility for the care of their drains (and keep the drainage bottle below the level of the drain entry site at all times).

Caring for the Patient With a Chest Drain

Air, fluid, blood or pus in the pleural space can result in an acutely ill patient who is severely breathless and requires an urgent chest drain. The small Seldinger drains (10–14 F) are easy to use, generally well tolerated and are increasingly used in preference to large bore tubes. There are still occasions, however, when a large (24–28 F) tube may be required.

Few procedures in the AMU cause as much fear and anxiety to the patient and the staff as the insertion of a large intercostal drain. Under stress, they are put in and under darkness, they fall out.

Prepare your patient for the procedure. The patients are often young and distressed and will need a lot of reassurance, with an honest explanation of what to expect: 'There may be initial discomfort and a sensation of pushing, but the local anaesthetic will deaden any pain; if the pain is severe, tell us and we will put in more anaesthetic'. Explain that the breathlessness will go away as soon as the tube is in place. It is wise to be non-committal about how long the tube will stay in. A sizeable proportion of pneumothoraces need prolonged drainage and surgical intervention: 'If things go according to plan, it will be removed in a few days, but if it is less straightforward, the tube will need to stay in longer until the lung goes up and stays up'.

Positioning the patient. The patient needs to be in a position exposing the 'triangle of safety' at the base of the axilla, the area chosen for the majority of drains. The patient can sit in bed at 45 degrees with the appropriate arm behind his or her head. Alternatively, the patient can sit in or out of bed and lean forward with their head bent across their folded arms, resting either on a bedside table or, if the patient is in a chair, across the bed.

Alleviate the pain of the intercostal drain. If there is no contraindication, a small dose of IV midazolam administered at the time of the skin incision may make the difference between a tense, panicking patient and one who is relaxed and cooperative. Check whether your patient is being given sufficient analgesia. Many doctors underestimate analgesic requirements in medical conditions.

Problems with intercostal drains falling out or falling apart. There should be a local protocol for a standardised technique for placing and securing a chest drain. Common problems that you will see include the following:

- Sutures that are too small (1–0 silk is ideal) and are badly tied around the tube
- The weight of the connecting tubing pulls the drain out of the chest
- Untaped connections coming apart
- Failure to recognise and act on a displaced or disconnected tube (clamp an open-ended tube, seal over a sucking chest drain site)

Try to use transparent dressings so that you can assess the state and site of the tube on at least a twice-daily basis. Simple follow-up measurements of how much of the tube is visible will warn of imminent displacement. If a tube is on suction and works its way out of the chest cavity, constant bubbling will be seen as soon as the drainage holes are exposed to the air. Important observations are: the amount of fluid drained (effusions), whether the tube is bubbling (pneumothorax) and whether the fluid level in the tube is swinging (confirming the tube is patent and remains in the pleural cavity). Increasingly, tube blockage is being minimised by the aseptic instillation three times daily of 10 to 20 mL of sterile saline via a three-way tap between the drain and the tubing.

Three simple tube rules:
- Bubbling tubes need to stay in and should never be clamped.
- Swinging tubes can probably be removed if the lung has expanded.
- Non-swinging tubes are often blocked (hence the failure to re-expand?)

IMPORTANT CLINICAL OBSERVATIONS
- Is the tube bubbling (continuous bubbling means a large leak in the lung or a leak in the circuit)?
- Is the tube swinging (it is in the pleural cavity and is patent)?
- Are the connections intact and the tube unkinked (it can twist at the entry point)?
- Is the rigid tube under the water level in the bottle?
- What is the volume of drainage (in an effusion)?

Thoracic Suction
At times, thoracic suction is applied to the underwater drain bottle to encourage the lung to re-expand. This requires a *wall-based Thoracic Suction Unit* rather than standard suction, as the pressure has to be restricted (maximum 7 kPa) to avoid serious lung damage. These units are usually confined to the respiratory wards. Fortunately, the introduction of digital suction units (e.g., the Thopaz system), which also measure the air leak (rather than looking for bubbles), will greatly simplify chest drain management.

COVID-19 and the Lungs
In severe COVID-19, the viruses spread from the nose and throat to the lungs, where they infect the small airways and alveoli. There they induce intense inflammation which floods the alveoli, leading to x-ray changes (COVID-19 pneumonitis), hypoxia and eventual respiratory failure. In addition, the body's immune system responds to this insult with a 'cytokine storm' whose aim is to fight off the infection, but it often compounds the situation as the exaggerated immune response itself augments the direct damage caused by the virus.

Clinically, COVID-19 pneumonitis presents as a 'viral pneumonia syndrome' with a cough, breathlessness, flu-like symptoms, muscle aches, fever and diarrhoea. In the elderly, it is a particular cause of delirium.

The process by which COVID-19 pneumonitis develops underpins its management. The mainstay of treatment is therefore to ensure:
- **Adequate oxygenation**, either by conventional oxygen masks, CPAP, high-flow nasal oxygen (HFNO) or ultimately ITU intubation and ventilation
- **Antiviral medication** to prevent viral replication (remdesivir)
- **Synthetic antibodies** to prevent the virus from attaching itself to the airway cells (tocilizumab)

- **Steroids** to counteract the intense inflammation (dexamethasone)
- **Inflammatory pathway inhibition** (baricitanib)

Despite this multi-pronged approach, some patients still do badly—those with significant comorbidities (diabetes, heart disease, frailty, severe COPD, obesity and chronic neurological disease) and patients over the age of 70.

Principles of oxygen treatment in COVID-19 pneumonitis

The oxygen target is 94% (88%–92% in patients with COPD). If this cannot be maintained on a Venturi mask up to 40% (red nozzle), patients move on to CPAP or HFNO.

There needs to be a clear escalation and ceiling of care plan before this happens.

CPAP

CPAP is delivered with a tight-fitting mask, through which a constant flow of pressurised oxygen is conveyed. CPAP splints the airways open and provides the alveoli with high concentrations of oxygen. The apparatus has safeguards to minimise viral spread.

HFNO

HFNO is used most commonly when CPAP has been unsuccessful. It is delivered through specially designed nasal prongs from a device (usually the Optiflow), which heats and humidifies oxygen at a flow rate of 30 to 60 L/min.

Awake proning

In patients on HFNO in whom it is difficult to maintain target oxygen saturations, awake proning can be very helpful. Proning opens up the lungs and helps mobilise secretions.

The suggested sequence (which requires physiotherapy input) is:

30 min to 2 h fully prone—bed flat

30 min to 2 h on the right side, bed flat

30 min to 2 h sitting up at 45 degrees

30 min to 2 h on the left side—bed flat

Repeat the sequence; check after 15 in each position that the oxygen saturations have not fallen.

If the oxygen saturations cannot be kept at 94% or above with these measures, depending on the escalation and ceiling of care plans, discussions should be opened with ITU regarding future management.

Further Reading

Asthma

Pavordet, I.D., et al., 2018. After asthma: redefining airway disease. The Lancet 391, 350–400.

COPD

Davidson, A.C., Banham, S., Elliott, M., et al., 2016. BTS/ICS guideline for the ventilatory management of acute hypercapnic respiratory failure in adults. Thorax 71 (Suppl 2), ii1–35.

Echevarria, C., Steer, J., Heslop-Marshall, K., et al., 2016. Validation of the DECAF score to predict hospital mortality in acute exacerbations of COPD. Thorax 71 (2), 133–140.

Chronic obstructive pulmonary disease in over 16s: diagnosis and management. NICE guideline [NG115].

Pneumonia

Eccles, S., Pincus, C., Higgins, B., Woodhead, M., 2014. Diagnosis and management of community- and hospital-acquired pneumonia in adults: summary of NICE guidance. British Medical Journal 349, 33–35.

Pneumonia in adults: diagnosis and management (see also COVID-19 NICE rapid guideline: managing COVID-19). https//www.nice.org.uk/guidance/ng191.

Pneumothorax

Bintcliffe, O., Maskell, N., 2014. Spontaneous pneumothorax. British Medical Journal 348, 27–31.

Website

Access to all the British Thoracic Society Guidelines (Asthma, COPD, NIV, Pneumonia, Pneumothorax): https://www.brit-thoracic.org.uk/standards-of-care/guidelines/.

Acute Neurological Problems

Introduction

The major issue in the patient who presents a neurological problem is to decide whether the patient needs supportive care or whether the patient needs active intervention. Many cases that present as neurological emergencies will recover fully, given time and good supportive treatment, because their underlying disorder is fully reversible. Examples include coma due to self-poisoning and the confusional states that follow an epileptic fit. Other cases require a much more active approach: typical examples are antibiotics for acute meningitis, glucose for hypoglycaemia and neurosurgery for subarachnoid haemorrhage. Therefore management decisions can only be made safely if the correct diagnosis has been established. Time is critical in neurological cases, as the nervous system has limited powers of recovery—the diagnostic path has to be followed with an appropriate degree of urgency. The acute medical unit (AMU) has a duty to ensure the safety of the patient during this time and the clinical team has a key role in this process (Box 4.1).

BOX 4.1 ■ Role of the Acute Medical Unit in Acute Neurological Problems

1. Ensure the safety of the patient
2. Prioritise the initial management
3. Differentiate and manage 'medical' and 'neurological' coma
4. Identify and respond to neurological deterioration
5. Reach appropriate outcomes

Role of the Acute Medical Unit in Acute Neurological Problems

ENSURING THE SAFETY OF THE PATIENT

There must be confidence in the ability to support the patient while the correct diagnosis is being reached. The role of the AMU at this stage is to prioritise the initial management. It may, for example, be necessary to stabilise the patient's condition before attempting to take a history.

There are four critical initial observations:

- Is the airway secure and is ventilation adequate?
- Are the vital signs stable?
- Is there a non-neurological condition that needs immediate attention?
- Is there anything neurological that needs urgent active intervention?

The most important examples in this latter category, and the ones we most fear missing, include the following:

- Intracranial infection (most notably, meningitis)
- Subarachnoid haemorrhage
- Expanding intracranial masses (bleeds in and around the brain, tumour, abscess)

It is critical that the patient reaches the appropriate service in the best possible condition, be it the acute neurosurgical unit, the stroke unit, the general medical wards or the intensive therapy unit (ITU).

Prioritising the Initial Management

GLASGOW COMA SCORE (GCS) AND ABCDE: ASSESSING AND KEEPING THE PATIENT ALIVE

Protection of the airway, ensuring adequate ventilation and maintaining circulation are the immediate priorities in any patient. At the most basic level, this means the following:

- Ensuring the upper airway is patent
- Giving sufficient oxygen
- Securing IV access and maintaining the blood pressure

Warning: At this first stage, if meningococcal meningitis is suspected, appropriate IV antibiotics must be given *straight away*.

If there is any suspicion of a neck injury (an example would be a patient who has been found at the bottom of some steps, having had an apparent fall), the neck must be protected and CT scanned immediately. If there is a cervical spine fracture, manipulating an unsupported neck either to establish an airway or to move a patient around in bed can damage the spinal cord beyond repair. At least be aware of the risk, know how to apply a stiff collar and use sandbags to support the neck, and if there is any doubt, protect the neck and logroll the patient until the neck images have been cleared by a radiologist.

CRITICAL CLINICAL OBSERVATIONS

Blood sugar. Hypoglycaemia is the most important cause of a fully reversible neurological disorder. At blood sugars below 3 mmol/L, the patient becomes comatose and may fit, but any neurological picture can be caused by hypoglycaemia. Providing the patient has not suffered irreversible damage from sustained hypoglycaemia, correction of the blood sugar will lead to a full and rapid recovery.

Response of the pupils. The size, symmetry and reactivity of the pupils are fundamental neurological observations. The most common cause of bilaterally fixed and dilated pupils is self-poisoning with tricyclic antidepressants, whereas poisoning with both opiates and diazepam-like drugs produces fixed constricted pupils.

CRITICAL CLINICAL OBSERVATIONS

- Blood sugar
- Pupillary responses
- Temperature
- Pulse
- Blood pressure
- Respiratory rate
- Oxygen saturation
- Glasgow coma score
- Top-to-toe examination
- Reliable history

The major reason for following the change in the pupils is to identify 'uncal herniation': a shift of the brain because of cerebral oedema that results in the third cranial nerve being 'pinched' between the brain and part of the skull (see Fig. 4.3). As the third nerve is responsible for pupillary constriction, an early warning of uncal herniation is pupillary dilatation followed by loss of the light reflex.

Any suspicion that a pupil is dilating and losing its light reflex must be reported to the senior medical staff for action to reassess the neurological status of the patient. This is a particular issue in the first 24 h after a major stroke when acute brain swelling can occur.

Temperature. In the right context, an increased temperature should be considered strong evidence of intracranial sepsis: meningitis, more rarely meningo-encephalitis, or even a collection of intracranial pus (intracerebral abscess).

Not every fever in a neurological emergency is due to intracranial sepsis, as there may be infection elsewhere such as aspiration pneumonia. High temperatures also characteristically occur in brainstem strokes. Nonetheless, intracranial infection should be the first consideration because of the need for immediate action.

Pulse. The rhythm and rate of the pulse are important. They may draw attention to non-neurological problems that need to be addressed. Extreme bradycardia, for example, may be the cause of an unexplained blackout. Atrial fibrillation is recognised by the irregularity of the pulse, and its presence increases the likelihood that an acute stroke is due to a clot of blood finding its way from the left atrium (a fibrillating atrium encourages clot formation) to the brain, which causes an embolic cerebral infarction. Changes in the pulse can be important: progressive slowing can indicate increasing intracranial pressure (ICP) and is often accompanied by increasing blood pressure.

Blood pressure. *Hypotension* must be evaluated in detail because it has several causes: heart problems, hypovolaemia due to dehydration, shock, sepsis and so forth. As a rule, in a patient with an impaired conscious level, hypotension suggests a metabolic cause such as sepsis, diabetes or hepatic encephalopathy. Postural hypotension (defined as a decrease in systolic pressure of more than 20 mm Hg or a fall in the diastolic pressure of more than 10 mm Hg 1 min after standing when accompanied by appropriate symptoms) is common especially in the elderly, it is often drug related and is a frequent cause of admissions with dizziness and unexplained falls.

Hypertension is commonly seen as an acute response to neurological events such as intracranial haemorrhage or large cerebral infarction. Severe hypertension can also complicate coma caused by self-poisoning with sympathomimetic recreational drugs such as ecstasy, amphetamines and cocaine and may need urgent correction. However, in most neurological conditions, including stroke, lowering the blood pressure acutely to 'normalise' it is fraught with danger. The brain is usually fairly impervious to changes in blood pressure as the cerebral blood flow 'autoregulates': if the blood pressure drops, the vessels open up to allow greater flow through them. If there is a major neurological insult, this autoregulation is lost, so if the blood pressure falls the blood supply also decreases, which may worsen the neurological deficit. Therefore in acute situations, especially in strokes, the temptation to 'treat' a high blood pressure should usually be resisted. There are important exceptions. In the first few hours after a cerebral haemorrhage, a systolic blood pressure of 150 mm Hg or more (confirmed on duplicate readings 10 min apart) needs urgent reduction—as does a systolic blood pressure of 185 mm Hg or more in a patient with a cerebral infarct, who is otherwise suitable for thrombolysis.

Immediate treatment with intravenous labetalol or glyceryl trinitrate (GTN) aims to reduce the blood pressure within an hour.

As already explained, the combination of a progressively falling pulse and increasing blood pressure may, in the appropriate circumstances (such as the aftermath of a major intracranial bleed), be a sign of increased ICP.

Respiratory rate. The respiratory rate remains an essential observation in the patient who is critically ill, whatever the cause. It is particularly important to document any changes in respiratory rate. Thus in the neurological emergency, a falling respiratory rate may reflect a deepening coma. If the change in conscious level is due to increasing ICP, the slowing respiration is accompanied by a falling pulse and rising blood pressure. **It is instructive to contrast this with the signs that are seen in shock, in which a change in conscious level is accompanied by an increase in the respiratory rate, an increase in the pulse and a decrease in the blood pressure.**

Oxygen saturation. Hypoxia remains a common, yet easily correctable, cause of avoidable death in acute emergency wards. The normal oxygen saturation is around 97%, and it must be appreciated that decreasing the saturation to 90% or less requires a major disturbance in ventilation that may be due to a deepening coma and a worsening neurological state. A fall in oxygen saturation needs careful reassessment:

- Is the airway secure?
- Is the coma deepening?
- What about the lungs and the circulation?
- Should blood gases be checked?
- What is the respiratory rate?

It must be remembered that the oxygen saturation does not always reflect the level of ventilation. If the patient is on a high concentration of oxygen, the saturation can be more or less normal even when the patient is hardly breathing. The saturations must not be interpreted in isolation. There would be no reassurance from an oxygen saturation that had stayed constant for 4 h at 95% if, during that time, the GCS had dropped from 12 to 4 and the respiratory rate had fallen from 15 to 8 breaths/min. This patient should be in ITU with a view to immediate ventilation.

Glasgow coma score. The GCS was described in 1974 as a way to assess any patient with an altered level of consciousness. It is based on three categories of response: eye-opening, the best motor response and the best verbal response (Table 4.1 and Fig. 4.1). The GCS is the universal measurement of the depth of coma. It is simple to carry out and score and, provided it is performed properly, the result should be the same whoever makes the measurement.

The GCS can be documented on a chart as the grand total from the three categories against time or as E4, M6, V5, etc. As a general rule, the scores reflect the severity of the neurological status:

Mild	13–15
Moderate	9–12
Severe	3–8

TABLE 4.1 ■ Glasgow Coma Score

Response	Score
Eye-Opening (E)	
Spontaneously	E4
To verbal command	E3
To pain	E2
No response	E1
Best Motor Response (M)	
Obeys commands	M6
Localises pain	M5
Withdraws to pain	M4
Abnormal flexion to pain	M3
Extension to pain	M2
No response	M1
Best Verbal Response (V)	
Orientated and converses	V5
Disorientated and converses	V4
Inappropriate words	V3
Incomprehensible sounds	V2
No response	V1
Total score (3–15)	

Coma is defined as a GCS of less than 9.

The initial GCS, often performed by the paramedics outside the hospital, acts as a baseline. A low initial GCS score (less than 9) will mean the airway is vulnerable and the patient is at risk from aspiration.

A change in the GCS is the single most important observation in the acute neurological patient. A fall in GCS needs immediate attention. Deepening coma may need increased supportive measures, perhaps involving a move to ITU with a view to ventilation. More critically, a fall in GCS is often the first sign of increasing ICP, which occurs in active intracranial bleeding, intracranial sepsis and during the development of brain oedema following a cerebral infarct.

Some triage systems use an abbreviated assessment of the conscious level based on the acronym AVPU:

A	Alert
V	Responds to voice
P	Responds to pain
U	Unresponsive

This is quick to perform and easy to recall. AVPU is part of the National Early Warning Score (NEWS) and has recently been updated. The importance of *new-onset confusion* as a sign of impending deterioration is now emphasised in the NEWS2 assessment of

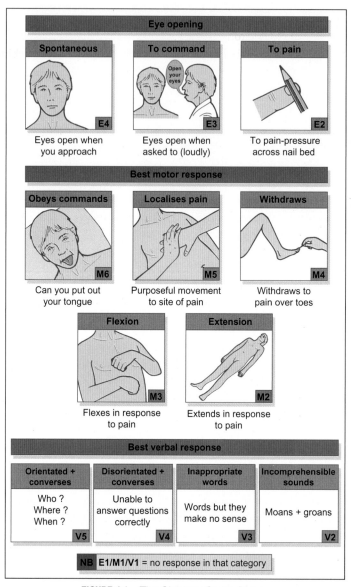

FIGURE 4.1 The Glasgow Coma Score.

consciousness (ACVPU) in which it is given a score of three. AVPU and ACVPU are insufficient where subtle changes in the neurological status (e.g., after a subarachnoid haemorrhage) need to be identified—the GCS is used in these circumstances.

Top-to-toe examination. Those closely involved with the care of acute neurological disorders should be aware of the importance of quite subtle physical signs in giving clues, particularly of head injury and infection. A head injury can result in local bogginess or scalp bruising, perhaps a palpable depressed skull and bleeding or loss of cerebrospinal fluid (CSF) from the ears and nose. Fractures to the base of the skull characteristically produce bruising around the eyes ('raccoon eyes') and behind the ears (Battle sign). All these can and will be missed by clerking clinicians, particularly if a 'stroke' label has been attached to the patient and the examination is less than thorough because of the pressures of time. Be particularly careful to look at any sites that appear to be the source of pain. Severe sinus sepsis is tender to the touch and very painful; falls from whatever cause lead to fractured hips and grand mal fits can produce shoulder dislocation. A widespread haemorrhagic skin rash will clinch the diagnosis of meningococcal septicaemia, but it can appear with alarming speed, sometimes even after the patient has been clerked in.

Observation frequency depends on the clinical situation: blood pressure every 5 min while it is being reduced urgently; blood pressure, pulse, GCS and pupillary responses every 15 min after thrombolysis, hourly GCS and pupils after a severe stroke.

A reliable history. One of the difficulties with neurology is the unreliability of the preadmission diagnosis. Unfortunately, diagnostic labels tend to stick and the consequences can sometimes be disastrous: the 'cerebrovascular accident' turns out to be a subdural bleed, 'off legs' a spinal cord compression, the 'well-known epileptic' a case of recurrent syncope due to intermittent heart block and so forth. Every neurological patient who is admitted to hospital should be looked at afresh, particularly where there is a 'known case of …' Known by whom and with what degree of certainty? Are we sure that the original diagnosis still applies?

It is not advisable to make 'stroke' the initial diagnosis in a patient in a coma, even if there is a history of cerebrovascular disease. This is particularly the case in elderly patients. It is a dangerous tendency to attribute all changes in the conscious level, all funny turns and all episodes of dizziness to a 'CVA' just because the patient is 80 years old.

Recent causes of coma initially labelled as stroke in our AMU included:
- Post-ictal state
- Respiratory failure
- Overdose
- Subarachnoid bleed

To make an accurate diagnosis, the history and eyewitness accounts are absolutely critical. By their nature, acute neurological problems are difficult to assess. The patients are often confused or uncooperative, making history taking and examination difficult. Nonetheless, these are the patients for whom a correct diagnosis is paramount. Skills that are needed to assess patients with confusion or impaired conscious levels must be perfected. Exact histories must be obtained from relatives and eyewitnesses, in particular, to establish whether there is a possibility of trauma to the head or cervical spine. The typical sequence of events leading to a post-traumatic brain haemorrhage is a head injury with transient loss of consciousness followed by amnesia for the event. The patient then becomes confused and aggressive and may fit. The GCS then starts to fall as a result of the haemorrhage. The patient may present at any of these stages. Intracranial infection is also easy to miss: here, the critical questions are concerned with recent sinus or middle ear infections. Collections of pus in and around the brain present with stroke-like illnesses and are frequently missed because a proper history has not been taken and the conditions have not even been considered.

Managing 'Medical' and 'Neurological' Coma

Coma is defined as a GCS of 8 or less. Broadly, there are two types: 'medical' coma, which is coma due to conditions such as liver failure, respiratory failure, septic shock and diabetic ketoacidosis (DKA), in which the management is primarily aimed at the underlying disease, and 'neurological' coma due to conditions such as stroke, subarachnoid haemorrhage and meningitis.

THE UNDERLYING MECHANISM IN COMA

Consciousness is maintained by a constant stream of neurological traffic in the form of nerve impulses that are sent from the brainstem upward into the two cerebral hemispheres. Loss of consciousness (coma) therefore has two general mechanisms that can form the basis of a practical classification of the causes of coma:
- Cerebral hemisphere malfunction
  - Drug and alcohol intoxication
  - Hypoxic brain damage (e.g., post-arrest)
  - Stroke
  - Metabolic disorders (DKA/hypoglycaemia, liver failure, respiratory failure)
  - Infection (meningitis, encephalitis, sepsis)
  - Inflammation (lupus, posterior reversible encephalopathy syndrome)
  - Post tonic–clonic convulsion
- Brainstem damage
  - Direct damage
    - Brainstem stroke
  - Indirect damage (from the downward shift of the cerebral hemispheres)
    - Cerebral mass (clot, tumour, abscess)
    - Cerebral oedema (due to stroke, anoxia, meningitis, etc.)

A coma that lasts more than 4 h is usually due to one of the four groups of conditions (Box 4.2). By far the most common cause is self-poisoning (40%).

Several features of the patient's initial observations can be used to identify a coma that is due to causes other than a stroke (Box 4.3). This has a practical purpose because

> **BOX 4.2 ■ Causes of Coma That Lasts 4 h or More**
>
> - Self-poisoning with sedative drugs 40%
> - Post-hypoxic cerebral damage 25%
> - Stroke 20%
> - Metabolic disorders 15%

> **BOX 4.3 ■ Features That Suggest That a Coma Is Not Due to a Stroke**
>
> - Deep coma
> - Reactive pupils
> - Pyrexia
> - No deviation of the eyes to one side
> - Moves all four limbs

> **BOX 4.4 ■ The Five S's: Critical Conditions That Must not Be Missed**
>
> - Sugar (high or low)
> - Sepsis
> - Sub- (and extra-) dural haemorrhage
> - Special causes of coma (respiratory failure, renal failure and liver failure)
> - Secret overdoses (late presentation of paracetamol/tricyclic overdose)

coma due to stroke has an extremely poor prognosis, whereas some of the other causes may be reversible.

There are five causes of coma that must not be missed as they are all treatable and relatively easy to diagnose, provided that they are considered at the time of the initial assessment (Box 4.4).

PRACTICAL MANAGEMENT OF COMA

The systematic way to approach a patient with a coma is to use the universal system of *primary assessment* based on the simple mnemonic ABCDE.

A is the airway. 'Are you all right?' If the patient responds appropriately, there is unlikely to be an airway problem. The airway can be maintained with a jaw thrust or chin lift. Placing the patient in the recovery position may be necessary (providing there is no sign or suspicion of spinal injury). Use a Guedel oropharyngeal airway if it can be tolerated or a nasopharyngeal airway. Administer high-flow oxygen immediately. Look, listen and feel for expired air.

B is the breathing

- Count the respiratory rate (breaths/min):

Less than 10	Imminent respiratory arrest
More than 20	Ill
More than 30	Critically ill

- Listen for noise (wheeze, upper airway gurgling, 'croup')
- Assess the effort
- Perform oximetry
- Continue high-flow oxygen
- Keep the saturations greater than 90%

C is the circulation

- Assess pulse rate and strength
- Assess capillary refill (press finger pulp for 5 s and release; refill should be less than 2 s). This gives an idea of the peripheral circulation
- Measure the blood pressure

D is the disability

- GCS
- Assess pupil size, equality and reaction
- Measure blood sugar (give sugar for hypoglycaemia and, if there is a suspicion of alcohol use disorder, thiamine)

E is the exposure

- Look for rashes and signs of trauma
- Check for hypothermia (core temperature)
- Look in the mouth (tongue biting)

IMPORTANCE OF AN EYEWITNESS IN COMA

Any relatives or eyewitnesses must be kept on the ward and interviewed (or if necessary telephoned). Their information may provide vital clues to the likely diagnosis. It is unacceptable for the doctor or the nurse ever to conclude that a history is either unobtainable or unavailable. Cerebral malaria is the classic example to emphasise this point: fatal if undiagnosed, curable with drugs, but too rare to remember to consider as a cause of coma. Only the patient's relatives will tell you of the safari holiday taken a week before the onset of headaches, fever and confusion. Patients who are most at risk are the least able to provide a good history for themselves. It is critical to ascertain whether there is a possibility of trauma. Patients with head injuries and trauma to the cervical spine are not usually admitted to the medical wards, but you should not lower your guard: in neurology, the most challenging and difficult problems are those in which a history is unavailable and for which preadmission clinical details are scanty. Review all the details in the paramedics' records. Their information is often comprehensive and systematic and dates from soon after the event. A good paramedic assessment will give you important data on the circumstances in which the patient was found, the initial GCS and NEWS2 score and their clinical course in the critical early stages of the illness.

Responding to Neurological Deterioration

It is not sufficient to document neurological observations. The reason for performing these time-consuming and exacting assessments is to act as soon as they change. The patient described below (Case Study 4.1) sustained traumatic intracerebral bleeding and was 'coning' (a shift of the brain as a result of raised ICP). The signs of increasing ICP were identified, but immediate action was not taken. A one-sided dilated pupil is often the earliest warning sign of elevated ICP which, if not corrected urgently, leads to a pressure cone.

HOW THE CLINICAL STATE CAN CHANGE IN THE FIRST HOURS OF ADMISSION

Case Studies 4.2–4.4 illustrate how the clinical state can change rapidly.

Other important examples include the following:

■ Deepening coma in an overdose
■ Deterioration due to missed infection elsewhere (blood, urine, chest, etc.)

CASE STUDY 4.1   **A Sudden Change at 04:00 h**

A 59-year-old male on warfarin for a valve replacement was taken to the accident and emergency department (AED) having collapsed and fallen backwards, striking and bruising his head. He appeared well, but x-rays showed a basal skull fracture. In view of his 'medical' problems, he was admitted to the AMU, where he was described as 'drowsy and vague, complaining of headache'. He was moderately over-anticoagulated (INR 4.9). Half-hourly, neurological observations recorded a systolic blood pressure increasing from 130 to 220 mm Hg and a sluggishly reacting right pupil which, over 3.5 h, became more dilated. He was responsive to commands until 4:00 h, 6 h after admission, when he suddenly vomited copiously and became unresponsive (GCS 3). At this stage, his right pupil was fixed and dilated. His anticoagulation was urgently reversed with prothrombin complex concentrate. He was intubated, ventilated and sent urgently to the neurosurgeons.

CASE STUDY 4.2   **Confusion Through Delirium to Coma**

A 55-year-old male became acutely confused the day after returning from a Turkish holiday. Over the next 48 h, his speech deteriorated and he became increasingly difficult to rouse. He then had a series of tonic–clonic convulsions. Investigations showed a severe viral encephalitis.

CASE STUDY 4.3	Fever to Skin Rash and Meningitis

A 19-year-old student was admitted on Christmas Eve with an acute abdomen. In the recovery room after a negative laparotomy, the anaesthetist noticed a petechial rash. Lumbar puncture was normal, but treatment for meningococcal infection was started. Repeat lumbar puncture 8 h later yielded ginger-beer coloured CSF which grew meningococci. He recovered fully.

CASE STUDY 4.4	Aspiration Pneumonia After a Stroke

An 80-year-old male developed dizziness and a mild hemiparesis. On admission, his GCS was 15, but he could not swallow at all. He would not tolerate an airway. Late the same night he vomited and dropped his GCS to 5. He became acutely short of breath and pyrexial. The cause of his deterioration was aspiration pneumonia. Despite physiotherapy and antibiotics, he deteriorated and died.

Reaching Appropriate Outcomes

The combination of good nursing and medical care should aim to reach an appropriate outcome for every patient. Important outcomes and the principles by which they can be achieved are listed below.

MAKING THE CORRECT DIAGNOSIS

- When is a CT scan needed?
  - To decide the type of stroke (block or bleed?)
  - To identify a major cerebral vessel blockage (CT angiogram)
  - To exclude tumour, abscess, haematoma
  - To diagnose a subarachnoid haemorrhage
  - To evaluate suspected increased ICP
  - Before a lumbar puncture (LP) if the patient is drowsy
- When is an LP needed?
  - To diagnose meningitis/encephalitis
  - To diagnose a subarachnoid haemorrhage if the CT is normal

URGENT ADMISSION TO THE ACUTE STROKE UNIT IN AN OPTIMUM CONDITION

- Coma management
- Swallowing assessment
- Early aspirin where indicated (transient ischaemic attack [TIA] and mild, non-disabling stroke)
- Emergency CT/MRI scanning and guideline-based interventions

AVOIDING A MAJOR STROKE AFTER A TRANSIENT ISCHAEMIC ATTACK

- Urgent investigation (within 24h) of suspected TIAs and minor strokes

SURVIVING INTRACRANIAL SEPSIS

- Early treatment of meningitis
- Recognising and managing complications

REACHING THE NEUROSURGEONS ALIVE AND ON TIME

- Recognising operable intracranial bleeds
- Diagnosing intracerebral masses
- Managing increased ICP
- Selection for decompression craniotomy (young patients with massive cerebral infarcts)

FULL RECOVERY FROM SELF-HARM

- Responding to a changing GCS

RECOVERY FROM REVERSIBLE CAUSES OF NEUROLOGICAL EMERGENCIES

- Rapid and effective primary assessment
- Good coma management

Stroke and Stroke-Like Emergencies

The World Health Organization's definition of a stroke is a syndrome of rapidly developing clinical signs of focal (e.g., hemiplegia) or global (e.g., coma) disturbance of function, with symptoms lasting 24h or longer (or leading to death) with no apparent cause other than of vascular origin.

The time frame of 24h is to differentiate a stroke from a TIA, which recovers rapidly but is an important risk factor for developing a subsequent completed stroke. There are around 2.4 strokes per 1000 population per year. Eighty per cent of these will be admitted as emergencies, but a significant number will occur in patients already in hospital. It is important, however, not to overuse the stroke label, as up to a fifth of all 'strokes' turn out to be something else: post-epileptic states, toxic states due to infection and metabolic problems such as respiratory failure.

In most hospitals, patients with stroke no longer go to the AMU. Guidelines now emphasise that all strokes should be admitted to a specialist stroke service within 4h of arriving in hospital. Terms used in current stroke guidelines such as 'Brain at Risk' and 'Next on Table' (for an urgent CT) illustrate the new approach to removing *any* treatment delays. There are three vital components to the service:

- A hyperacute service for urgent interventions in the first 72 h
- An acute stroke unit for intensive specialised multidisciplinary input
- Ongoing rehabilitation through a multi-agency team

Patients admitted straight to a stroke unit are more likely to be alive and independent 1 year after the event.

There are clear recommendations on early interventions, which improve the outlook of stroke and prevent further damage:

- Emergency intravenous thrombolysis (IVT)—using alteplase—within 4.5 h of the onset of symptoms improves the neurological outcome of cerebral infarction and is now a standard part of stroke care. In the United Kingdom, 10% of acute strokes receive thrombolysis.
- Consideration of urgent blood pressure management before thrombolysis and in cerebral haemorrhage.
- Carefully selected patients benefit from thrombectomy—mechanical clot extraction (a technique analogous to that used after an acute myocardial infarction (MI)).
- Selection of patients for potential neurosurgical intervention.

Causes

Most typical strokes are caused either by a cerebral infarction (an area of brain tissue death) or by an intracerebral haemorrhage (bleeding into and around the brain). Stroke-like illnesses are also caused by subarachnoid haemorrhage, subdural haemorrhage and extradural haemorrhage. Subarachnoid haemorrhage is an important cause of sudden severe headache and collapse and requires neurosurgical input. Subdural and extradural haemorrhages are rare but important causes of stroke-like illnesses that can be treated successfully if they are recognised in time.

There has been a recent increase in strokes in young patients due to carotid artery dissection associated with neck trauma, cocaine use and pregnancy. Early diagnosis is essential as the treatment is anticoagulation. Thrombosis of the cerebral veins can masquerade as a stroke and has been seen recently as a very rare complication of some COVID-19 vaccinations.

CEREBRAL INFARCTION (APPROXIMATELY 80% OF ALL STROKES)

A cerebral infarction occurs when the blood supply to part of the brain is cut off, resulting in a focal area of brain tissue death (an ischaemic stroke). There are two ways in which the blood supply can be interrupted: by a clot that travels through the arterial system and becomes lodged somewhere critical in the cerebral circulation (*cerebral embolus*) or by a clot that forms within the cerebral arteries themselves (*cerebral thrombosis*).

Cerebral Embolus

A fifth of ischaemic strokes are due to cerebral emboli. Cerebral emboli can come from anywhere from the left atrium to the carotid arteries in the neck. Rarely, clots can enter the arterial circulation from the venous side through a hole between the right atrium and the left atrium (termed a 'patent foramen ovale') and present as a young patient with a sudden unexplained stroke.

Left atrial clot. The most common cause of left atrial clots is atrial fibrillation. In atrial fibrillation, normal regular atrial contraction is replaced by irregular, uncoordinated atrial activity more akin to muscular shivering than proper contraction. As a result, blood stagnates and can form a clot within the atrium. There is a particular risk of this happening if there is also heart disease in the form of heart muscle damage (which leads to further stagnation) or diseased valves (which can act as a focus for clot formation). Atrial fibrillation is a common age-related arrhythmia. It is found in around 8% of people older than 80 years and constitutes a major risk factor for stroke. However, the risk can be significantly reduced by anticoagulating patients who have atrial fibrillation so that there is less chance of clot formation, by trying to restore a normal heart rhythm or, where anticoagulation is contraindicated, by percutaneous occlusion of the left atrial appendage—the site where 90% of atrial clots form.

Left ventricular clot. It is quite common for a clot to form on the inside of the heart chamber over the scar of a recent myocardial infarction. In most cases, the clot stays put, but there is always a risk of it breaking loose and travelling to the cerebral circulation. This is a particular problem in the first week or two after a myocardial infarction, when the clot is new.

Carotid artery clot. Atheromatous hardening of the carotid arteries has two relevant consequences for stroke formation. It may lead to critical narrowing (carotid artery stenosis) with a reduction in the blood supply to the brain. More importantly, blood clots form on the abnormally roughened arterial wall and can break off to lodge within the cerebral arterial tree. Small emboli produce minor stroke-like symptoms (TIAs), which are warning signs of a subsequent major stroke.

Cerebral Thrombosis

Hardening of the cerebral arteries (cerebral arteriosclerosis) leads to the narrowing of the vessels and can progress to atheromatous plaque formation and localised thrombosis with blockage. As with atheroma elsewhere in the body, there are several causes: these include smoking, high cholesterol and a positive family history.

The two most important risk factors are as follows:

- Hypertension
- Diabetes

Of the two, hypertension is the more significant: a diastolic blood pressure of 110 mm Hg or more increases the stroke risk 15-fold. This compares with an increase of two to three times normal in diabetes.

The important point about these two risk factors is that they are both reversible. Controlling blood pressure and controlling diabetes have a major impact on lowering the increased levels of risk.

Clinical Picture of a Cerebral Infarction

The clinical features depend on the site and extent of the infarct and range from immediate coma and death to minor short-lived clumsiness of a limb. It is helpful to use clinical features to divide cerebral infarctions into two categories: those affecting the circulation to the front of the brain (*anterior circulation infarcts*) and those affecting the back (*posterior circulation infarcts*) (Fig. 4.2).

Anterior circulation infarcts. Anterior circulation infarcts result in the picture of the 'classic' stroke with a variable combination of one-sided weakness (hemiparesis), one-sided sensory loss (hemianaesthesia), visual disturbance in the form of a gaze paralysis (the eyes are deviated away from the weak side) and partial loss of the visual field

Type	Site on CT	Deficit	1 year mortality %	1 year dependency %
TACI		One sided weakness/ sensory loss + Hemianopia + Cortical dysfunction	60	35
PACI		Two of the following • One-sided weakness or sensory loss • Cortical dysfunction • Hemianopia	20	30
LACI		One-sided weakness/ sensory loss	10	25
POCI		Slurred speech Dysphagia Double vision Dizziness Unsteadiness	20	20

FIGURE 4.2 Types of cerebral infarct. *LACI*, Lacunar infarct; *PACI*, partial anterior circulation infarct; *POCI*, posterior circulation infarct; *TACI*, total anterior circulation infarct.

(the patient cannot see toward the weak side). In addition, there is a variable disturbance of higher functions (termed 'cortical function'): language disturbance (if the dominant side of the brain is damaged), neglect of the affected side and incontinence.

Total anterior circulation infarct (TACI) is a combination of motor or sensory deficit, visual field loss and cortical dysfunction (e.g., language disturbance).

Partial anterior circulation infarct (PACI) consists of any two of the following:

- Unilateral weakness/sensory loss
- Visual field defect (hemianopia)
- Cortical dysfunction (language disorder or neglect)

Lacunar infarct (LACI) consists of very small infarcts within the anterior circulation that pick off single pathways at critical points in the brain. They are particularly associated with a history of hypertension. The clinical picture is of a 'pure' one-sided motor or sensory loss.

Posterior circulation infarcts (POCI), also termed a 'brainstem CVA', result in symptoms that often affect both sides of the body (the brainstem transmits information to and from *both* sides of the brain) and characteristically affect coordination in four vital functions: talking, swallowing, looking and balancing. These patients have combinations of dysarthria (slurred speech), dysphagia (difficulty swallowing), double vision and dizziness. The important combination of sudden loss of consciousness and brainstem signs would suggest a major posterior circulation occlusion and needs urgent imaging as the vessel should, if feasible, be unblocked.

Site of the Cerebral Infarction and the Outlook

Patients who suffer a TACI have a poor outcome: high initial mortality and high levels of long-term dependence. Some patients with an extensive TACI develop severe cerebral oedema and deteriorate 3 or 4 days after admission. If they are identified early, some of these patients can be salvaged by neurosurgical decompression to lessen the effects on the rest of the brain of the cerebral oedema. Patients who have suffered a PACI have a much better outlook, with low mortality but a high recurrence rate. An LACI is associated with a good outcome, low mortality and a low recurrence rate.

Posterior circulation strokes have the best overall outlook, although the swallowing difficulties need to be managed carefully to prevent the development of aspiration pneumonia. There is also a high recurrence rate.

TRANSIENT ISCHAEMIC ATTACKS AND MINOR ISCHAEMIC STROKES

Transient ischaemic attacks are minor strokes caused by the passage of small emboli that negotiate the cerebral circulation without producing any permanent damage. The clinical picture depends on the route the emboli take and varies from a paralysed or clumsy limb (Case Study 4.5) to an isolated speech or visual disturbance. By definition the symptoms

CASE STUDY 4.5	A 70-Year-Old Male With Episodic Numbness

A male was admitted with episodic weakness of the right arm and leg lasting 5 min and associated with difficulties finding the right words. He returned to normal between attacks. During the previous week, there had been four or five episodes. He had been treated for hypertension and a heart murmur. He was otherwise well. Subsequent urgent investigations showed a near-total blockage of the left common carotid artery. His hypertension was controlled, and he was started on aspirin and a statin and referred for consideration of surgery for the blocked carotid.

and signs of TIA last no longer than 24 h, but in practice the clinical picture is of an immediate onset with resolution within 5 to 20 min. It is unusual for any deficit to last longer than 1 h. Clearly, such short-lived symptoms can be confused with several other conditions, including epilepsy, migraine, hypoglycaemia, syncope (fainting) and acute vertigo (giddiness). A head CT is required if there are ongoing neurological signs or symptoms or if there are risk factors that this is a cerebral haemorrhage, not ischaemia (e.g., anticoagulant therapy). The term 'minor ischaemic stroke' is used where the symptoms persist longer than an hour but are not disabling, that is, no speech or visual field defect, no swallowing difficulty and no issue with walking or self-care. Thrombolysis in minor ischaemic strokes is not recommended as the risk outweighs the benefit. However, there is a risk of a further stroke so the approach is similar to that with a TIA including urgent carotid artery imaging and anti-platelet drugs (usually dual anti-platelet therapy, e.g., aspirin and clopidogrel).

The areas of narrowing and roughening within the carotid arteries from which the emboli usually arise can, in time, give rise to a major stroke. Someone who suffers a TIA is at more than 10 times the normal risk of having a major stroke, and the risk is highest immediately after the event. As an approximate guide, the chances of a major stroke after a TIA or minor stroke are 4%–6.5% at 7 days and 11%–15% at 1 month. Treatment can significantly reduce these chances, but the situation is urgent and systems should be in place for those with TIAs and minor ischaemic strokes to have specialist assessment within 24 h.

It should be noted that patients who have had two or more TIAs within a period of 7 days carry a 30% risk of stroke within the subsequent week. However, all patients with a suspected TIA should be considered high risk for a stroke—they should receive 300 mg aspirin and be seen by a specialist within 24 h. If subsequent investigations show significant blockage (50%–99%) of the carotid artery, patients need surgical endarterectomy within a maximum of 2 weeks of the TIA to lessen the risk of an early and disabling stroke.

INTRACEREBRAL HAEMORRHAGE (APPROXIMATELY 10% OF ALL STROKES)

Intracerebral haemorrhage occurs when the wall of an abnormally weak cerebral artery suddenly bursts and releases blood into the brain tissue with the formation of a clot (intracerebral haematoma) (Fig. 4.3). The weakened areas consist of small outpouchings

FIGURE 4.3   Types of brain haemorrhage.

of the vessels, termed microaneurysms, which are the result of damage from chronic hypertension. As with cerebral thrombosis, controlling hypertension has a major role in primary prevention by reducing arterial damage.

Clinical Features

A severe intracerebral haemorrhage presents as a dramatic collapse with headache and vomiting, leading rapidly to coma and then death. This is by no means the rule, however, and in many cases, there are no clinical features that reliably differentiate a stroke caused by haemorrhage from that due to a cerebral infarct.

The distinction is critical because aspirin and, increasingly, thrombolytic drugs are being used to treat cerebral infarction, and they would be absolutely contraindicated in cerebral haemorrhage. For this reason, early CT or MRI scanning has become an important part of acute stroke management, as it will show a haemorrhage within minutes of it happening. The longer the CT scan is delayed, the more difficult it is to distinguish a haemorrhage from an infarct. Patients with acute stroke must have a scan within an hour of arriving at hospital. If this shows a cerebral haemorrhage, significant hypertension is treated urgently and any anticoagulants are reversed immediately.

SUBARACHNOID HAEMORRHAGE (APPROXIMATELY 5% OF ALL STROKES)

The arachnoid is a double-layered membrane that coats the surfaces of the brain and forms the subarachnoid space through which the cerebral arteries pass. Due to a genetic predisposition, some patients develop berrylike aneurysms on these vessels. The aneurysms are prone to rupture, particularly during periods of physical exertion and after binge drinking. Hypertension and especially smoking are also important reversible risk factors for a subarachnoid. If an aneurysm bursts, there is acute haemorrhage that spreads throughout the subarachnoid space, typically causing intense meningeal irritation with severe sudden headaches and vomiting (see Fig. 4.3).

The major complications are as follows:

- Increased ICP
- Spasm of the cerebral arteries, leading to further damage
- Re-bleeding

The aneurysms are often multiple, so management is based on supporting the patient through the first episode and taking urgent neurosurgical advice on the preventative options of surgery to clip the aneurysms or, more commonly, embolization with coils to clot them off. The optimum time to intervene to prevent further bleeding is within 48 h of the haemorrhage so there is urgency to establish the diagnosis.

The drug nimodipine—60 mg 4 hourly given either orally or by nasogastric tube—is used to lessen the risk of cerebral arterial spasm and must be started as soon as the diagnosis is confirmed.

SUBDURAL HAEMORRHAGE

This is a low-pressure venous 'ooze' that slowly enlarges within the confines of the subdural space. The slowly forming haematoma presses on the brain and causes a progressive or fluctuating neurological deficit. Subdurals are usually caused by minor and frequently forgotten trauma, particularly in patients with other risk factors, most notably, anticoagulant therapy or frequent falling (Case Study 4.6). The classic presentation is with fluctuating drowsiness and rather vague one-sided weakness. In the elderly the clinical features can be non-specific: confusion, delirium, behavioural changes and 'dementia'. The diagnosis is confirmed by a CT scan.

EXTRADURAL HAEMORRHAGE

This is a high-pressure arterial bleed virtually always associated with a fractured skull (see Fig. 4.3). The rapid development of a large extradural clot compresses and shifts the cerebral hemisphere, producing coma and pupillary changes. Characteristically, but not always, there is a lucid interval after the head injury before the patient suddenly starts to deteriorate. It is the fear of a delayed extradural haemorrhage that keeps patients in hospital after head injuries.

In theory, extradural haemorrhages should not be seen on the medical wards, but an occasional patient may be admitted with an unrecognised head injury who suddenly deteriorates as a result of an extradural bleed. These patients survive only if the condition is recognised and they are sent for urgent neurosurgery.

The patients themselves may simply appear confused and aggressive after a head injury of which they have no recollection. The key, as with many of these neurological disorders, is to remember the possibility of the diagnosis, particularly where there is a dramatic change in the level of consciousness. It is, of course, critical to take a full history from the patient and witnesses with regard to possible head injury. It is also helpful to remember that vomiting after a head injury is a warning symptom of a skull fracture and these are the patients who are at risk of an extradural haemorrhage.

CASE STUDY 4.6 Subdural Haemorrhage

CASE 1
An 84-year-old female was admitted from a nursing home where she was normally mobile, conversant and continent. Four days previously, she had fallen out of bed and banged her head. She was discharged from AED with a GCS of 14. The following day she became drowsy and incoherent. Her GP diagnosed a urinary infection. She deteriorated and was admitted. Her GCS was 8. There was bruising around the left eye. Her CT scan showed a large subdural haematoma. She was referred to neurosurgery to aspirate the haematoma.

CASE 2
A 75-year-old male was knocked down by a slowly moving bus and sustained a glancing blow to the side of his head, with transient loss of consciousness. On admission to the surgical ward, his GCS was 13. He remained 'mildly' confused but was discharged after 3 days. The relatives rang the surgical ward to say his mobility and confusion were worsening, but no action was taken. A week after discharge, he was readmitted to the medical ward. He was difficult to rouse: he had a GCS of 8 and was still confused. A CT scan showed a large subdural haemorrhage, with a shift of the brain to the opposite side. Despite neurosurgical intervention, he made very poor progress.

Care of the Patient With a Stroke: The First 24 H

The nature of the emergency initial assessment of a patient with a stroke is determined by the patient's condition. When there is impairment of the conscious level, the immediate assessment and management is that of any patient in a coma, with the focus naturally being on securing the airway and performing resuscitation (ABCDE). When there appears to be a less severe disability such as a weak arm or speech disturbance in an alert and stable patient, the assessment may concentrate on the functional capacity of the patient, in particular vision, communication, balance and swallowing.

CRITICAL CLINICAL OBSERVATIONS AND IMMEDIATE MANAGEMENT

The immediate management of the stroke is that of coma and has already been described. The primary aim is to maintain oxygen delivery to the brain. The initial examination should concentrate on the vital signs, the conscious level (GCS) and the swallowing:

- Assess the security of the airway (recovery position ensures the safety of the airway)
- Maintain an oxygen saturation (94%–98%)
- Pulse (atrial fibrillation?)
- Temperature (aspiration pneumonia? hypothermia?)
- Blood pressure—after a cerebral infarction a blood pressure above 185/110 will need urgent reduction before alteplase can be given. After a cerebral haemorrhage a systolic blood pressure above 150 needs intensive treatment aiming for a controlled reduction to 140 or less.

Avoiding aspiration pneumonia and assessing the swallow. About one in three stroke patients will have at least temporary swallowing problems after a stroke and will be at risk from aspiration; if they are also kept 'nil by mouth', there is the added problem of avoiding dehydration and even malnutrition. The fact that the conscious level is normal does not reliably predict that the swallow is safe (Case Study 4.7). There must be a formal swallowing assessment in every patient with acute stroke within 4 h of admission and before oral fluids are allowed. The initial assessment will identify some of the features that are seen in patients who are at risk from aspiration:

CASE STUDY 4.7	Loss of Swallowing

A 74-year-old male was admitted to hospital because he awoke and found that he could not swallow. He tried to get to the phone, but was unable to stand because of unsteadiness. On admission, he had slurring of his speech and was unable to sit unsupported without toppling over. His arm movements were very uncoordinated; when he tried to touch his nose he was in danger of damaging his eyes. His blood pressure was 180/120 mm Hg, and he had loud bruits over both carotid arteries, suggesting arterial disease. He insisted he was well enough to go home but could not stand. On testing his swallow there was immediate choking and coughing. Investigations confirmed a posterior circulation cerebral infarct.

- Low GCS (less than 8)
- The voice sounds wet and rough and the gag reflex is reduced
- The cough is weak and the tongue mobility is impaired
- The larynx (Adam's apple) does not move upwards on swallowing
- The patient is elderly and frail
- Previous stroke
- Patients who are unable to sit upright and who have a loss of balance

A simple water test must be carried out to identify disordered swallowing:

- Support the patient in the sitting position
- Give 5 mL of water and look for choking, coughing, dribbling, wet voice
- If swallowing is satisfactory, repeat the test with 50 mL of water
- If the test fails, keep the patient nil by mouth, start IV fluids and refer for advice

If the swallow is unsafe, maintain the fluid intake with IV fluids. Refer the patient to the specialist team (either the dietician or the speech and language therapist) and consider retesting in 24 h. As there is a risk of inhalation of oropharyngeal contaminants, particular care should be taken to ensure good oral hygiene. Adequate hydration and nutrition are critical to ensuring the patient's recovery: if the swallow is not secure the decision on a nasogastric tube should not be delayed beyond 24 h after admission at which point feeding should be started.

History. The basis for making the correct diagnosis is the history of the patient and their relatives. It is important to evaluate pre-existing dependency using measures such as the Barthel ADL index (Box 4.5) or the National Institutes of Health Stroke Scale (NIHSS) to find out the home situation, for example, carers, independent housing, warden control, residential care or nursing home. The NIHSS is also used to assess stroke severity.

If there has been a previous stroke, how much of the present problem is due to residual disability and how much is new will have to be established. Risk factors for stroke can be identified from the history: hypertension, atrial fibrillation, diabetes and heart disease.

BOX 4.5 ■ Barthel ADL Functional Assessment Scale

- Bowels
- Mobility
- Bladder
- Transfer
- Grooming
- Dressing
- Toilet use
- Stairs
- Feeding
- Bathing

Managing urinary incontinence. Urinary incontinence suggests disordered higher (cortical) function and is common in anterior circulation strokes. Catheterisation causes infection and leads to a reduction in the bladder capacity; it must therefore be avoided, as it reduces the chance of the spontaneous recovery in bladder function that usually occurs after a stroke. Urge incontinence is a common early problem and is not helped by problems with communication and mobility. The focus for the ward team should be on the use of simple communication aids and in trying to anticipate or respond as rapidly as possible to the patient's toileting needs (do not use pads, employ timed toileting and prompted voiding). If the patient develops acute retention a quick 'in-and-out' catheterisation is the preferred option.

The return of independent mobility is often associated with improved continence.

Communication. During the initial assessment, it will be apparent if there is a communication problem other than that due to an impaired conscious level. The three basic aspects of communication *must* be evaluated and documented at an early stage: this must be interpreted in light of the relatives' description of the patient's pre-existing cognitive function.

Vision. The more extensive strokes are often complicated by visual disturbance. The pattern of visual loss that is usually seen is termed a hemianopia. This is a loss of the left or right visual field and involves both eyes. As a rule, the visual loss is toward the paralysed side, so, for example, a patient with left hemiplegia would not be able to see toward the left. A person standing and talking from the patient's left-hand side will therefore not be seen and will often be ignored by the patient. Similarly, food and fluid placed to the left of the patient will not be seen. A hemianopia has to be specifically looked for because many stroke patients will be unaware of its presence. It is also important to note if the patient is unable to move his eyes to one or other side (gaze palsy).

Hearing. Perhaps surprisingly, the most common cause of poor communication in the acute medical ward is a failure to appreciate simple deafness in an elderly patient. Hearing loss itself is not usually caused by stroke.

Speech and language. Slurring of the speech may be a problem, particularly after a POCI, but it is usually not a major barrier to communication. Much more importantly, stroke may be complicated by a problem with language: finding, using and understanding words, known as dysphasia (*dy*sphasia is *d*ifficulty with speech; *a*phasia is *a*bsence of speech). There are two types of dysphasia:

1. **Motor dysphasia.** There is a block in getting the words out, despite the patient understanding everything and knowing what he wants to say. This is most frustrating for the patient. Motor dysphasia is often accompanied by a hemiplegia.
2. **Sensory dysphasia.** The patient has difficulty finding the right words and understanding what is being said. The patient's speech is jumbled and senseless, although the patient may not appear distressed by it. Sensory dysphasia is often accompanied by a hemianopia.

INTERVENTIONS IN THE FIRST 24H

Diagnosis. The **FAST** test (Facial droop–Arm weakness–Slurred speech Test) has been promoted to speed up the referral of stroke victims to hospital. Initial hospital assessment is dependent on the Rosier scale (Fig. 4.4) to differentiate stroke from 'look-alikes' including hypoglycaemia, syncope and epilepsy.

Imaging. Emergency stroke care is dependent on a head CT scan to show whether the patient has had a cerebral infarction, a cerebral haemorrhage or a stroke 'look-alike'— subarachnoid, subdural or extradural haemorrhage. The scan must be done immediately (within an hour of admission) to inform the management plans especially where:

- Thrombolysis—with or without subsequent thrombectomy—is a potential therapy
- The patient is on anticoagulants and may need reversing
- The GCS is less than 13 or the picture is progressing or fluctuating
- The onset was with a sudden severe headache (subarachnoid?)
- There is fever, neck stiffness or raised intracerebral pressure (papilloedema)

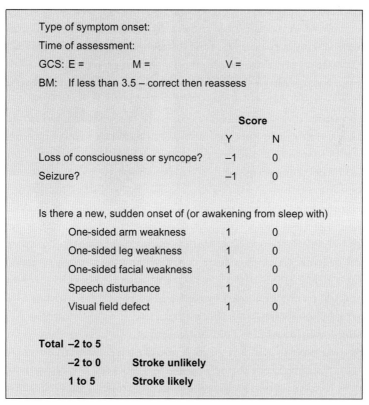

FIGURE 4.4 Rosier scale to diagnose stroke. *BM*, Blood glucose; *E*, eye response; *GCS*, Glasgow Coma Score; *M*, motor response; *V*, visual response.

It is no longer acceptable to 'scan strokes within 24 h', the approach is now 'next in scanner'.

Acute drug intervention. Acute stroke services are now organised so that immediate (within 30 min of admission—often giving the first dose in the CT suite) thrombolysis ("clot-busting") with intravenous alteplase can be given to those cases with a non-haemorrhagic stroke who would benefit in terms of reduced disability and better survival. The critical issue is that an improved outlook has only been shown if alteplase is given within four and a half hours of the onset of symptoms to patients with a proven ischaemic stroke. Outside this time frame, the risk of causing intracerebral bleeding may outweigh the benefit of reducing ischaemic brain damage so specialised imaging with CT and magnetic resonance imaging (MRI) are used to see the extent of any salvageable brain tissue. All patients with an acute ischaemic stroke should receive high-dose statin therapy as soon as they can swallow safely and, if they are not to receive thrombolysis, 300 mg aspirin as soon as possible after the onset. Initiatives around early recognition, referral and accelerated assessment are aimed at achieving thrombolysis rates of at least 10% of patients with stroke. For patients with ischaemic strokes, selected patients may be suitable for thrombolysis followed by mechanical clot extraction.

After thrombolysis, aspirin 300 mg should be given after 24 h or as soon as possible if not thrombolysed. Anticoagulation reduces the recurrence of stroke in patients with atrial fibrillation. However, because of the risk of bleeding into the softened and damaged area affected by the stroke, most clinicians prefer to wait at least 14 days before starting anticoagulants after a thrombotic stroke and, as with aspirin, only after cerebral haemorrhage has been excluded with a CT.

Blood pressure. The blood pressure needs to be less than 185/110 before alteplase can be given, so immediate intervention may be needed. A systolic blood pressure of greater than 150 mm Hg in the first 6 h after a cerebral haemorrhage requires urgent and sustained reduction—usually with intravenous antihypertensives, either nicardipine or labetalol.

Temperature. Pyrexia during the first 72 h of hospital admission is associated with early worsening of the neurological status. Apart from excluding infection, paracetamol can be used to bring the temperature down to normal (less than 37.2°C).

Cerebral oedema. Cerebral oedema may develop after a severe cerebral infarction and produce a deterioration in the conscious level after 3–5 days. Preventative referral for neurosurgical intervention (decompressive hemicraniectomy) within 24 h of a very large infarct in selected cases can be life saving.

Reversing warfarin and direct oral anticoagulants (DOACs). Patients on warfarin, particularly those where the INR is too high, and to a lesser extent those on DOACs, are at risk of an intracerebral (or subdural) haemorrhage. Should this occur, the anticoagulants must be reversed immediately as the mortality from an anticoagulant-associated cerebral haemorrhage approaches 50%.

For warfarin, prothrombin complex concentrate (PCC) 20–50 IU/kg (depending on the INR) combined with intravenous vitamin K 5 mg will normalise the INR within 10 min and (because of the vitamin K) the INR will remain normal for at least 24 h. Intravenous idarucizumab reverses the DOAC dabigatran. Intravenous andexanet alfa reverses the effects of apixaban and rivaroxaban. If these drugs are not available, four-factor PCC can be used.

Blood sugar. Maintaining a blood sugar between 6 and 10 mmol/L during the acute phase is recommended although, unlike post-MI, the outlook is not affected by very tight blood sugar control. A variable rate intravenous infusion will be needed in most insulin-dependent diabetics.

Avoiding pressure sores. Many elderly patients who suffer a stroke do so alone, and they may have been lying in one position for many hours, putting pressure on the skin and setting the scene for skin breakdown. This can be alleviated with appropriate physical measures such as the correct pressure-relieving mattress, combined with attention to nutrition and hydration. Specialist advice on appropriate positioning, taking into account limb paralysis, must be obtained within 4 h of arrival on the ward.

The philosophy in an acute stroke unit (and in the AMU) should be based on initiating preventative measures and on starting to address nutritional issues as soon as the patient is admitted. In the past, hydration, nutrition and their effects on the risk of complications have been neglected. Not uncommonly, patients would be admitted and find their way to a rehabilitation unit over the course of 2 weeks or more, without having received any proper food. In these cases, patients lose weight and are at a major risk from pressure sores. As a rule, although fluids are appropriate for 24 h while the swallowing is assessed, after that nutrition is required. This often means passing a fine-bore nasogastric tube.

Resuscitation status. A judgement must be made and explicitly stated on the resuscitation status of the patient. This is based on a number of important factors that include the following:

- The wishes of the patient (in practice, these will seldom be known, and in the patients for whom the decision is most relevant—those who are critically ill—it is unlikely to be ascertainable)
- The chances of survival (as an example, patients who are comatose 24 h after a stroke have only a 20% chance of survival)
- The pre-existing dependency of the patient (the Barthel score will give an accurate picture of the patient's level of independence)
- The perceptions of close relatives and carers (due weight is given to their views, although ultimately the decision rests with the clinical staff in the absence of the patient's own views)
- Coexisting diseases, for example, advanced malignant disease
- The opinion of the relevant medical and nursing staff

Any resuscitation decision must be reviewed at predetermined intervals so it would be appropriate to revisit the question of resuscitation at least 12 hourly during the first 2–3 days.

It should be noted that around 1 in 20 strokes will receive end-of-life care within 72 h of admission.

Early mobilisation. Very early mobilisation (within 24 h for those who need little or no assistance) improves the longer-term outlook in stroke. For those with more difficulty, daily mobilisation should be started within 48 h of onset. These time intervals also apply to speech therapy.

Avoiding venous thromboembolism (VTE). Stroke victims are at risk from VTE: deep vein thrombosis (DVT) and pulmonary embolus. Of the possible preventative measures, anti-embolus stockings probably do more harm than good. If the patient's mobility is impaired, intermittent calf pneumatic compression is preferable to prophylactic low-molecular-weight heparin and must be started within the first 3 days of admission.

Answering Relatives' Questions on Stroke

Will the patient recover? The answer to this depends on the severity of the stroke. Patients who are comatose on admission or who persistently ignore or neglect their paralysed side do badly. Stroke patients who start to recover within hours, particularly in terms of sitting balance, will do well. A 'cover-all' answer for all cases soon after admission would be to say that two out of every three stroke victims regain more or less full independence after a stroke. The patients who do badly are those with severe motor and sensory impairment, especially combined with hemianopias and urinary incontinence.

Why cannot we simply dissolve the clot as in a heart attack? Clot busters work in about one in 10 strokes but if they are given more than 4½ hours after the onset they sometimes do more harm than good. Outside of this time frame, we rely on our specialised scans and stroke experts to decide if it is safe and beneficial to give clot busters (if it is available and the stroke specialists think the patient may be suitable, you may be able to discuss possible clot removal at this point as it can be used up to 24 h after the stroke).

Why have you not done an MRI? We need to tell whether the stroke is caused by a bleed or a blockage. The CT is the easiest test to do this. The MRI is reserved for particular types of stroke, but it is much less easy to do and the patient can find it quite an unpleasant test.

Why can't you operate? Surgery can only rarely help a stroke patient—if there has been a large cerebral haemorrhage that has blocked the internal circulation of spinal fluid or if a young patient has a massive cerebral thrombosis and there are signs of increasing pressure inside the brain. Even in these cases, there is a risk that surgery can make the situation worse.

What has happened? Part of the brain has been damaged and the function of that area has been affected. This explains why there is paralysis/speech problems/confusion. The cause is a blockage to the blood supply or a sudden leak of blood into the brain tissue from a leaking artery.

Is it a heart attack–is the heart affected? Although sometimes a clot causing the stroke comes from the heart, the heart itself is not affected. Nonetheless, the risk factors for stroke and for heart attack are the same, so any preventative measures we recommend, such as smoking cessation, will have a dual benefit.

When will we know the amount of damage? The main recovery takes place over the first days or weeks after a stroke, but some further more limited recovery is possible over a much longer period.

What happens in a specialist stroke unit? Initially, we do whatever we can to reduce the damage and, if possible, remove any blockage. We provide a combined approach to early rehabilitation and preventative measures to stop it from happening again.

What physiotherapy will the patient need? The immediate emphasis is on positioning the limbs and body correctly and on assessing balance, rather than on simply seeing if the patient can walk. Unless the patient has little difficulty with walking, we start mobilisation at 24–48 h after the stroke. If you wish, you can talk to the physiotherapists about it.

What about feeding? At present the patient's swallowing is not particularly good, so we are using a drip and restricting any oral intake for a day or so to allow time for it to improve.

What is in the drip? This is dextrose, which provides fluid and some calories. If we cannot feed the patient orally within 24 h, we will need to consider a thin feeding tube, possibly as a short-term measure, to give some nutrition. If the swallowing remains unsafe we will start tube feeding at around 24 h after admission.

Was it stress that caused the stroke? No, there is no relationship between the two.

How much can the patient understand?

1. This is motor aphasia, which means the patient can understand but cannot find the right words.
2. This is sensory aphasia, so there is quite a problem at present with understanding as well as with the use of words.
3. The patient is in a coma, so at present, we are unclear how much can be taken in, but the patient may be able to hear and understand you.

Will it happen again? There is a chance of a further stroke if the patient has suffered one already, but we will do whatever we can to lessen the risks of recurrence. This will involve aspirin, smoking cessation, blood pressure control, etc.

Were there any warning signs we/the GP could have seen? Unless there were mini-strokes, there are few if any warnings of this sort of thing.

Will the patient always have a disability? The degree of disability cannot be accurately predicted at this early stage. (However, if the patient is recovering already or has retained good power in the legs and has a clear understanding of the situation, you can be reasonably encouraging, particularly if the patient was not previously dependent for his care.)

Is there anything we can do? Once we know the patient's level of ability with feeding and personal needs, you can assist with meals and other care if you wish.

Excellent Acute Stroke Care

Documentation of:
- Conscious level
- Eye movements
- Swallowing
- Communication
- Understanding
- Vision (field and gaze)
- Sensation
- Neglect of the affected side (is there correct positioning of a paralysed arm?)
- Classification of the type of stroke
- Documentation of pre- and post-stroke functions (Barthel Index/pre- and post-NIHSS scores)

Early:
- Direct admission to the acute (or hyperacute) stroke unit
- CT scan and assessment for immediate thrombolysis
- Physiotherapist assessment
- Speech therapy assessment

Acute Meningitis in Adults

In adults, acute *bacterial* meningitis is seen predominantly in two age groups—meningococcal meningitis in the late teens/early 20s and the over-60s who are also at risk from listeria, *Streptococcus pneumoniae* and *Haemophilus influenzae*.

There are often additional risk factors:
- Immunosuppression (AIDS, sickle cell anaemia, immunoglobulin deficiency, etc.)
- Overcrowded or institutional accommodation (halls of residence)
- Preceding sinusitis or middle ear infection (especially *H. influenza*)
- Travel to high-risk areas (Middle East and Sub-saharan Africa)

Viral meningitis is more common but less severe and is usually caused by enteroviruses (gut originated). Should the virus spread to the brain (meningo-encephalitis), as may occur with herpes simplex (cold sores) and herpes zoster (chicken pox and shingles), the situation is more serious.

General management overview of bacterial meningitis:
- Patients can deteriorate rapidly developing cerebral oedema or septic shock
- Initial systematic management is based on ABCDE, the GCS and NEWS2
- NEWS2: 5 or 6, or 3 in a single category, requires urgent senior review
- NEWS2: 7 or more needs critical care (CCU) Outreach involvement
- GCS less than 12 or a fall of 2 or more—call CCU outreach with a view to transfer/intubation
- Intravenous antibiotics need to be administered in the first hour of admission
- IV ceftriaxone or cefotaxime are the key antibiotics, adding amoxicillin in the over-60s
- If it is safe (i.e., initial urgent CT not indicated) an LP is done in the first hour

- Appropriate diagnostic tests on blood and CSF are critical to a successful recovery
- Urgent IV steroids for suspected bacterial meningitis *unless* the patient is shocked or septic
- The management principles are illustrated by those used in meningococcal meningitis

Meningococcal Meningitis

Meningococcal meningitis is one of the most feared neurological emergencies: it affects children and young adults, it carries a 5% mortality rate and, even with treatment, patients can be moribund within hours of its onset. The AMU will admit one to two cases per month, but many more patients than this will be admitted for investigations, including LP, to exclude the diagnosis.

There are several strains of meningococcal bacteria, Groups A, B, C, W135 and Y cause most cases. In the United Kingdom, groups B and C cause virtually all meningococcal infections, although W135 is increasing and, often complicated by pneumonia and septic arthritis, is particularly severe. In the Middle East and the tropics, group A has been responsible for major outbreaks of meningitis—until vaccination was made compulsory, Hajj pilgrims were particularly susceptible to W135.

Group B, which causes 60%–65% of the cases in the United Kingdom, affects babies and toddlers, while group C causes the remaining 35%–40% and particularly affects young adults around university age. In recent years, the proportion of cases caused by group C (specifically the C2a serotype) has reduced due to the introduction in the United Kingdom of an effective vaccine. Fourteen-year-olds are now offered a combined vaccination against A, B, C, W and Y.

There are important public health implications when a case of meningococcal infection is admitted. It is an infectious disease that can be spread to close contacts, particularly in semi-closed communities such as university halls of residence. Close contacts of isolated cases receive prophylactic antibiotics to eradicate any meningococcal bacteria colonising the oropharynx. In meningitis outbreaks, whole groups may require prophylaxis and, in the case of group C infections, vaccination.

Clinical Picture

Meningococcal bacteria normally live quite naturally in the oropharynx of about 10% of the healthy population. This figure rises to 25% in those living in close proximity, particularly when they are of school and university age. In meningococcal disease, for some unexplained reason, the bacteria become virulent and invade the bloodstream. The result is meningococcal septicaemia and, if the nervous system is also invaded, meningococcal meningitis (Fig. 4.5).

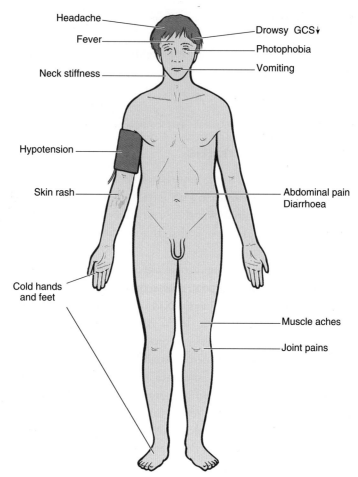

Headache

Fever

Drowsy GCS↓

Photophobia

Neck stiffness

Vomiting

Hypotension

Skin rash

Abdominal pain
Diarrhoea

Cold hands
and feet

Muscle aches

Joint pains

FIGURE 4.5   Clinical features of meningococcal septicaemia.

There are, therefore, two components to meningococcal infections, either of which may dominate the clinical picture:

- Septicaemia alone (mortality 30%) 10% of cases
- Meningitis alone (mortality 5%) 50% of cases
- Mixed features of meningitis and septicaemia 40% of cases

The key features of meningococcal infection are (Box 4.6):

- Headache and fever
- Haemorrhagic rash
- Altered level of consciousness

However, the early symptoms can be non-specific ones of fever, lethargy, abdominal pain, vomiting, joint pains and diarrhoea. The rash is caused by meningococcal infection within the skin and is the major feature of septicaemia, but it can be difficult to recognise at first. It may start off as a red discolouration that blanches on pressure and only later develops into the non-blanching haemorrhagic spots that are so characteristic of meningococcal

---

BOX 4.6 ■ Clinical Features of Meningococcal Infection

Septicaemia
- Influenza-like symptoms
- Vomiting
- Muscle pain
- Drowsiness
- Shock

Meningitis
- Headache
- Fever
- Neck stiffness
- Confusion/coma
- Photophobia
- Vomiting
- Seizures

---

infection. Patients often have an extensive rash and an impaired conscious level during the septicaemic phase, with headache, photophobia and neck stiffness developing with the onset of meningitis. Patients with meningitis alone may not have a rash at all.

Clinical deterioration can be extremely rapid—of patients who die, almost a fifth die at home or on the way to the hospital and, overall, 50% of the deaths occur in the first 48 h. Antibiotics must be given within an hour of the first suspicion of meningococcal infection (and preferably after an LP and blood cultures have been taken)—2 g of IV cefotaxime or 2 g of IV ceftriaxone. Over a few hours, the patient with septicaemia can become confused, tachycardic, peripherally shut down and acutely hypotensive. The respiratory rate increases, the conscious level falls and the patient develops profound shock.

The patient with meningitis can develop acute elevation of the ICP, with deepening coma, fitting, hemiparesis, pupillary signs and a combination of bradycardia and hypertension. The causes of death in meningitis are as follows:

- Septicaemic shock
- Increased ICP

Caring for the Patient With Suspected Meningococcal Meningitis

If a patient is admitted to hospital with suspected meningococcal meningitis, there are a number of immediate critical clinical tasks that must be carried out. There are also a number of important clinical tasks.

IMMEDIATE CRITICAL CLINICAL TASKS IN MENINGOCOCCAL MENINGITIS

- Assess ABCDE
- Give oxygen
- Check vital signs NEWS2
- Secure IV access and careful fluid resuscitation
- Septic shock? Follow surviving sepsis guidelines
  - 500 mL crystalloid IV bolus if septic or a rapidly evolving rash
- Administer *immediate* IV antibiotics (ceftriaxone or cefotaxime)
- Measure GCS: record serial data on a flowchart
- Note any rash
- Discuss isolation for 24 h with control of infection

IMMEDIATE IMPORTANT NURSING TASKS IN MENINGOCOCCAL MENINGITIS

- Detain any relatives for further history and advice on contacts, and ask about recent travel
- Ensure there are no drug allergies
- Blood gases, blood for FBC, renal function, glucose, clotting and lactate
- Ensure immediate specimens are taken for bacteriology
  - Blood cultures
  - EDTA blood sample for urgent PCR (a test to establish the cause of the meningitis)
  - Oral or per nasal posterior pharyngeal wall swab (immediate culture)
- Preparations should be made for an LP, should it be needed to confirm a diagnosis of meningitis. Contraindications to an LP include neurological deterioration such as fits or a GCS of less than 13. LP is also not advisable if the patient is severely shocked or septic or if increased ICP is suspected

---

CLINICAL CARE

The prime aims of clinical management are as follows:

- To support the patient while the antibiotics take effect
- To be vigilant in recognising complications

The patient with meningococcal infection can be mildly unwell, extremely ill with classic features of meningitis (headache, fever and neck stiffness) or ill in extremis with septicaemic shock. Most cases need intensive input during the first few days of admission. Fortunately, most patients respond rapidly to IV antibiotics, high-dose IV steroids (dexamethasone 10 mg qds) and supportive care—volume resuscitation and high-flow oxygen—but in a minority, the course will change rapidly with worsening septicaemia or a progressive increase in ICP. This is why sequential NEWS2 and GCS scores play a critical role in management.

Changes in the observations, particularly in the GCS, the pulse and the blood pressure, are vitally important. If the patient is doing badly, the GCS drops below 13, the pulse increases and the blood pressure falls (shock), or the pulse falls and the blood pressure increases (increased ICP; Box 4.7). These patients need to be moved to an ITU.

Shock needs to be managed with inotropic support (dopamine or adrenaline (epinephrine)), invasive monitoring, and, probably, ventilation. Increased ICP caused by severe meningitis requires interventions to bring the pressure down, including raising the head of the bed by 30 degrees, reducing external stimuli, IV mannitol, corticosteroids and ventilation (see Box 4.7). The role of urgent use of steroids (dexamethasone 0.15 mg/kg qds) for 4 days, starting with the first dose of antibiotics is now clearly recommended in current guidelines (provided the patient is not in septic shock). In common with other patients with septicaemia, there is increasing evidence that good control of the blood sugar during the critical stage improves the outlook.

BOX 4.7 ■ Recognising and Managing Raised Intracranial Pressure

Clinical Features

- Persistent vomiting
- Falling Glasgow coma score
- Falling pulse
- Rising blood pressure
- Unilateral dilated pupil

Management

- Raise the head 30 degrees
- Intravenous mannitol 20% solution 250–500 mL
- Dexamethasone 10 mg IV qds
- Reduce external stimuli, adequate pain relief
- Ventilation to correct oxygen and blow off carbon dioxide
- CT scan and urgent neurosurgical opinion

CRITICAL CLINICAL OBSERVATIONS IN THE FIRST 24 H

The frequency of observations should be modified according to the patient's condition.

CRITICAL CLINICAL OBSERVATIONS IN THE FIRST 24 H IN MENINGOCOCCAL MENINGITIS

- Half-hourly Glasgow coma score (fluctuation or deterioration are bad signs)
- Half-hourly pupillary responses (increased intracranial pressure [ICP])
- Half-hourly pulse, blood pressure, state of extremities (capillary filling) (shock/increased ICP)
- Half-hourly respiratory rate and saturations (shock/pulmonary oedema)
- Hourly urine volumes and strict fluid balance (shock/correcting hypotension)
- Two-hourly temperature (response to antibiotics)
- ECG monitoring (arrhythmias due to septicaemic shock/heart muscle toxicity)
- Progression of any rash (worsening septicaemia)

OVERVIEW: THE SIGNS OF WORSENING MENINGITIS

- Rapidly progressing rash
- Poor peripheral circulation
  - Capillary refill >4 s
  - Systolic blood pressure <90 mm Hg
  - Falling urine output (less than 0.5 mL/kg/h)
- Respiratory rate <8 or >30 breaths/min
- Pulse <40 or >140 beats/min
- Falling (less than 12) or fluctuating (by more than 2) GCS
- Development of a focal limb weakness
- Fitting
- Falling pulse and climbing blood pressure
- pH <7.3, Lactate greater than 4 mmol/L white cell count less than 4.0×10^9
- Poor response to fluid resuscitation

CLINICAL MANAGEMENT APART FROM THE CRITICAL TASKS AND OBSERVATIONS

- Managing a confused, restless or aggressive patient
- Comforting and reassuring a critically ill young patient
- Antiemetic treatment
- Antipyrexia measures: tepid sponging, fan, adequate fluids
- Explaining the various observations and interventions
- Assessing headaches, joint pains, neck stiffness, muscle pain
- Ensuring adequate analgesia is prescribed and given (dihydrocodeine by choice)
- Using appropriate handling manoeuvers to minimise patient's discomfort (e.g., log rolling)
- Minimising external stimuli: light, noise, visitors
- Source isolation of the patient
- Ensuring a fully informed ward handover, including a shared GCS and NEWS2 assessment
- Ensure relevant Public Health officials know about the case; they will be responsible for dealing with contacts
- Appropriate management plan for anticipated complications (e.g., fitting)

Answering Relatives' Questions in Meningitis

The relatives of a young patient with meningococcal infection are understandably among the most distraught that will be encountered in the AMU. The lay perception is that young people are struck down *en masse* at the threshold of their adult life by a 'killer infection' (there are currently around 260 deaths per year from meningococcal meningitis in the United Kingdom). The first task will be to reassure the family that 90% of all cases of meningococcal infection make a complete recovery.

Should we have acted any sooner? The early symptoms of meningitis are notoriously difficult to spot and can be confused with flu or gastroenteritis, even by experienced doctors.

When will we know whether the patient will pull through? Complications, by which we mean shock and worsening of meningitis with increased pressure on the brain, usually occur within the first 48 h. We are aiming to head off complications by giving potent antibiotics to clear the infection before it spreads.

What are the signs of improvement we should expect? The patient will become less drowsy and the observations will stabilise, with a return to normal pulse, breathing rate, and blood pressure.

What are the signs that things are not going so well? Drowsiness will increase and the patient may become more restless and confused. We may have to move the patient to ITU if we think ventilation (life support machine) and other forms of intensive support may be needed to get the patient through the next few days while the antibiotics get to work.

Could there be any permanent brain damage? Permanent damage is unusual but not unknown. The most common damage is hearing disturbance, but this is seen more commonly in children. Most adults make a full recovery. We can do further assessments if necessary, with special tests such as a CT scan at a later stage if we suspect complications.

Are we all at risk now? Yes, there is a 10% risk that close contacts, those who live with the patient and who may perhaps have been kissing their mouth, may develop symptoms of meningitis. The risk is greatest over the next week but remains high for several weeks. We will arrange for you to have urgent antibiotic treatment (usually rifampicin 600 mg 12 hourly for 2 days) to kill any bacteria that may be living at the back of your throat and reduce the risk of you getting meningitis. If you are worried about your symptoms, you must see your doctor urgently.

What about the patient's friends? Household contacts and 'kissing contacts' will be given preventative antibiotics and vaccination. We will need their details.

Should we all be vaccinated? Vaccinations against meningitis are now effective in preventing meningococcal infections. Close domestic contacts (of group C cases) will be offered a vaccine.

What vaccination is available? Vaccination is available for groups A and C and two strains that cause occasional infections in travellers: W135 and Y. The original C vaccination is not suitable for children under 18 months and its protective effect is short lived. The recent introduction of a new group C conjugate vaccine (MenC), which gives long-term protection and is suitable for babies and toddlers, heralds the start of a routine vaccination programme against meningitis in the general population, in contrast to previous vaccinations that were used to protect household contacts and to control outbreaks when there were clusters of group C cases. Meningitis B vaccinations are only given to adults who are at particular risk (e.g., sickle cell anaemia and certain immune deficiencies/immunosuppressant drugs) or during an outbreak.

What about the university/school? If this is a single case, preventative antibiotics are only recommended for close contacts (flatmates, girlfriends/boyfriends, etc.). If the case proves to be part of a cluster (more than one case from the same group or class within 4 weeks), then preventative treatment may have to be given to a wider population. This is a matter for the public health specialists.

Are the nurses and doctors at risk? Nurses and doctors are only at risk if they have performed prolonged mouth-to-mouth resuscitation or have inhaled oral secretions during, say, attempts at intubation.

Acute Severe Headache

Patients are admitted to the AMU with headache because of two primary concerns:
- Is this meningitis?
- Is this a subarachnoid haemorrhage?

The three most common 'benign' causes of acute severe headache are as follows:
- Migraine
- Tonsillitis/pharyngitis with meningism
- Stress headache

However, the stakes are high, and most of us remember at least one case of 'missed subarachnoid' and 'missed meningitis' in our clinical practice. As with most neurological problems, the patient's history is important.

Bacterial meningitis has already been described in detail. Viral meningitis has a similar, although less severe picture and the patients are not usually critically ill unless the inflammation has spread to the brain tissue (encephalitis).

Subarachnoid Haemorrhage

Subarachnoid haemorrhage occurs with the speed of a lightning strike: 'like a brick', 'like a sudden blow', 'like an explosion inside my skull'. It does not build up over an hour or so—it drops the patient in seconds. The headache is extremely severe, peaks at between 1 and 5 min and often spreads to the neck. There may be immediate loss of consciousness followed by immediate recovery or prolonged coma. The patient does not wake up with pain, struggles to work and has to come home to lie in the dark: that is migraine.

There are catches and exceptions: occasionally, patients with a subarachnoid haemorrhage have little warning bleeds in the days leading up to the major event, whereas some patients without a subarachnoid suffer so-called 'thunderclap headaches' that can be as severe as a subarachnoid but are entirely harmless. As a rule, however, a description of the exact onset will be the main way in which a provisional diagnosis is reached, to be confirmed or refuted by a CT scan and LP. Of the true explosive headaches, around one in eight patients will have had a subarachnoid haemorrhage. Interestingly, up to a fifth of all cases of meningitis are initially thought to be a subarachnoid haemorrhage.

THE COMPUTED TOMOGRAPHY AND LUMBAR PUNCTURE IN SUBARACHNOID HAEMORRHAGE

It is critical not to miss a subarachnoid haemorrhage. The 30-day mortality rate is 45%, and most of this is due to re-bleeding. In view of the uncertainty of making a firm clinical diagnosis, a CT scan is always required to confirm a subarachnoid bleed. If the scan is done within 12 h, around 98% of the bleeds will be found and in 2% the scan will look normal. If the CT is delayed by 72 h, only 75% of the bleeds will be found and in 25% the scan will look normal, even though the patient has bled. Thus if there is a suggestive history but a negative scan, the patient will need an LP to look for blood and xanthochromia in the CSF.

Caring for the Patient with Subarachnoid Haemorrhage

The aim of the management is to keep the patient in the best possible condition until the patient can be transferred for neurosurgical assessment. The management principles are the same as those for a conventional stroke or a patient with coma: primary assessment with ABCDE and subsequent clinical care with attention to fluid balance, pressure areas and adequate pain relief. Stool softeners will prevent unwanted straining. Compression stockings and intermittent pneumatic calf compression lower the risk of a DVT. Heart monitoring is required as the shock of a subarachnoid haemorrhage can cause cardiac complications.

Headache and neck stiffness. These symptoms are severe in patients with a subarachnoid and need powerful regular analgesia, conventionally using intramuscular dihydrocodeine and an antiemetic such as cyclizine. Opiates tend to be avoided because of their effects on the pupils but may be required occasionally. Patients will be severely photophobic and will be most comfortable in a quiet, darkened room with a minimum of visitors.

Neurological observations. After a subarachnoid haemorrhage, the main complications and their warning signs include:

- Re-bleeding
  - Further headache
  - Falling GCS
  - Seizures
- Bleeding into the brain tissue (intracerebral haematoma)
  - Falling GCS
  - Development of stroke-like features (unilateral weakness, etc.)
  - Seizures
- Spasms of the cerebral arteries
  - Falling GCS
- Increased ICP
  - Falling pulse, rising blood pressure
  - Falling GCS
  - Pupillary changes

Sequential neurological assessment. GCS and pupillary responses, pulse and blood pressure and general clinical observations will identify the warning signs of complications. Any change in these parameters should be reported so that the overall clinical state can be reassessed with a view to repeat CT scanning and perhaps accelerate a transfer to the neurosurgeons. A fall in the GCS to 8 or less requires an immediate ITU transfer with a view to ventilation.

Answering Relatives' Questions in Subarachnoid Haemorrhage

Where is the bleeding? The blood has escaped from a ruptured artery on the surface of the brain. It has spread around the brain and into the spinal fluid.

Why is the patient unconscious? The bleeding can cause the brain to go into 'shock', which we are hoping will be temporary. We are supporting the breathing at present, but we are hoping there will be signs of recovery within the next 24–48 h.

Will the patient recover? The prospects of recovery depend on the extent of the bleeding and also on two other factors: whether there are spasms of the cerebral arteries and whether there is a second bleed.

Why this patient? The usual cause is an unexplained weakness in the artery wall that suddenly ruptures.

Could the doctor not have seen the warning signs? Occasionally there is a warning bleed, but these are often like migraine attacks. In most patients, there is no warning at all.

Was it all stress? There is no relationship to stress.

What about the well-man clinic visits, blood pressure, etc.? There are no warning signs of a subarachnoid haemorrhage, and it is not directly related to high blood pressure.

Will there be brain damage? That depends on whether there is bleeding into the brain substance itself and also whether the treatment we are using (nimodipine) is successful in preventing spasms of the leaking artery.

Can you operate? If the situation stabilises, we will transfer the patient to the neuro-surgeons, who will assess whether surgery or blocking off the bleeding site with coils is needed to prevent further bleeding. These procedures are preventative and are unlikely to improve the patient's present condition.

Will it happen again? Sometimes there is more than one area of weakness or the weakened spot can itself leak again. About 10% of patients with aneurysms re-bleed within hours and, if untreated, up to 30% re-bleed within a few weeks.

Can the patient drive again? Non-vocational driving can be resumed in due course, providing recovery is complete. There will, however, need to be a certain period before driving can resume. You may need to inform the Driver and Vehicle Licensing Agency and check with your insurance company if you have any doubts.

Can't you just send the patient to a specialist unit straight away and they can operate? The best time to operate is when the patient is in the best possible medical condition but before the peak time for re-bleeding. We are working with the specialist unit and have taken their advice on the best time for a transfer.

Lumbar Puncture

The LP has a justified reputation as an unpleasant and potentially dangerous procedure. The main danger is inadvertently doing an LP when there is an acute increase in the ICP, so that CSF is forced out of the breach in the subarachnoid space. The sudden release of increased CSF pressure sucks the brain in a downward direction and can cause a dramatic deterioration in the neurological state (termed a 'pressure cone').

CONTRAINDICATIONS TO A LUMBAR PUNCTURE

- Suspected increased ICP
- A cerebral mass (abscess, haemorrhagic stroke or tumour)
- Patients in a coma who have not had a CT scan
- Suspected cord compression
- Local sepsis over the proposed LP site
- Abnormal clotting including anticoagulant treatment

INDICATIONS ON THE ACUTE MEDICAL UNIT

- Suspected meningitis and encephalitis
- Suspected subarachnoid haemorrhage (after a negative CT)
- Suspected Guillain–Barré syndrome

Suspected meningitis and encephalitis. Although the LP is important in the diagnosis and management of meningitis, **it should not lead to a delay in giving antibiotics.** Modern techniques identifying the DNA fragments of infecting organisms (polymearse chain reaction [PCR]) give positive results up to 4 days after antibiotics have been given.

In patients who are drowsy or with clinical signs of increased ICP or a possible cerebral abscess, the LP is only performed once a normal CT scan has been obtained.

Suspected subarachnoid haemorrhage. The LP is done to find the few cases of subarachnoid bleeding that the CT has missed. In a suspected subarachnoid bleed with a normal scan, fewer than 1 in 20 LPs will be positive.

Suspected Guillain–Barré syndrome. The CSF is examined to look for the characteristic changes seen in the Guillain–Barré syndrome (a high protein and few or no cells).

PROCEDURE

A full explanation of the reason for doing the LP and a description of what discomfort to expect will help to allay the anxiety of most patients. The very restless and agitated patient may need cautious sedation with IV midazolam (IV flumazenil, which will reverse midazolam immediately, must be on hand in case of oversedation).

The patient should be warned of the following:

- The position
- The cold skin preparation
- The poking around to find the correct entry spot over the back
- The burning of the local anaesthetic
- The pushing sensation in their back
- The possibility of acute shooting pain in either leg
- The possibility of post-LP headache due to a low-pressure CSF leak

The position. It cannot be overstated that the correct positioning of the patient makes the difference between success and failure in performing an LP.

The patient must be lying right on the edge of the bed curled up (comfortably, not forcibly) in the foetal position with the back and both shoulders perpendicular to the mattress. This position is easiest to achieve with a pillow under the head and two pillows between the knees and pushed into the abdomen, across which the patient can rest his upper arm (Fig. 4.6).

The two common mistakes are for the top shoulder to roll over rather than remain vertical and for the spine to be curved rather than straight.

The equipment. The advice is to use a small (22 G) atraumatic (Sprotte) LP needle to reduce the risk of post-LP CSF leak and headache. A CSF leak is less likely if the stylet is reintroduced before the needle is removed. The manometer is used to record the CSF pressure (normally 6–20 cmH$_2$O; if it is above 30 cmH$_2$O there is significantly increased ICP).

In suspected subarachnoid haemorrhage, three sequential bottles are needed (labelled 1, 2, 3) to identify the progressive decrease in blood staining of a traumatic tap. In addition, one specimen is sent for microbiology, one for biochemistry, one for cytology and a fluoride oxalate (yellow label) tube is used for sugar. CSF and simultaneous blood sugar levels are compared. In suspected meningitis, samples are sent for PCR (looking for DNA fragments of *Pnemococcus*, *Haemophillus*, herpes simplex, herpes zoster and

Indications	Contra-indications
• Suspected meningitis	• Suspected raised intracranial pressure
• Suspected subarachnoid	• Coma (GCS < 12)
• Suspected Guillain-Barré	• Cord compression
	• Local sepsis over back

FIGURE 4.6   Positioning for a lumbar puncture. *GCS*, Glasgow coma score.

enteroviruses such as coxsackie—which can all give meningococcal-like illnesses) and for lactate (an indicator of severity). A CSF lactate of >4.0 mmol/L indicates bacterial meningitis and its level is an indicator of severity.

In cases in which subarachnoid bleeding is not an issue, the three sequential bottles may not be used but should always be on hand.

Five drops (1 mL) is sufficient in each bottle in a suspected subarachnoid haemorrhage, whereas the multiple tests in suspected meningitis require around 15 mL.

Analysis of the results is summarised in Table 4.2.

Aftercare. Patients should stay flat on one pillow for 3 to 4h after an LP. Any post-LP headache should be recorded, analgesia will be needed and the patient should be reassured but kept flat until the headache improves.

If the CSF pressure is found to be very high, urgent neurosurgical transfer may be required. In these circumstances, frequent neurological observations (pupils, GCS, pulse and blood pressure) should be started as soon as the LP has been completed. Measures to lower the pressure may be instituted before transfer. In the meantime, any changes in the neurological status must be recorded and reported.

XANTHOCHROMIA: A PRACTICAL GUIDE TO INTERPRETING THE CSF RESULT IN SUBARACHNOID HAEMORRHAGE

- Blood in the CSF from a recent subarachnoid haemorrhage can only be distinguished from a traumatic tap caused by the LP needle by the finding of red/yellow pigmentation in the CSF specimen, due to breakdown within the CSF of the red blood cells which releases bilirubin. This process takes 12h to occur. Bilirubin appears as a yellow tinge (xanthochromia) after the CSF has been spun down in the laboratory. Xanthochromia can be seen with the naked eye or, in more subtle cases, by spectrophotometry. In traumatic bleeding caused by the LP itself, this breakdown does not have time to occur and xanthochromia is absent.

TABLE 4.2 ■ **Diagnosis From Analysis of LP Results**

Condition	CSF	Cell Count (Cells/µL)	Protein (g/L)	CSF Sugar/ Blood Sugar (%)
Normal	Clear	Less than 5 cells	0.2–0.5	>50
Bacterial meningitis	Cloudy	Neutrophils >100	0.5–2.0	<50
Viral meningitis	Clear	Lymphocytes 5–1000	<0.8	>50
Subarachnoid	Bloody	More than 100 red cells	>0.2	>50
Guillain–Barré syndrome	Clear	Fewer than 3 cells	0.5–3.5	>50

CSF, Cerebrospinal fluid; *LP*, lumbar puncture.

- To allow breakdown to occur, 12 h should elapse between the subarachnoid haemorrhage and the LP. Before then, especially within 4 h of a subarachnoid, it may be difficult to differentiate between a bleed and a traumatic tap. (One consequence of this is that the LP does not usually need to be done during the night). If there is no xanthochromia, three sequential CSF specimens from the LP will show a progressive fall-off in the amount of blood if the tap was traumatic. However, this is not as reliable as finding xanthochromia.

- The CSF (at least 1 mL of it) must be spun immediately, otherwise, blood will start to break down in the tube, giving a false positive result; this means that the specimen must be dealt with urgently, day or night. The CSF sample should be protected from the light when transported to the laboratory. LPs are a major intervention and handling of the specimens cannot be left to chance. Careful liaison is needed with the porters and the laboratory staff.

- If the CSF is 'gin-clear' but the history is very suspicious, the specimen should be stored in darkness until it can be checked by the laboratory for xanthochromia using a spectrophotometer.

- Xanthochromia will be found in the CSF at LP, even if it is performed 2 weeks or more after a subarachnoid haemorrhage.

Sudden Loss of Consciousness: Faints and Fits

Sudden loss of consciousness followed by recovery is usually due to a faint (syncope) or a fit (tonic–clonic convulsion). These patients are frequently admitted to the AMU with a variety of labels (Case Study 4.8). Provided that the underlying mechanisms and clinical features of epilepsy and syncope are understood, a correct diagnosis can usually be made without too many investigations, once a good eyewitness account has been obtained.

The history will differentiate fits and faints in 80% of cases. A witnessed account is vital and may have to be obtained by a phone call from the ward if necessary. The paramedic record is particularly important.

Triggers. Syncope will often be triggered by standing upright, pain, strong emotion and heat, particularly in crowded places. Fits do not have specific triggers—they occur anywhere, at any time.

CASE STUDY 4.8   Sudden Collapse: Was This a Fit or a Faint?

A 50-year-old female was admitted with a 'fit'. She had awoken with severe abdominal colic and while being comforted by her husband turned ashen grey, started to sweat profusely, and collapsed on the bed 'as though she had died'. She stopped breathing for a few seconds and then slowly came round over 2–3 min. On close questioning of the husband, there had been no convulsive movements, no confusion after the event, no incontinence and no tongue biting. A similar episode had occurred during a severe attack of calf cramp some years before. The diagnosis was of a vasovagal attack triggered by pain (a simple faint).

Onset. Fits have an aura: often a feeling of anxiety or fear building up in the pit of the stomach. Faints start gradually and share a number of typical warning features: nausea, dimming of the vision, roaring in the ears, sweating and a feeling of heat and a sense of slipping away.

The attack. Generalised tonic–clonic attacks are accompanied by rapid, grunting respirations, foaming at the mouth and self-injury. In syncope, the patient is cold, grey and clammy. There may be isolated convulsive jerkings, but not as the main feature of the attack. In a fit, the loss of consciousness may last for more than 5 min.

Recovery. Recovery is slow after a convulsion, with drowsiness and confusion lasting at least 30 min. This is followed by a headache and generalised limb pains. Syncope recovers in a few minutes with no confusion but is often accompanied by a bout of vomiting. Patients can faint a second time if they sit up or stand up too soon. Self-harm is rare in syncope, in contrast to the tongue biting seen with many convulsions.

The Basic Mechanisms: Syncope

Syncope (fainting) is due to a sudden reduction in the blood supply to the brain. In most cases, provided that the patient is allowed to stay horizontal, there is a full and rapid recovery. Sometimes the blood supply does not return rapidly—typically this is seen if the patient is wedged upright during a faint. As a result, the syncope may progress to an anoxic convulsion (termed *convulsive syncope*).

The reduction in cerebral blood supply has two possible causes:

- A sudden change in heart rate, for example,
  - Heart block
  - Ventricular tachycardia
  - Acute atrial fibrillation
  - Acute coronary syndrome
- A sudden change in blood pressure, for example,
  - Reflex syncope
  - Acute gastrointestinal haemorrhage
  - Acute pulmonary embolus
  - Drug side effect (postural hypotension)

CARDIAC SYNCOPE

Syncope due to heart disease is a medical emergency: it has a poor prognosis if it is not recognised—the next attack may be fatal. A history of sudden death in family members under 40 is an important clue to inherited cardiac abnormalities. In cardiac syncope, unlike reflex syncope, there is either no warning at all or it occurs in a setting of recent onset 'cardiac' symptoms—chest pain, breathlessness and palpitations. Syncope which occurs during exertion strongly suggests a cardiac cause and requires urgent specialist assessment.

A 12-lead ECG with automated interpretation must be done after any syncopal episode. Conduction problems on the 12-lead ECG require urgent referral (abnormal prolongation of the QT interval is usually missed as a cause for serious cardiac arrhythmias and yet the measurement, which should be less than 450 ms, is automatically calculated and printed out on the traces from most modern ECG machines). Further tests of the heart rhythm are vital if a cardiac cause is suspected. These can include bedside monitoring, 24-h tapes (Holter monitor), external event recorders (1–2 weeks) or implanted loop recorders (months) depending on how often the events are occurring.

REFLEX SYNCOPE (ALSO TERMED 'NEURALLY MEDIATED SYNCOPE')

This is increasingly recognised as a cause for both sudden faints and misdiagnosed epilepsy. There are two forms of reflex syncope: *vasovagal syncope* and the *carotid sinus syndrome*. Vasovagal syncope includes the 'classic' faint commonly triggered by the sight of blood, intense pain, and emotion, and the less common form of vasovagal syncope—orthostatic hypotension—in which the pulse or blood pressure drops acutely in an upright individual. This diagnosis is suggested by a fall in the systolic pressure of 20 mm Hg or more within 3 min of standing.

The carotid sinus syndrome is syncope due to pulse or blood pressure changes in response to stimulation of the carotid sinus (an area of the carotid artery) resulting from sudden head movements or pressure from a tightly fitting collar.

Tilt table testing, which examines the effect of posture and sublingual GTN on the pulse and blood pressure, has revolutionised the diagnosis of these various forms of syncope and is an important part of the follow-up of unexplained blackouts and 'drug-resistant' epilepsy (Case Study 4.9).

SITUATIONAL SYNCOPE

This is syncope triggered by a spasm of coughing (cough syncope) or by passing water, usually in men arising in the night from a warm bed to urinate (micturition syncope). These patients can be reassured and given simple preventative advice.

CASE STUDY 4.9 | **Blackouts**

A 75-year-old male was admitted to hospital with blackouts. He had suffered a number of fainting attacks in recent months. His ears would start buzzing and he would blackout 'for a few seconds'. In the past, he had suffered two mild heart attacks and a small stroke. He had had negative tilt table studies when the blackouts had been investigated previously.

On admission, he had fully recovered, but his pulse was 34 beats/min. His ECG showed that the atria and ventricles were beating independently (complete heart block). After settling into bed, he called the nurses suddenly and said he was 'going'. His ECG monitor showed ventricular standstill.

An urgent temporary pacemaker was inserted before his referral for a permanent device.

Postural Orthostatic Tachycardia Syndrome (POTS)

There is increasing recognition of this disabling condition in which an inappropriate increase in the pulse rate (typically 30 bpm or more) within 5 min of standing results in dizziness and syncope. Recently an association with recent COVID-19 infection has been identified.

DRIVING

The regulations for driving after a transient loss of consciousness are complex and there are major implications for the patient and public safety, particularly for vocational drivers. A safe course of action is to advise the patient to obtain medical advice after any form of blackout before recommencing driving.

The Basic Mechanisms: Epileptic Seizures

Two broad types of epilepsy are seen in adults: partial seizures and generalised tonic–clonic convulsions.

PARTIAL SEIZURES

Partial seizures arise from a single electric focus in the brain and produce a localised focal fit during which the patient is usually conscious (Case Study 4.10). There is usually a 'march' of localised twitching, starting from a single area and spreading up a limb or from the face onto the same side of the body. At times the fit can become generalised into a classic tonic–clonic attack.

The clinical picture can be very similar to, and must be distinguished from, those seen in TIAs and in the initial stage of a migraine attack.

GENERALISED CONVULSIONS (TONIC–CLONIC FITTING)

In adults over 25 years, first-time generalised fits usually have an underlying cause— either a structural abnormality such as vascular disease or a brain tumour, or a metabolic cause such as alcoholism or hypoglycaemia (Case Study 4.11).

CASE STUDY 4.10	Partial Seizure in a Female With Diabetes (Not Hypoglycaemia)

A 45-year-old female was admitted following two transient episodes of numbness and tingling of the right side of her face and right arm. There was slight slurring of her speech. Each episode lasted 15 min and cleared completely. She was a patient with insulin-dependent diabetes with good control and had normal blood sugars on admission. A CT scan showed a focal abnormality in the left cerebral hemisphere in the area concerned with movement to the face and arm. At surgery, a large meningioma was found and successfully removed.

CASE STUDY 4.11	Generalised Convulsions

CASE 1: EPILEPSY DUE TO OLD CEREBROVASCULAR DISEASE

A male aged 55 years with a known previous stroke was admitted to hospital, having collapsed at home. The assumption was that this was another stroke. On admission, his GCS was 6. He had bitten his tongue and both plantars were upgoing (suggesting some disturbance to both sides of the brain). He made a full recovery after a period of confusion over the next 24 h but had a witnessed grand mal fit 3 days after admission. The diagnosis was epilepsy triggered by the scar of an old stroke. After a stroke, 10% of patients will have a seizure within the first 5 years.

CASE 2: POST-TRAUMATIC EPILEPSY

A male with a learning disability was admitted after his first generalised convulsion. Three years previously he had suffered a single fit a few days after a blunt head injury with a depressed skull fracture. On admission to hospital, he had a GCS of 13 and had bitten his tongue. A diagnosis of post-traumatic epilepsy was made. He had a further three fits after admission and was started on carbamazepine.

CASE 3: THE IMPORTANCE OF A DRUG HISTORY

A 60-year-old female with residual hemiplegia from a past cerebral haemorrhage was admitted with confusion. Several hours after admission she had a generalised convulsion followed by a series of rapidly recurring convulsions, with no period of recovery between them. She was intubated and ventilated, but continued to fit on weaning despite diazepam, chlormethiazole and phenytoin. Five days after admission, her GP informed us that she had recently discontinued long-term phenobarbitone. A diagnosis of barbiturate withdrawal-induced fits was made.

CASE 4: UNEXPLAINED CONVULSION

A 45-year-old male collapsed at the wheel of his car while driving to the local shops, and collided with a roundabout. He had no memory of the event and was still confused when he was seen in AED. When he was admitted, it was noted he had a fine petechial rash over his upper torso and had bitten his tongue. These changes were consistent with the effects of a major convulsion. There was a past history of ischaemic heart disease and mild angina.

A diagnosis of epilepsy was made. He was also investigated to exclude a cardiac cause, in particular an abnormal heart rhythm, for the collapse.

CASE 5: EPILEPSY DUE TO ALCOHOL?

A 68-year-old female was admitted with a 4-day history of rigours and confusion. There had been a single convulsion immediately before admission. On examination, she had a GCS of 14 and a fever. The suspicion was of heavy alcohol consumption, with fitting precipitated by abrupt alcohol withdrawal. Twenty-four hours after admission, she remained pyrexial and mildly confused. She then had a series of tonic–clonic convulsions. The patient was sedated and investigated by an urgent CT scan and LP. The scan was normal and the CSF showed a protein of 0.8 g/L. Urgent tests on the CSF showed a positive result for the herpes simplex virus, confirming viral encephalitis. She was treated successfully with acyclovir.

Caring for the Patient Who Has Sudden Loss of Consciousness

CLINICAL TASKS

Patients who have regained consciousness:

- Primary assessment ABCDE
- Blood sugar measurement

- Measure the blood pressure lying and either sitting or standing
- 12-Lead ECG and cardiac monitor/telemetry for arrhythmias
- Look for injuries, painful areas, bruising and swelling (document on a chart)
  - Wrists (commonly fractured by falls in the elderly)
  - Ankles
  - Hips
  - Shoulders (can be dislocated during convulsions)
- Look for signs of upper gastrointestinal blood loss
  - Coffee-ground vomit around mouth
  - Melaena (inspect first bowel movement after syncope)
- Look for signs of DVT (pulmonary embolism as a cause of syncope)
- Detain the relatives, telephone witnesses, contact nursing home/GP, etc.
- Obtain a drug history (postural hypotension due to drugs, hypoglycaemics, etc.)

Patients who are fitting (Fig. 4.7):

- Primary assessment: ABCDE
  - With the emphasis on the airway and good venous access (wide bore)
  - Do not insert anything in the mouth
- Ensure the patient cannot injure himself; stay with him, summon help
- Give high-concentration oxygen with a non-rebreathing mask at 15 L/min
- Place the patient in the recovery position, cushion the head, do not restrain
- Carry out blood sugar measurement, bloods for drug levels, toxicology, biochemistry, clotting, etc.
- Initiate anticonvulsant drugs: IV lorazepam 4 mg (buccal midazolam or rectal diazepam if there is no venous access)
- If there is a history of alcohol abuse or impaired nutrition, consider IV thiamine (250 mg) as Pabrinex and/or 50 mL of 50% glucose
- Take a full history, especially concerning drugs and alcohol, from a relative

Patients with status epilepticus. Status epilepticus is defined as fits that last for 5 min or more *and is a medical emergency*. Without treatment, there is a risk of brain damage, hypoxia, shock, other major complications and death. Three groups of patients with pre-existing epilepsy are at particular risk of status epilepticus: those with a severe learning disability (who often have structural brain damage and are on complex therapeutic regimens), those undergoing anticonvulsant withdrawal and those who are not compliant with their treatment.

However, a third of patients with status epilepticus have no previous history of fitting. Occurring de novo status epilepticus can be triggered by stroke, intracranial infection, brain tumour, head injury, hypoxia and metabolic disturbances such as electrolyte abnormalities and alcohol abuse.

The management is the same as for a single fit—resuscitation and preventing harm to the patient. Because intensive drug therapy is required, there is also a risk of drug-induced respiratory depression. Close monitoring is therefore needed, particularly of the

Do cushion the head with hands/forearms if nothing else available

Do administer oxygen via a face mask

Do turn them over into the above position once it is over–it will help them breathe

Do have suction available

Do not move them during the seizure unless in danger

Do not put anything between the teeth

Do not restrict their movement

Do not leave them until fully recovered

FIGURE 4.7　First aid for seizures.

respiratory rate. If alcohol withdrawal or malnutrition is suspected, give high-potency Pabrinex IV with or without 50 mL of 50% glucose.

DRUGS COMMONLY USED IN STATUS EPILEPTICUS
Lorazepam
- *This is now the drug of choice for status epilepticus*

- *4 mg IV to be repeated after 10 min*
- *If there is no response, move to second-line treatment*

Midazolam

- Given buccally as Buccolam 10 mg in a pre-filled syringe
- Only used if no IV access
- Potential of using it intramuscularly

Levetiracetam (Keppra)

- Safe and quick-acting second-line treatment
- Safe in pregnancy
- 20 mg/kg diluted with saline
- Administer over 15 min

Sodium Valproate

- Alternative to phenytoin and levetiracetam as second-line treatment
- Unsafe in pregnancy
- 10 mg/kg diluted with saline
- Administer over 5 min

Phenytoin

- Slow onset, so give with a bolus of midazolam
- Safe in pregnancy
- 1000 mg intravenously (18 mg/kg) over 20 min is a typical dose for an adult
- Must be given with ECG and blood pressure monitoring

Phenobarbital

- Effective, but slow onset, can be combined with phenytoin
- 700 mg (10 mg/kg) over 7 min IV is a typical dose for an adult

COMMON REASONS WHY MANAGEMENT IS UNSUCCESSFUL

- Prescribed drug doses are inadequate (continue full doses of the patient's usual anticonvulsant regimen)
- Initial IV drugs not followed up by maintenance therapy
- Uncorrected hypoxia, acidosis, hypotension
- Missed underlying cause, for example, encephalitis, drug withdrawal
- Complications of status epilepticus, for example, disseminated intravascular coagulation, hyperpyrexia
- Pseudoseizures rather than true convulsions

Sudden Unexplained Death in Epilepsy

Sudden unexplained death in epilepsy (SUDEP) is of increasing concern because it reflects an overall picture of suboptimal epilepsy care and may therefore be avoidable. SUDEP is particularly associated with long-standing, early-onset epilepsy in patients with multiple disabilities who are not under epilepsy specialists and whose drug regimen is disorganised, outdated or both.

Pseudoseizures (Non-Epileptic Seizures)

Pseudoseizures are similar to and can be confused with true tonic–clonic fits. The attacks represent conscious or unconscious manipulative behaviour, simple malingering, or are a manifestation of an underlying psychiatric disorder. Pseudoseizures are commonly misdiagnosed, particularly by inexperienced staff in emergency situations. The diagnosis can be particularly difficult in patients who have a combination of true and pseudo-fits. However, there are several characteristics that help to identify pseudoseizures:

- Pseudoseizures can be of gradual onset with a fluctuating course
- The movements are semi-purposeful and include kicking out
- The head thrashes from side to side; there are often pelvic thrusts
- The posture is often a hyperextended back with the patient lying on his side
- Examination is resisted and the eyes remain tightly screwed up
- Incontinence and tongue biting can occur in pseudoseizures
- Some patients with pseudoseizures just collapse limply to the ground
- Cyanosis occurs only in true tonic–clonic convulsions
- True convulsions last between 50 and 90 s
- Pseudoseizures last between a few seconds and many minutes
- Patients with pseudoseizures can recall the period of unconsciousness

MANAGEMENT

Once pseudoseizures are suspected, anticonvulsant medication should be cautiously tailed down and the patient referred to a neurologist with a special interest in epilepsy. It is not helpful to confront the patient at this stage. A simple explanation that further tests are needed is sufficient, particularly as the diagnosis may not be straightforward.

Non-convulsive status epilepticus

A patient with known epilepsy who fails to recover fully from a series of fits may be suffering from ongoing non-convulsive seizure activity. The features include confusion, personality change and even acute psychosis. The diagnosis is notoriously difficult as it mimics other neuro-behavioural conditions.

Acute Paralysis of the Lower Limbs

Patients who are admitted to hospital with sudden weakness in both legs are a rare but important group, as misdiagnosis can leave the patient paraplegic. For practical purposes, there are two basic conditions that need to be considered:

- Spinal cord disorders
- Guillain–Barré syndrome (ascending polyneuropathy)

SPINAL CORD COMPRESSION

Acute diseases of the spinal cord are compressive (e.g., spinal secondaries or spinal abscess) and need urgent surgery; inflammatory (e.g., multiple sclerosis; Case Study 4.12) and may need specific drug therapy; or vascular (spinal cord stroke; Case Study 4.13). Urgent MRI will differentiate between the three groups.

The key for the AMU is to recognise that a patient who comes in 'off his legs' could well have a progressive neurological problem in both lower limbs. The ward team are well placed to assess lower limb movement, power and sensation when they first expose the patient during the primary assessment. Patients who have acutely weak legs, bladder dysfunction and escalating back pain (characteristically worse on lying flat) need to be taken particularly seriously, for they are the ones with probable cord compression. The site of the problem can often be identified from the site of the back pain and any points of maximum tenderness over the spine. It is important to look at bladder function in such cases, as painless urinary retention may be one of the early warning signs and always needs urgent investigation.

CASE STUDY 4.12	Cord Compression or Multiple Sclerosis

A 30-year-old female awoke with non-specific lumbar pain that progressed over a few hours to involve numbness of both legs and difficulty passing urine. Within 48 h of the onset, she had painless retention and weakness of both legs.

On examination, the legs were weak and she could not stand. Her bladder was palpable, and there was loss of sensation from her upper abdomen down to her feet. An emergency MRI was normal, so the provisional diagnosis was not cord compression but an inflammatory lesion, probably multiple sclerosis.

CASE STUDY 4.13	Diabetic Lady 'Off Her Legs' With a Vascular Cord Lesion

A 65-year-old obese type II diabetic was admitted with acute 'left-sided stroke'. On the consultant's round, it became clear that the weakness involved the extensor muscles of both arms as well as the left leg. She could not stand, and the pattern of the change in her reflexes suggested a high cord lesion. An urgent MRI scan showed a vascular lesion (acute spinal cord ischaemia) in the midcervical cord. She remained immobile and was referred for rehabilitation.

Malignant spinal cord compression: escalating back pain in a patient with cancer must be taken seriously, particularly if it is described as 'band-like' or 'constricting'. Pain is the red flag symptom in malignant cord compression–the next stage is paralysis so immediate action (high-dose dexamethasone and an MRI of the whole spine) is required.

GUILLAIN–BARRÉ SYNDROME

The Guillain–Barré syndrome is an ascending paralysis that starts in the feet and moves progressively up the body, to the extent that the respiratory muscles are often involved. The disease can progress rapidly over a matter of hours and put the patient's breathing at risk.

Respiratory monitoring is particularly important in Guillain–Barré syndrome. Impending critical respiratory muscle involvement is suggested by breathlessness and an inability to cough and perhaps swallow effectively. The best way to monitor for deterioration is to take serial forced vital capacity (FVC) measurements with a spirometer (the peak flow rate is not a useful test in this particular situation). As a general rule, once the FVC decreases to 1 L the patient needs ventilation, although a downward trend on hourly readings should prompt a transfer to an high-dependancy unit or ITU.

Recognising Acute Illness in Patients With Chronic Neurological Disability

Acute medical illnesses in the presence of chronic neurological disability can be difficult to diagnose. Cognitive impairment and aphasia can impair history taking, it is therefore vital to interview family and professional carers. Frequently acute illness presents not with classic symptoms, but with a sudden worsening of the underlying neurological condition. This takes the form of a sudden reduction in functional ability, increased spasticity and muscle spasms, sudden cognitive changes, and acute agitation/confusion. The source of the sudden change ranges from a urinary tract infection to infected bedsores or even to the sudden withdrawal of medication. The classic case of the neurological condition masking an acute illness occurs in chronic paraplegia in which an intra-abdominal catastrophe (e.g., perforated ulcer) presents with sympathetic over-activity: headache, sweating, high blood pressure and vomiting. The abdomen, however, remains soft and non-tender.

COVID-19 AND THE NERVOUS SYSTEM

SARS-CoV-2 readily infects the brain, probably via the nervous pathway responsible for the sense of smell. Once there the virus, as it does elsewhere, can directly damage and clot off small blood vessels and trigger intense, unwanted inflammation. In a proportion of patients, around 10%, this leads to neurological complications. Headache, 'brain fog' and delirium are the commonest neurological problems but in the more severe COVID-19 cases, there is a significant risk of stroke, generalised encephalitis (coma and convulsions) and psychiatric syndromes, notably acute psychosis. Risk factors are predictable—COVID-19 severity, age, co-morbidities and pre-existing cognitive dysfunction. The clinical challenge is to recognise a specific neurological problem among the various other manifestations of COVID-19—hypoxia, confusion, shock and multi-organ failure.

Further Reading

Coma

Addison, C., Crawford, B., 1999. Not bad, just misunderstood— Glasgow coma scale. Nursing Times 95 (43), 52–53.

Shah, S., 1999. Neurological assessment. Nursing Standard 13 (22), 49–56.

Stroke

National Clinical Guidelines for Stroke, 2023. Up-date. Royal College of Physicians, London. www.strokeguideline.org.

Meningitis

Mc Gill, F., et al., 2016. The UK joint specialist societies guideline on the diagnosis and management of acute meningitis and meningococcal sepsis in immunocompetent adults. Journal of Infection 72, 405–438.

Epilepsy

NICE, 2022. Epilepsies in children, young people and adults. NICE guideline [NG217]. NICE. org.uk/guidance/ng217.

NICE, 2010. Transient loss of consciousness ('blackouts') in over 16s. NICE clinical guideline. NICE.org.uk/guidance/cg109.

Chronic Neurological Disability

Bakheit, A.M.O., 2006. Recognition of acute illness in people with chronic neurological disability. Postgraduate Medical Journal 82, 267–269.

Websites

Guidelines for managing meningitis in adults. www.meningitis.org.

NICE, 2008. Metastatic spinal cord compression. https://www.nice.org.uk/Guidance/CG95.

Gastroenterology

Introduction

It is common for patients in the acute medical unit (AMU) to have gastrointestinal (GI) symptoms either as their presenting complaint or complicating another medical condition. The common medical gastroenterological emergencies are upper GI bleeding—haematemesis and melaena—and acute infective diarrhoea. The issues in GI bleeding are those of adequate resuscitation and the problems caused by re-bleeding; those in acute diarrhoea are of distinguishing simple viral gastroenteritis from bacterial diarrhoea and its associated complications. Unfortunately, both groups of emergencies are still mismanaged and associated with an unacceptable mortality rate. Owing to the overwhelming influence of alcohol abuse on the pattern of acute medical admissions, there will also be a significant number of emergencies in which liver disease is the dominant problem. These admissions pose a major nursing and medical challenge, with issues concerned with fluid balance and transfusion in the sick, bleeding patient who may be confused, septic and in impending liver failure.

Other medical conditions also present with GI symptoms. In our unit, we have recently seen two young patients presenting with acute abdominal pain, one with diabetic ketoacidosis (DKA) and the other with meningococcal meningitis. Acute myocardial infarction, basal pneumonia and pulmonary embolus are all known to masquerade as an acute abdomen from time to time. More commonplace is the problem of nausea and vomiting—common diagnostic dilemmas in themselves, but also occurring as accompanying symptoms in diseases as diverse as cerebral haemorrhage and septicaemia.

The AMU Clinical Team must be familiar with the causes and clinical course of the common acute GI emergencies, particularly with the complications that can occur in the first 24 h and which often determine whether the patient will recover. Clinicians must also have a working knowledge of the common GI symptoms that they will encounter—what will be the likely cause and what will be the best form of management?

Nausea and Vomiting: Underlying Mechanisms

Nausea is one of the most distressing acute symptoms, but it is easy to relieve, provided that:

- The underlying mechanism is understood.
- The cause is identified and corrected.
- The appropriate drugs are used.

Vomiting is a common but potentially serious problem:

- It can occur in response to a minor illness, but it can indicate serious disease.
- It can itself lead to metabolic problems.

The Patient Who Is Vomiting: The General Approach

CONSIDER THE UNDERLYING MECHANISMS AND POTENTIAL CAUSES

Severe pain, particularly when associated with anxiety, causes nausea through a direct effect on the cerebral cortex. Chemical toxins, notably, opiate drugs, ketones and urea, act through chemoreceptors in the brainstem, the area of the brain that can also be affected by increased intracranial pressure and posterior circulation stroke, both of which can present with nausea and vomiting (Fig. 5.1).

Local GI causes include acute gastritis and gastroenteritis (especially staphylococcal food poisoning), liver inflammation, acute pancreatitis and cholecystitis.

ESTABLISH THE HISTORY

- When and how did it start?
- Did it occur in the setting of another illness?
- Is there pain anywhere?
- What other symptoms are present (e.g., headache, giddiness, abdominal pain)?
- Has it happened before?
- Has anyone else got the same symptoms?
- Date of the last menstrual period

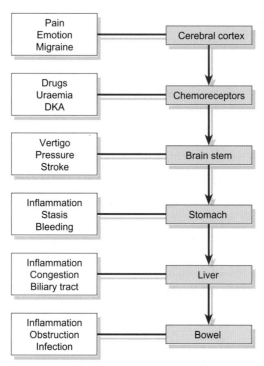

FIGURE 5.1 Underlying mechanisms and causes of nausea and vomiting. *DKA*, Diabetic ketoacidosis.

IS THIS GASTROINTESTINAL DISEASE?

- Is there any diarrhoea?
- Is there or has there been any abdominal pain? (Try to identify abdominal pain other than that due to the mechanical effects of retching.) Vomiting is a common feature of cholecystitis and pancreatitis.
- Are there any features of obstruction? (Absolute constipation, cramps, abdominal distension and a tender lump in the groin may be a strangulated hernia.)
- Is the cause acute liver damage? (Hepatitis or paracetamol overdose.)
- Is there an alcohol use disorder?
- Is there anorexia and weight loss? (Suggesting advanced malignant disease.)

IS THIS DRUG RELATED?

- What drugs have been started or increased in recent days?
- Is this digoxin toxicity/opiate side effect?
- Is there chronic cannabis use disorder? (Typically severe chronic vomiting relieved by hot baths.)

COULD THIS BE RAISED INTRACRANIAL PRESSURE?

- What is the accompanying clinical setting?
  - Headache? (Meningitis/subarachnoid haemorrhage)
  - Malignant disease? (Cerebral secondaries)
  - Altered conscious level (Cerebral mass/encephalitis, etc.)
  - Disturbed vision and balance? (Brainstem tumour or stroke)

COULD THIS BE METABOLIC?

- Is there renal failure?
- Are the sodium and calcium levels normal?
- Could this be ketoacidosis? (The patient may be diabetic.)
- Acute adrenal insufficiency—low blood pressure, low sodium (easily treated, fatal if missed).

Nausea and Vomiting in Acute Medical Conditions

MIGRAINE

Migraine is commonly accompanied by vomiting. Other more worrying causes of headache—meningitis, increased intracranial pressure and subarachnoid haemorrhage—are also associated with vomiting, so the symptom itself is of little diagnostic help in this setting. In these situations, other features such as a skin rash or stroke-like symptoms help to clarify the underlying diagnosis.

MYOCARDIAL INFARCTION

Vomiting is an important feature that distinguishes the pain of myocardial infarction from that of angina and is often accompanied by nausea and sweating. In the elderly patient, vomiting may be the only symptom of a myocardial infarction.

SEPSIS

Vomiting can be the only symptom of hidden infection, even of frank septicaemia, particularly in the elderly or immunocompromised patient. This is particularly the case in infections in the kidneys and lower urinary tract.

ACUTE GASTRIC DILATATION

Acute gastric dilatation is important because it is an easily preventable cause of sudden death. In this condition, gross gastric distension leads to upper abdominal swelling associated with nausea, often accompanied by hiccups and belching. These patients are often already unwell and a common outcome is sudden vomiting, aspiration and cardio-respiratory arrest. Factors that can trigger acute gastric dilatation include electrolyte disturbance, bacterial toxins and, most commonly, DKA. Treatment is simple—anticipate the possibility (in DKA, in severe infection and in any critically ill patient), recognise the condition and prevent aspiration by decompressing the stomach with a nasogastric tube.

Acute Upper Gastrointestinal Haemorrhage

Acute upper GI bleeding is a common cause of acute admission. In a catchment population of 200,000, around 300 acute GI bleeds will be admitted per year. Some will be trivial (a young male who has light blood streaking after repeated vomiting the 'morning after') and can be discharged home very quickly. The majority will be of moderate severity, can undergo endoscopy on the next available list and will stop bleeding of their own accord. A minority, however, will be life threatening and complex: a truly multidisciplinary approach will be needed, involving gastroenterologists, radiologists, surgeons and several members of the ward clinical team.

At the centre, in the severe cases, is the ward clinician. It is they who will be the first to assess the initial blood loss, who will personally witness any re-bleeding and who will be on the ward at critical times—when the patient returns from endoscopy, when the consultant surgeon arrives seeking an urgent update and in the early hours when the observations deteriorate. Also caught up in the frenetic activity will be a critically ill patient who, possibly in a confused and agitated state, may be frightened and uncertain about what is going on. The clinician's role is as follows:

- To ensure the immediate safety of the patient
- To assess the degree of initial blood loss
- To collect information for assessing the risk to the patient of the bleed
- To identify the earliest signs of re-bleeding
- To coordinate the management of fluid replacement, transfusions and fluid balance
- To reassure the patient and ensure that there is appropriate symptomatic relief

There are some critical issues in the presentation and management of GI bleeding on the AMU:

- Early diagnosis and adequate resuscitation are the keys to successful management.
- Patients with significant haemodynamic disturbance or who need transfusion will need urgent endoscopy.
- Patients who do badly are older, lose a larger quantity of blood and either continue to bleed or stop and then bleed again.
- There is an overall mortality rate of 8%–10%, which has not improved in recent years.
- The mortality risk is almost entirely confined to patients over 60 years and with significant co-morbidity.
- Close surgical involvement is critical in a large haemorrhage and particularly where there is re-bleeding.

Causes of Acute Bleeding

The success of the management of acute GI bleeding lies in making an early diagnosis of its likely source. Unfortunately, there are several potential bleeding sites: from the oesophagus to the duodenum in patients with haematemesis and from the oesophagus to the beginning of the colon in patients with melaena. The cause of the bleeding determines the outlook: some types (e.g., gastric erosions) will always stop bleeding on their own; some will often need intervention (e.g., varices) (Fig. 5.2). Once the initial bleed has settled, some lesions will have resolved completely (e.g., Mallory–Weiss tear), whereas others have a high risk of re-bleeding (e.g., arterial bleeds from a peptic ulcer). Diagnosis rests on knowing the likely source, bearing in mind the patient's age (Box 5.1) and history and, most importantly, the findings at early endoscopy—which ideally means within the first 24 h of admission.

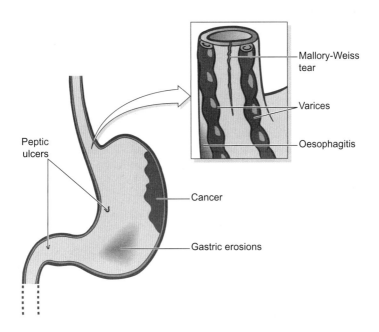

FIGURE 5.2 Common causes of upper gastrointestinal bleeding.

BOX 5.1 ■ Age and the Common Causes of Upper Gastrointestinal Bleeding	
Young	**Old**
Mallory–Weiss tear - - - - - - - - Varices - - - - - - - - - -	Gastric/oesophageal cancer
Duodenal ulcer	Gastric ulcer
Acute gastritis	Oesophageal ulcer
Acute duodenitis	Oesophagitis

PEPTIC ULCER DISEASE (25%)

Duodenal and gastric ulcers are the causes in a quarter of all cases of acute upper GI bleeding. Most ulcers (8 out of 10) stop bleeding of their own accord; the remainder need intervention at endoscopy (injection of the ulcer base with adrenaline (epinephrine) and coagulation with a heat probe or laser/clipping), in the radiology department (embolisation) or possibly by surgery. After a bleed, patients require a 3-week ulcer-healing course of lansoprazole or omeprazole followed, if the patient has to restart on non-steroidal anti-inflammatory drugs (NSAIDS) or aspirin, by maintenance therapy.

HELICOBACTER PYLORI INFECTION AND BLEEDING PEPTIC ULCERS

About 60%–70% of all gastric ulcers and 80% or more of all duodenal ulcers are caused by *H. pylori* infection within the stomach (most of the remainder are associated with the use of NSAIDs). Eradication of the infection speeds ulcer healing and, of importance to the AMU, if the ulcer has bled, eradication lessens the risk of re-bleeding. Eradication therapy is simple—a week of ampicillin, omeprazole and clarithromycin—and should be started once the patient returns from endoscopy if the patient has a duodenal ulcer and tests on the endoscopic specimens are *H. pylori* positive. This aspect of management is frequently neglected. The situation with bleeding gastric ulcers is more controversial and in most cases, re-endoscopy is advisable 6 weeks after the initial bleed, at which time tests for *H. pylori* can be performed and eradication therapy given if necessary.

ACUTE OESOPHAGITIS, GASTRITIS, DUODENITIS AND ACUTE EROSIONS ('STRESS ULCERS') 40%

Acute gastric and duodenal erosions are common in patients taking NSAIDs and aspirin. Although they can cause massive blood loss, the bleeding will stop provided the patient survives the initial event. The two major issues are adequate resuscitation and ensuring that the blood loss is not arising from a more serious source such as a chronic ulcer or varices.

MALLORY–WEISS TEAR 3%

Acute oesophageal mucosal tears can be diagnosed from the history: patients retch and vomit several times before noticing that one of their vomits contains a varying amount of fresh blood. The patients are usually young and acute alcohol intake is often involved. The bleeding can be heavy and the patients can be very alarmed. The outlook is almost universally excellent, with the bleeding stopping of its own accord and the tear healing completely within 24 h.

GASTRO-OESOPHAGEAL VARICES 8%

In practical terms, acute upper GI haemorrhage is split into two categories: non-variceal and variceal bleeding—their outlook and management are entirely different. Blood loss from variceal bleeding can be massive and can itself result in death, but more commonly it triggers acute liver failure—in patients whose livers are already performing badly. Varices need active intervention to stop the bleeding and to reduce the risk of a re-bleed. Overall death rates are high, up to 30%. Fortunately, there have been important improvements in the field using endoscopic (variceal band ligation) and radiologic (transjugular intrahepatic portosystemic anastomosis) techniques. It is to the general relief of many that the Sengstaken tube is now making progressively fewer appearances in the medical ward.

GASTRIC AND OESOPHAGEAL CANCERS 3%

Gastric and oesophageal cancers occur in older patients, and the bleeding is often preceded by a history of weight loss, anorexia and, in the case of oesophageal cancer, a swallowing difficulty.

DIEULAFOY EROSION 2%

This rare cause of massive bleeding is due to erosion of a congenitally abnormal artery in the lining of the stomach. Emergency surgery is often required.

Management of Upper Gastrointestinal Haemorrhage

ENSURING THE SAFETY OF THE PATIENT: ABCDE

Patients with major GI bleeding need instant assessment and urgent resuscitation.

The conscious level may be impaired, either as part of shock (poor cerebral blood supply) or because the bleeding has occurred in a patient with liver disease and has triggered liver failure. However, unless the bleeding has taken place, say, as a stress reaction to an acute stroke, the airway is unlikely to be at risk.

Administer high-flow oxygen immediately if the patient is hypotensive or has a pulse over 100 beats/min—on the assumption there has been a major bleed. Monitor the oxygen saturations to assess the response.

Check the patient for any pain: severe abdominal pain is unusual in upper GI bleeding and needs urgent medical assessment. In the elderly, blood loss can readily trigger an anginal attack or even cause myocardial infarction.

Anticipate that large-bore IV cannulae will be inserted into both arms and that either immediate saline or polygeline (Haemaccel) may be needed. As in all acutely ill patients, the patient's condition and the response to deterioration are based on the use of National Early Warning Score 2 (NEWS2).

If there is haemodynamic disturbance (e.g., pulse 110 beats/min, systolic blood pressure (SBP) 100 mm Hg, respiratory rate 30 breaths/min), it would be appropriate to give 500 mL of isotonic saline rapidly (over less than 15 min) and then, if there is no improvement, consider polygeline (Haemaccel), as at least 20% of the blood volume will have been lost. Patients who are actively bleeding and have abnormal clotting may need it corrected with fresh frozen plasma (FFP), prothrombin complex concentrate or, if indicated, (platelets under 50,000) a platelet transfusion.

WHO NEEDS URGENT ENDOSCOPY?

At presentation, before endoscopy, all patients are assessed with the Glasgow-Blatchford Score which predicts the need for transfusion, endoscopic intervention and death. The score is derived from the pulse, systolic blood pressure, clinical features, basic blood tests and a history of liver or heart disease.

Patients with minor GI bleeding with no change in pulse or blood pressure (and a low Glasgow-Blatchford Score) can be safely discharged and do not require endoscopy. Most other patients with GI bleeding can safely be endoscoped on the next available endoscopy list, which should be within 24h of admission. Indeed, the risks of emergency endoscopy in an inadequately resuscitated patient in the middle of the night can outweigh the potential advantages. However, urgent endoscopy (within an hour post-resuscitation) to establish the site of blood loss, assess the risk of re-bleeding and attempt endoscopic haemostasis is required:

- When gastro-oesophageal varices are suspected
- After severe bleeding
- In the high-risk elderly
- When the problem is a re-bleed
- With a high pre-endoscopy Glasgow-Blatchford Score

ASSESSING THE DEGREE OF BLEEDING

The history is invaluable in assessing blood loss:

- Haematemesis with melaena indicates greater bleeding than either alone.
- Clots in the vomit and recognisable blood in the stool both indicate heavy bleeding.
- Bleeding accompanied by syncope is an ominous sign.
- Postural dizziness and overwhelming thirst suggest a major bleed.

The examination adds supporting evidence to the history. However, the patient's age will influence the signs—a young person can lose 500 mL or more of blood before any of the observations change, but a similar loss in an elderly person would have a major impact. The patient with major bleeding characteristically:

- Is pale and clammy
- Has a tachycardia of more than 100 beats/min

- Has an SBP of less than 100 mm Hg
- Shows postural hypotension, with a 20+ mm Hg fall in the systolic pressure on sitting

ASSESSING THE RISK TO THE PATIENT FROM THE BLEED

Age—is the patient over 60 years of age? The mortality rate for upper GI bleeding is 20 times higher in the elderly than in the young (Case Study 5.1):

- The underlying causes are more serious (e.g., gastric ulcers and gastric cancer).
- Ageing arteries do not stop bleeding so readily.
- Pre-existing heart disease may complicate the effects of acute blood loss.
- The patients are more likely to be on anticlotting drugs.

Amount—small, moderate or large? The initial assessment of pulse and blood pressure and direct observation should be interpreted in combination with the results from the endoscopy. Clearly, the finding of 'a spurting arterial bleed from the base of a chronic gastric ulcer' is much more significant than 'no visible blood in the stomach or duodenum.'

Is there another complicating condition present? The three most important diseases that will influence the chances of recovery are:

- Liver failure (abnormal clotting, varices, encephalopathy)
- Kidney failure (worsened by acute blood loss and reduced renal blood flow)
- Heart failure (impairs the corrective responses to blood loss, increases the risks of transfusion)

CASE STUDY 5.1	Death due to Re-bleeding in a High-Risk Patient

An 84-year-old independent male presented with two syncopal episodes followed by a large vomit of recognisable blood. He had a 1-week history of upper abdominal pain and was taking regular low-dose aspirin. There was a past history of chronic angina and Type II diabetes.

On admission, the patient was pale, alert and orientated with blood visible around the mouth. The pulse was 80 beats/min and the blood pressure 135/65 mm Hg lying and 80/35 mm Hg sitting. There was mild epigastric tenderness and rectal examination revealed soft brown stool. His Hb was 105 g/L and urea 15 mmol/L.

The initial assessment was of an acute upper GI bleed in an elderly male with ischaemic heart disease and a high Glasgow-Blatchford Score, putting him in a high-risk category. Five hundred millilitres of saline was given over 10 min.

While awaiting the first of six units of blood that were ordered, the surgeons were contacted and agreed to visit 'if there was a second bleed.' A central line was inserted.

Three hours after admission the patient vomited 500 mL of fresh blood. Emergency endoscopy showed a 1.5-cm-deep gastric ulcer. This ulcer was not actively bleeding and was injected with adrenaline (epinephrine). Twenty-four hours later the patient appeared to be stable, having had a total of 5 units of blood. A second endoscopy was ordered by the surgeons and showed a 'spurting vessel'; this was reinjected. After this, the patient's condition remained stable. Surgery was planned in the event of further bleeding.

Six days after admission the patient had a sudden massive bleed and suffered a cardiac arrest. The patient aspirated blood into the lungs. Resuscitation was unsuccessful and the patient died.

Is there an underlying malignancy? This may be the direct source of the bleeding, or the bleeding may be from stress ulceration caused indirectly by a malignancy elsewhere. Upper GI bleeding is quite a common problem in terminal malignant disease.

RISK ASSESSMENT WITH THE GLASGOW-BLATCHFORD AND FULL ROCKALL SCORES

All patients with an acute upper GI bleed must have a formal risk assessment before (Glasgow-Blatchford Score) and after (Full Rockall Score) endoscopy. Both scores reflect the size of the bleed and the presence of shock, significant co-morbidity and, in the case of the Rockall Score, endoscopic findings. The Glasgow-Blatchford Score identifies low-risk cases (scores 0 and 1) who can be discharged immediately without endoscopy. High scores indicate that intervention is likely and that there is a risk of re-bleeding and death. The post-endoscopy Full Rockall Score is an important measure of severity and the risks of re-bleeding and death (Table 5.1).

A Full Rockall score of <3 indicates a low risk of re-bleeding or death, and these patients can be considered for accelerated discharge. In contrast, a score of 7 carries a 25% chance of death within 30 days of the bleed.

LOOKING FOR EVIDENCE OF RE-BLEEDING

Patients who stop bleeding initially and then re-bleed are at special risk. They will need further endoscopic intervention and if unsuccessful, radiologic intervention (embolisation) and possibly surgery. The initial endoscopy report should contain an explicit management plan to be followed in the event of a re-bleed.

TABLE 5.1 ■ Risk Assessment with the Rockall Score

	Score 0	1	2	3
Age	≤60	60 to 79	80+	
Shock	Pulse<100 SBP>100	Pulse>100 SBP>100	SBP<100	
Co-morbidity	Nil		CCF, IHD, other major conditions	Renal failure, liver failure, metastases
Diagnosis	Mallory–Weiss	All other	GI cancer	
Endoscopic signs of bleeding	No bleeding		Fresh blood, clot, spurting	

CCF, Congestive cardiac failure; *GI*, gastrointestinal; *IHD*, ischaemic heart disease; *SBP*, systolic blood pressure.

There are several endoscopic features that predict a high risk of re-bleeding:

- Active arterial bleeding (24% risk)
- A vessel visible at the base of an ulcer (20% risk)
- An adherent clot over an ulcer crater (20% risk)

Features that indicate re-bleeding are fresh haematemesis or melaena associated with disturbed haemodynamics—a pulse rate over 100 beats/min, a systolic pressure less than 100 mm Hg, a fall in central venous pressure (CVP) more than 5 cmH$_2$O or a fall in haemoglobin of more than 2 g in 24 h. Depending on the underlying diagnosis, patients who re-bleed will need further endoscopic procedures and, if these are unsuccessful, a second re-bleed will almost certainly lead to emergency surgery. Reliable, well-charted observations are critical in the close monitoring of these patients during the first 48 h of their admission. The pulse rate is the single most useful measurement, as it is the first to change if the patient re-bleeds (or remains high if bleeding does not stop in the first place). The drop in blood pressure lags behind the increase in pulse rate, although a postural decrease also provides a useful early warning. Half-hourly NEWS2 observations are needed in the first 4 h after an acute bleed.

In major bleeds, the CVP provides the most reliable guide to re-bleeding because it falls before there is any increase in the pulse rate. It is invaluable in the elderly in whom the risks are high and other factors such as β-blocker therapy and cardiac arrhythmias render the pulse rate unreliable as a sign of blood loss (Case Study 5.2).

The patient described in Case Study 5.1 is typical of the type of patient who is commonly admitted to the acute medical wards. He was at high risk because of:

- Age
- Existing health
- Blood loss degree
- Source of the bleeding
- Early re-bleeding

Many personnel were involved, and the patient needed extremely close monitoring. Characteristically, there was uncertainty over the indications and timing of surgery—in circumstances in which a clear management plan from the outset is a fundamental requirement. An early, combined and well-documented consultation between the

---

| CASE STUDY 5.2 | Re-bleeding in the Early Hours? |

An 87-year-old female was admitted with haematemesis and melaena. Endoscopy showed oesophagitis, pyloric stenosis and a bleeding duodenal ulcer, which was injected, with apparent success. At 1:00 a.m., her pulse suddenly increased from 100 to 140 beats/min and her blood pressure fell acutely. There were no external signs of further bleeding. Her electrocardiogram (ECG) showed rapid atrial fibrillation at 140 beats/min. She remained hypotensive for half an hour before she reverted spontaneously to a normal rhythm, when her pulse and blood pressure also normalised. She did not re-bleed after admission and made a good recovery. Any acute illness in the elderly can trigger rapid atrial fibrillation, which in itself can lead to a sudden, but reversible, deterioration in the patient's condition.

physicians, surgeons and ward team is invaluable in cases such as this, in which the risks of major complications can be anticipated from the moment the patient is first seen.

While difficult management decisions are being considered, it is also critical that the ward team are focused on the immediate condition of the patient:

- Quarter-hourly observations may be necessary during the first few hours after a massive bleed to determine whether the bleeding has stopped. These can be rein-stated at the first sign of re-bleeding (e.g., a fall in a previously stable CVP or a large fresh melaena stool).
- Reassuring signs are a decrease in the pulse rate and a reduction in any postural hypotension.
- The respiratory rate is raised in shock, but will also increase if the patient develops pulmonary oedema due to over-transfusion—this is a particular risk in an elderly patient with pre-existing heart disease who has needed vigorous resuscitation with fluids and blood. Current recommendations are for a conservative transfu-sion policy aiming for an Hb of 70 to 100 g/L—possibly higher if there is cardiac co-morbidity.

Intensive monitoring and urgent investigative procedures are likely to lead to disori-entation and distress in these elderly patients. Constant reassurance is needed, combined with careful explanations of the various interventions and staff that the patient is suddenly encountering. It will be a great comfort to the patient to be able to identify at least one familiar face among the frenetic activity of the first 12 to 24 h. Patients with significant blood loss are extremely weak and debilitated. If there is frequent melaena, the effort of calling for, and using, a commode at short notice will be exhausting (and often extremely embarrassing) for the patient. Ward staff have to be readily available to assist the patient and to deal with the distress of melaena or haematemesis with sensitivity and professionalism.

INTRAVENOUS PANTOPRAZOLE/OMEPRAZOLE

High-dose IV proton pump inhibitors (PPIs) pantoprazole/omeprazole 80 mg stat and 8 mg/h for 72 h are used in patients who have had non-variceal bleeding and have endo-scopic evidence of recent bleeding which has required active intervention. Treatment is started after the patient has returned from endoscopy and reduces transfusion require-ments, hospital stay and the risk of re-bleeding.

ROLE OF THE CLINICAL TEAM IN FACILITATING COMMUNICATION

Case Study 5.3 illustrates how poor communication can affect a patient's treatment. This was a very high-risk case due to the bleeding source, the age of the patient and the pre-existing health of the patient. There was good early liaison with the surgeons, but the problems arose because of the quality of the communication. An issue as simple as the

CASE STUDY 5.3 Unusual Cause of Bleeding Hindered by Problems with Communication

A 71-year-old female was admitted with major upper GI bleeding: there were large fresh clots in her vomit bowl and dark red blood mixed in with melaena. A week before admission an exercise test had been aborted because of early ischaemic changes on her ECG. She had also suffered a myocardial infarction 6 months previously. Emergency endoscopy revealed a typical Dieulafoy anomaly with a visible arterial bleed, high in the lesser curve.

After unsuccessful attempts at endoscopic injection and embolisation, she was taken as an emergency to the operating theatre. There was no direct communication between the senior surgeon and the endoscopist; much of the information transfer was either through a third party or from the endoscopy form, which itself was filled out ambiguously. Furthermore, the first operation, a partial gastrectomy, was performed under adverse conditions with the patient actively bleeding and hypotensive. The lesion was not included in the resected gastric tissue. She continued to bleed after surgery and so further surgery with a total gastrectomy was performed. She made an uneventful recovery after this.

orientation of an endoscope photograph had serious consequences and underlines the enormous value of effective communication. In this case, it would have been invaluable to have had a senior member of the surgical team present at the endoscopy.

The ward team are in an ideal position to facilitate the liaison between surgeons and physicians.

- Are the observations and transfusion charts clearly documented and displayed so that the surgeons can judge whether the patient is still bleeding or is re-bleeding?
- Is the most recent bowel action/vomit available to be seen and documented in the clinical notes?
- Are the most up-to-date blood results available (especially the blood count and clotting studies)? Ideally, they should be displayed on a flow chart.
- Is there an informed member of the medical team (e.g., the endoscopist or the registrar) available on the ward?
- Are the case notes available and, most importantly, is the endoscopy record available? Is there a re-bleed management plan?
- Does the patient understand why a surgeon has been involved?
- Has an ECG been performed and seen by the medical team?

Excellent Care for Acute Upper Gastrointestinal Bleeding

- Following an established management protocol based on national guidelines
- Intensive clinical input during the initial period of instability
- Clear guidelines for the changes in observations to be reported to medical staff
- Combined medical and surgical input in high-risk patients
- Use of central venous lines in high-risk patients
- Good liaison with the gastroenterology team
- Access to early endoscopy and endoscopic haemostatic techniques
- Appropriate monitoring, including clotting studies in all high-risk patients
- Patients for emergency surgery to see the senior surgeon preoperatively
- Early ITU/outreach liaison in high-risk patients

Answering Relatives' Questions in Acute Upper Gastrointestinal Bleeding

How serious is the bleeding? The answer depends on the patient. Although the average mortality risk from upper GI bleeding is 10%, it varies by a factor of 20 between the young and the elderly, and from extremely low rates in acute gastritis to perhaps 20%–30% in acute bleeding varices.

Will the ulcer stop bleeding of its own accord? Eight out of 10 ulcers stop bleeding on their own; the rest are treated at endoscopy with injection or coagulation. In these cases, nine out of 10 will stop bleeding, but a very small number will need to go on to urgent surgery, either because the procedure does not work or because it is only temporarily successful.

How will the endoscope examination help? It will tell us the cause of the bleeding and will give us some idea if it will stop. Heavy bleeding from an artery, for example, is more likely to need surgery than a superficial area of inflammation in the gullet. It may be necessary to try and seal off the bleeding at the time of the examination, using locally applied heat or an injection into the bleeding point.

What is the outlook in bleeding from oesophageal varices? Although treatments have improved greatly in recent years, this remains a very serious condition. Much will depend on whether the bleeding can be stopped and, if it can, whether there is further bleeding in the first 2 to 3 days. About a fifth of all patients who bleed from varices re-bleed in the first few days, and for them, the outlook is not particularly good.

Can the patient eat and drink? The patient will need to remain nil by mouth in preparation for an urgent endoscopy. Depending on the findings and the subsequent progress, they may then be able to start fluids and a light diet.

Important Questions to Ask the Patient or Relatives

- What is the patient's alcohol intake?
- Is the patient on NSAIDs, low-dose aspirin, steroid tablets or warfarin/direct acting oral anti-coagulants?
- Is there a history of abnormal bruising or bleeding?
- Has there been previous surgery, and if so what was it?
- Has there been a problem with blood transfusions?
- In a frail and vulnerable patient—is there an advanced care plan?

Reassessing the Patient on Return From Endoscopy

Patients will have been away from the ward for an hour or more undergoing endoscopy. Systematic clinical observations may have been curtailed during and after the procedure. Fluid balance charts and transfusion needs may not be correctly documented and the patient, who is already sick, has the after-effects of the procedure and sedation to over-come. It is vital to reassess the patient on return to the ward.

- Is the airway secure (most patients will have been sedated for the endoscopy)?
- Is the patient in the recovery position while the sedation wears off?
- Is the patient oxygenated?
- Has resuscitation been adequate (pulse, blood pressure, CVP, capillary filling) NEWS2?
- Are the management plans clear (particularly should the patient re-bleed)?
  - What did endoscopy show (spurting/oozing arterial bleed, varices)?
  - Are there prescriptions for fluids and blood?
- Are there any special requirements (octreotide, omeprazole infusion, platelets, FFP, antibiotics)?
- Can the patient eat and drink? Patients who remain stable 4h after endoscopy can usually drink and start a light diet.
- Is the fluid balance chart accurate and is adequate blood available?
- Ensure that the post-endoscopy Full Rockall Score is calculated and document as there been liaison with the relatives?

CRITICAL CLINICAL TASKS IN UPPER GASTROINTESTINAL BLEEDING

- Ensure the safety of the patient
- Correct the oxygen saturation
- Secure the venous access
- Measure the pulse, blood pressure and respiratory rate - NEWS2
- Identify the signs of shock—pallor, sweating, restlessness, confusion
- Ask about liver disease and clotting disorders

IMPORTANT CLINICAL TASKS IN UPPER GASTROINTESTINAL BLEEDING

- Assess the likely severity of the initial blood loss and chart further loss
- Take an appropriate history
- Complete baseline observations
- Reassure the patient and attend to the patient's basic comforts
- Follow the vital signs at appropriate intervals
- Ensure accurate fluid balance charts
- Report signs of re-bleeding/changes in the vital signs
- Save any important evidence (vomited blood, fresh melaena)
- Warn the patient about the likely need for an endoscopy
- Report any abdominal pain
- Initiate careful oral hygiene measures

At this point, the intensity of ward team input depends on whether the patient is in a high-risk category. A sick patient with heavy blood loss (more than 4 units of blood transfused in the first 12 h) and with a high chance of re-bleeding will require continuous and close observation; a young patient with superficial gastritis and little evidence of bleeding will need much less intensive input.

Portal Hypertension and the Management of Oesophageal Varices

Nutrients, drugs and potential toxins are carried in the *portal vein* from their main site of absorption, the stomach and small intestine, to be processed and detoxified within the liver. To enable these substances to reach the liver cells, the portal vein divides into small capillaries (venules), which form a delicate network throughout the substance of the liver. The branches of the portal vein are vulnerable to any disease process such as cirrhosis or severe hepatitis that causes structural damage within the liver—the venules become obliterated and the portal venous blood flow is obstructed. If the venous drainage from the upper intestine to the liver is obstructed, pressure builds up behind the blockage (*portal hypertension*; Fig. 5.3) and the blood is forced into finding an alternative route. In this situation, veins at the lower end of the oesophagus, which drain into the inferior vena cava (part of the systemic venous system) and normally only carry small amounts of blood, become the main route of venous traffic from the upper GI tract (*portosystemic shunting*). These veins have to enlarge and in doing so form *oesophageal varices* (Fig. 5.3).

There are two consequences of portosystemic shunting for the patient as follows:

- Substances absorbed from the gut bypass the liver and pour straight into the vena cava. The resulting accumulation of toxic dietary components, in particular ammonia, can lead to increasing confusion, drowsiness and ultimately coma—*hepatic encephalopathy.*
- The varices enlarge progressively and may rupture and bleed.

The logical way to stop bleeding from oesophageal varices is either physically to obliterate the varices themselves or to reduce the pressure in the portal vein. Varices can be obliterated by oesophageal banding, which uses an endoscopic device to lasso the varices with small elastic bands. Varices within the stomach respond best to endoscopic injections of a strong adhesive glue—cyanoacrylate These two techniques have largely replaced the use of direct oesophageal compression with an inflated balloon (the Sengstaken tube).

There are two important drugs, terlipressin and octreotide, which will stop variceal bleeding by lowering the portal pressure and reducing the flow of blood through the varices. Terlipressin, 1 to 2 mg IV prior to endoscopic treatment and at 4 h and at 8 h is the preferred initial treatment and will stop the bleeding in 8 out of 10 patients. In patients with known liver disease, terlipressin or octreotide is often given at the first sign of significant upper GI bleeding, to be discontinued later if endoscopy does not confirm that the blood is coming from varices. Treatment is then continued with either terlipressin for 48 h (2 mg IV every 6 h) or octreotide (50 mcg IV bolus then 50 mcg/h for 5 days).

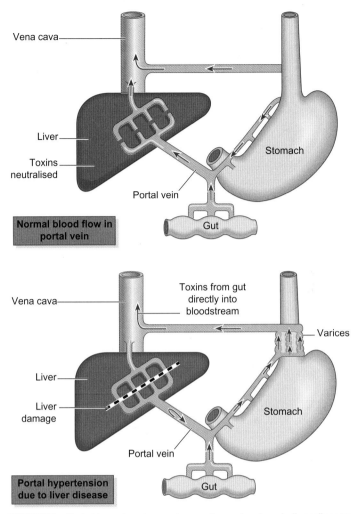

FIGURE 5.3   Portal hypertension and oesophageal varices in liver disease.

*T*ransjugular *i*ntrahepatic *p*ortosystemic *s*huntin is a new radiological technique for reducing the portal pressure when other methods to stop the bleeding fail. The procedure, performed through a cannula inserted into the jugular vein, involves making a channel within the substance of the liver between the portal vein and the systemic veins—an artificial portosystemic shunt—which reduces the pressure in the portal vein (although the extra shunting may trigger or worsen hepatic encephalopathy).

PREVENTATIVE ANTIBIOTICS

Patients who have bled from gastro-oesophageal varices are at a high risk from serious bacterial infection. Prophylactic antibiotics (e.g., IV ceftriaxone which is active against gut organisms) improve the chances of survival and must be started at the first suspicion of variceal bleeding.

Fresh Rectal Bleeding

Melaena (black tarry stool) indicates that the site of the bleeding is the stomach or duodenum—occasionally it is in the small bowel or the first part of the colon. In contrast when fresh blood is passed, unless there is catastrophic upper GI bleeding, the site is usually the colon. The principles of clinical care and resuscitation of the hypovolaemic patient are the same irrespective of the bleeding site. Colonoscopy replaces gastroscopy as the urgent intervention of choice.

Acute Liver Failure, Jaundice and Hepatic Encephalopathy

Two groups of patients present with acute liver failure: those in whom it is precipitated by an acute event such as viral hepatitis, and those in whom the episode occurs on a background of chronic (most commonly alcoholic) liver disease with portal hypertension. Acute liver failure has a number of components that make it a particularly challenging clinical problem (Fig. 5.4).

IMPAIRMENT OF THE CONSCIOUS LEVEL

The combination of poor liver function and portosystemic shunting means that toxic substances from the gut, in particular ammonia, are either dealt with ineffectively by the liver or bypass it altogether. The result is a toxic encephalopathy with impairment of the conscious level that can progress rapidly from confusion and agitation to deep coma. When it does, the patient has usually developed cerebral oedema and requires intensive care, preferably in a specialist liver unit. It is vital to assess and follow changes in the hepatic encephalopathy using a standard scoring system (Box 5.2) as even small changes in the mental state can be a warning of catastrophic deterioration in the patient's condition.

BLEEDING VARICES AND CLOTTING ABNORMALITIES

Patients in acute liver failure are at great risk from upper GI bleeding due to the combination of varices and impaired clotting. Not only will this cause cardiovascular instability, but blood in the gut provides a source of toxins that can worsen hepatic encephalopathy. Changes in abnormal clotting tests are a fundamental part of assessing a patient's clinical progress and the need for transfer to a specialist centre. Therefore clotting should not be corrected unless there is active bleeding (and only after specialist advice).

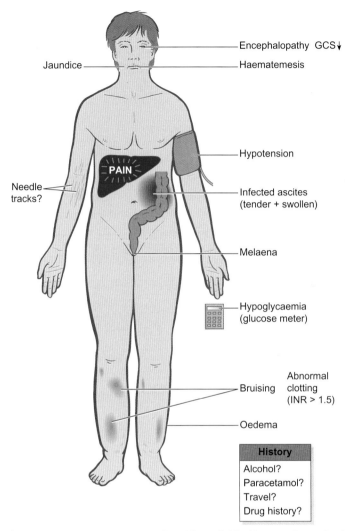

Encephalopathy GCS↓

Haematemesis

Jaundice

Hypotension

Needle tracks?

Infected ascites (tender + swollen)

PAIN

Melaena

Hypoglycaemia (glucose meter)

Abnormal
Bruising   clotting
(INR > 1.5)

Oedema

History
Alcohol?
Paracetamol?
Travel?
Drug history?

FIGURE 5.4   The features of acute liver failure. *GCS*, Glasgow Coma Scale.

BOX 5.2 ■ Hepatic Encephalopathy Scoring System	
0	Normal
1	Mood change
2	Drowsy
3	Confused/disorientated
4	Coma/unrousable

SEPSIS

Infection can trigger or complicate acute liver failure and can be difficult to recognise. Systemic fungal infections occur in up to a third of patients. Blood, urine, ascitic fluid and any sputum are routinely cultured. Pleural effusions may need drainage to help respiration and to exclude empyema.

METABOLIC ABNORMALITIES

The main problems are hypoglycaemia, low sodium levels, and renal failure. Hypoglycaemia is important because it will contribute to confusion and can be readily corrected. Sodium levels need to stay between 140 and 145 mmol/L. Patients in liver failure who develop renal failure do particularly badly. At presentation, these patients are often hypovolaemic: careful early fluid replacement (monitored with a CVP line) can improve their renal function. Hypotension unresponsive to fluid replacement may require inotropic support with norepinephrine.

Management of Acute Liver Failure in the First 24 H

Patients with acute liver failure need supportive care until there is either spontaneous improvement or they are transferred to a specialist unit with a view to more intensive treatment; this may include transplantation. All patients with acute liver failure should be considered as potential transplant candidates.

HEPATIC ENCEPHALOPATHY

Hepatic encephalopathy is managed according to its severity and its mode of onset. Acute liver failure with grade 3 or grade 4 encephalopathy (confusion or coma) is usually associated with cerebral oedema. The patient needs to be sedated, paralysed, and ventilated, as agitation and restlessness increase intracranial pressure. Intravenous mannitol (0.5 mg/kg) can be used in the emergency situation to reduce cerebral oedema. Acute on chronic liver failure with encephalopathy (such as may occur in decompensating alcoholic liver disease) can be treated less aggressively: the intake of protein, the main source of ammonia, is reduced and the bowel is cleared using lactulose, which reduces production of ammonia in the bowel and also empties it through its action as a laxative. The dose of lactulose is adjusted until there are between two and four soft stools per day. Oral neomycin, or rifaximin, which sterilise the bowel of all ammonia-producing gut bacteria, can also be used. If there is a history of heavy alcohol consumption, intravenous Pabrinex (high strength) is started to treat potential thiamine deficiency, which can lead to permanent neurological damage.

BLEEDING

Active bleeding can be minimised by correction of any clotting abnormality. However correction can be problematic as the uncorrected INR (international normalised ratio) is the best indicator of liver recovery or deterioration. Usually platelets and FFP are only indicated if there is active bleeding.

The safest way to monitor bleeding and fluid replacement in the unstable phase is to use a CVP line. There is a fine line between under- and over-transfusion in these patients, with the constant risk of pulmonary oedema (particularly when saline is infused) to be balanced against the deleterious effects of undertransfusion on kidney function. If variceal bleeding is suspected intravenous terlipressin is started.

SEPSIS

Bloodstream infection and peritonitis are common in patients with acute or chronic liver disease, particularly after acute GI bleeding, and can precipitate encephalopathy. Gut bacteria are usually to blame, so most regimens for liver failure include aggressive targeted antibiotic therapy aimed at these organisms if infection is suspected. Alcoholics with liver disease are often heavy smokers and are prone to respiratory infection, particularly pneumonia.

METABOLIC PROBLEMS

Hypoglycaemia must be avoided by 2 hourly checks on the glucose stix and the appropriate use of IV 10% or 20% dextrose. Patients with acute on chronic liver disease have often been on diuretics for ascites and may have acutely low potassium and sodium levels that need to be corrected. Patients with acute liver failure are 'hypermetabolic'—burning up calories and protein—so nasogastric feeding must be considered early. If there is an excessive gastric aspirate, it can be reduced using metoclopramide and clarithromycin (acting as prokinetic drugs to aid gastric emptying).

CRITICAL CLINICAL TASKS IN ACUTE LIVER FAILURE

Ensure the safety of the patient: ABCDE. The airway is at risk in grade 4 encephalopathy, although most patients with acute liver failure will be confused and restless rather than comatose. Oxygen is administered and oxygen saturations are monitored. A baseline respiratory rate is required because hypoxia and an increase in respiratory rate are early signs of pulmonary oedema, but could also indicate aspiration pneumonia. The pulse and blood pressure are critical for assessing blood loss and septicaemic shock—septicaemia from gut organisms often gives a picture of hypotension, increased respiratory rate, fever, and warm vasodilated extremities. Measure the BM stix urgently:

hypoglycaemia is the one important cause of reversible neurological disturbance. The patient should be rapidly assessed for signs of GI bleeding (nature of the stool, evidence of haematemesis).

 CRITICAL CLINICAL TASKS IN ACUTE LIVER FAILURE

- Ensure the safety of the patient: ABCDE
- Gain venous access
- Carry out head-to-toe examination
- Liaise with the patient's family
- Ascertain the possible causes of liver failure
- Explain the likely interventions in the first 48 h
- Obtain a drug history

Gaining venous access. Large peripheral venous cannulae will be inserted using a careful aseptic technique (these patients are, in effect, immunosuppressed). Most patients with complex liver failure will need CVP monitoring.

Carry out head-to-toe examination. Examine for signs of sepsis, infected needle tracks (hepatitis) and tender abdominal distension (infected ascites).

Liaise with the patient's family. It may not be possible to obtain the necessary details from the patient. It is critical to try and obtain some form of psychosocial history. If emergency transplantation becomes an issue, a major determinant of likely success is the patient's pre-existing psychological status.

Ascertain the possible causes of acute liver failure. The most common causes of acute liver failure are paracetamol poisoning and acute viral hepatitis (hepatitis A,B,C and E, herpes simplex and zoster, cytomegalovirus and the glandular fever virus, Epstein-Barr virus). It is critical to exclude the possibility of a paracetamol overdose: by the time the patient presents with liver failure, the drug may be undetectable in the blood, and yet specific intervention with the antidote, N-acetylcysteine (Parvolex), can be life-saving even at this late stage. The various forms of hepatitis can be suspected from the history: recent travel, pregnancy, IV drug abuse, transfusions, mushroom ingestion and drug history (notable NSAIDS and antibiotics). Include recreational drugs (ecstasy) and over-the-counter medications (health food preparations). Acute on chronic liver failure is most commonly seen in alcoholic liver disease, but other causes include various forms of non-alcohol-related cirrhosis such as primary biliary cirrhosis and autoimmune liver disease. The blood tests will supplement the history in establishing the cause; for example, in paracetamol poisoning the liver enzymes are massively elevated, whereas with ecstasy it is the muscle enzymes which are increased.

Explain the likely interventions in the first 48 h.

- **Endoscopy**—this will be carried out urgently if there is active bleeding
- **Radiology**—possible interventions to control bleeding
- **Transfusions**—blood products and clotting factors may be necessary

- **Multiple infusion lines**—central and peripheral infusions, urinary catheter to monitor output
- **Transfer**—some patients with acute severe liver disease may need intensive care, either locally or at a regional liver unit. The patient will need to be stabilised before transfer can be considered or safely undertaken. Fulminating acute liver failure may require emergency transplantation.

Obtain a drug history. It is vital to obtain an accurate drug history. Some drugs are directly toxic to the liver (anti-TB drugs are notoriously hepatotoxic) or may have important side effects—hypokalaemia associated with diuretic use is a common problem in liver disease. Non-steroidal drugs increase the risk of GI bleeding and also increase the likelihood of problems with kidney function. Intravenous drug abuse increases the risk of both acute and chronic hepatitis.

Important Clinical Tasks in Acute Liver Failure

Determine accurate fluid balance. Fluid balance in acute liver failure is complex, but its management is made easier if there are accurate input and output charts. Several infusions can be running simultaneously: dextrose, N-acetylcysteine (Parvolex), clotting factors, and central lines. Vomit and any bowel action must be strictly documented. Hourly urine output measurements are critical to the assessment of kidney function: an output of less than 30 mL/h is a cause for concern. Acute kidney injury is common in decompensated liver disease and is treated along conventional lines—stop all nephrotoxic drugs, fluid resuscitation, and the maintenance of an acceptable blood pressure.

IMPORTANT CLINICAL TASKS IN ACUTE LIVER FAILURE
- Determine accurate fluid balance
- Identify sepsis
- Reassure the patient and manage confusion and disorientation
- Carry out general caring measures

Identify sepsis. Primary bacterial peritonitis—infection of the patient's ascitic fluid—is a common problem in liver failure and can be difficult to diagnose. All patients with ascites should have it tapped and sent for bacteriologic investigations. Patients with peritonitis may complain of generalised abdominal pain, associated with tenderness and discomfort when they are moved around the bed. There may be a fever. Chronic liver disease, especially in malnourished alcoholic patients, is often associated with skin sepsis as infected abrasions, skin abscesses or infected pressure sores. The mouth is also an important focus of infection.

Reassure the patient and manage confusion and disorientation. Patients with acute liver disease are often distressed and agitated. There may be hepatic encephalopathy and some may be suffering from alcohol withdrawal. Sedation has a limited role to play, unless the patient is a danger to himself, as it can worsen liver failure. In the less confused patient, simple measures such as nursing the patient in a well-lit room, constant reassurance and explanation, and bringing in close relatives are often sufficient. In severe encephalopathy, however, sedation and ventilation may be the only option in the face of worsening cerebral oedema. It is important to exclude a reversible cause for the restlessness, such as hypoxia, hypoglycaemia, pyrexia or acute urinary retention. Venous access is often difficult, so infusion sites should be well protected.

Carry out general caring measures. The safety of these acutely ill patients is at risk. Pressure areas and the skin in general are often poorly nourished and in poor condition. Oral hygiene is usually poor and needs careful attention. Restless patients will need close observation, which may have to incorporate safety measures such as cot sides.

Example Cases in Acute Liver Failure and Hepatic Encephalopathy

Case Studies 5.4 and 5.5 give examples of management of cases of acute liver failure.

CASE STUDY 5.4	A 34-Year-Old Female With Jaundice and Abdominal Swelling

A 34-year-old female was admitted to hospital with a 4-week history of abdominal swelling and a 3-day history of increasing jaundice. There had been a general deterioration in her health, with lethargy and anorexia. For the past 2 weeks she had been taking regular paracetamol for a constant headache, but she denied taking an overdose.

She had been a heavy drinker since the age of 16 years, predominantly cider—between 6 and 10 cans every day. She had been tremulous in the morning for some time and was spending all her money on alcohol. She was unable to remember a day when she had not had a drink. She was married, with a 4-year-old son and smoked 25 cigarettes per day.

On admission the patient was jaundiced and smelt of alcohol. The patient was agitated but not confused or drowsy and there was a fine tremor. The BM stix reading was 6 mmol/L. Temperature was normal, pulse 110 beats/min and blood pressure 130/70 mm Hg, with no postural drop. Her abdomen was distended but not tender, but both her liver and spleen were enlarged. There was no melaena on rectal examination.

The working diagnosis was acute alcohol-induced liver damage, possibly associated with an additional insult from excess paracetamol ingestion.

Blood samples were taken for:
- Liver function tests
- Clotting studies
- Haemoglobin (to exclude bleeding), WCC (to exclude infection) and platelets (low in alcoholics)
- Blood sugar
- Kidney function (the kidneys are very vulnerable in liver disease)
- Alcohol level
- Paracetamol level (to exclude acute paracetamol toxicity)
- Culture (infection can trigger off liver failure if there is pre-existing liver disease)

Ascitic fluid was tapped and cultured.

CASE STUDY 5.4 A 34-Year-Old Female With Jaundice and Abdominal Swelling—cont'd

IMPORTANT INITIAL QUESTIONS

- Why is she agitated?
  - Hypoglycaemia?
  - Alcohol intoxication?
  - Alcohol withdrawal?
  - Early hepatic failure (encephalopathy)?
- Sepsis?
- *Is there any GI bleeding (i.e., bleeding varices)?*

INITIAL AND SUBSEQUENT INVESTIGATIONS

The results of the investigations are shown in Table 5.2. Paracetamol levels were negative and alcohol levels were three times the legal driving limit.

PROGRESS

The patient was started on IV cefuroxime and metronidazole. Intravenous N-acetylcysteine (Parvolex) was given but discontinued once the paracetamol levels were available. She was prescribed intravenous thiamine-vitamin C combination (Pabrinex) and oral lactulose.

Half-hourly observations including BM stix were started. Four hours after admission, she became more drowsy and her BM stix fell to 4.5 mmol/L. Intravenous glucose 20% was started. After some discussion, she was given 10 mg vitamin K IV.

The patient was observed overnight and by the next day she was confused and increasingly restless in spite of normal blood sugars. Her liver function had deteriorated and she had developed a flapping tremor.

At this stage the differential diagnosis was between alcohol withdrawal and hepatic failure with encephalopathy. The liver function test results had deteriorated and the high liver enzyme findings suggested acute alcohol-induced liver damage: alcoholic hepatitis. There was neither evidence of acute infection nor active upper GI bleeding, both of which could have triggered liver failure in a patient with underlying liver disease.

Over the next 48 h, the patient's increasing confusion became difficult to manage and so she was cautiously given oral Heminevrin. Her renal function was noted to be deteriorating and her urine output had fallen to less than 20 mL/h. After discussion with the Liver Unit she was started on oral prednisolone (a treatment for alcoholic hepatitis). Twenty-four hours later, as her confusion had increased, she was transferred with a view to assessment and possible liver transplantation.

TABLE 5.2 ■ Results of Investigation

	Day 1	Day 2	Day 3
Bilirubin (mmol/L)	313	393	396
AST (IU/L)	623	1477	1282
Albumin (g/L)	33	28	26
Sodium (mmol/L)	132	121	124
Urea (mmol/L)	3.8	6.7	12.3
Creatinine (mmol/L)	45	87	148
Prothrombin time (s)	17	24	20

CASE STUDY 5.5   A Heavy-Drinking 55-Year-Old Male With Melaena

A retired 55-year-old male was admitted to hospital, having collapsed at home after passing a large amount of black stool. According to his wife, he had been unwell for 3 weeks since returning from a holiday in Spain: a graze on his leg had become infected, he had developed swelling of both ankles, and his motions had been very dark for a week. He had been drinking heavily for around 10 years to cope with business worries, and on the recent holiday had consumed between 5 and 10 pints of beer daily. He had previously been told that he was suffering from alcoholic cirrhosis.

On admission, he was drowsy but rousable and responding appropriately: Glasgow Coma Scale (GCS) = 14 (E3 M6 V5). His BM stix result was 8.5mmol/L. His pulse was 120 beats/min and his blood pressure was 105/80mm Hg lying down and 90/60mm Hg sitting up. He was apyrexial. Oxygen saturations were 94%. Capillary filling was normal. He was obviously jaundiced and had gross abdominal distension, with tense oedema of both ankles. There was an infected skin abrasion on his right calf and scattered bruising. While being admitted, he used a bedpan and passed 400mL of black stool containing fresh clots.

This man had the features of advanced (decompensated) liver disease. These are as follows:

- **Failure of the liver to manufacture enough albumin**—*ascites and oedema* and low serum albumin.
- **Failure of the liver to excrete bilirubin**—*jaundice* and a high bilirubin level.
- **Failure of the liver to manufacture enough clotting products**—*bruising or bleeding*. The liver is the main source of several important clotting factors and if, as a result of liver damage, these fall to a third or less of their normal levels, the patient will be at risk from bleeding. This results in spontaneous bruising and, more importantly, an impaired clotting response to any GI bleeding. Vitamin K, which is needed to activate these factors, may also be in short supply because, as one of the fat-soluble vitamins, it needs normally functioning bile for it to be absorbed from the diet. The prothrombin time tests these vital aspects of liver function: it should not normally exceed 11 to 13s.
- **Failure of the liver to destroy toxic products**—a major function of the liver is to break down the body's toxic products. In liver failure the accumulation of toxins, in particular ammonia, leads to increasing drowsiness, confusion, and ultimately coma—so-called *hepatic encephalopathy.*
- **Upper GI bleeding**—the main worry in this male's case is that he is bleeding from oesophageal varices, a common and potentially fatal complication of severe liver disease. Because of their lifestyle, patients with alcoholic liver disease are also prone to peptic ulcer disease: the management of a bleeding ulcer is so fundamentally different from that of bleeding varices that the exact source of the haemorrhage has to be identified as soon as possible.

ENSURING THE SAFETY OF THE PATIENT: ABCDE

The conscious level of the patient was impaired, but with a GCS above 8 the airway is not at risk. However, an abnormal GCS must always be monitored. In acute liver failure, for example, the GCS can fall abruptly due to complications: worsening encephalopathy and, in particular, the sudden development of cerebral oedema. The BM stix result of 8.5mmol/L excluded hypoglycaemia (a complication of liver failure) as the cause for the altered conscious level.

The circulatory changes suggest significant blood loss: tachycardia and postural hypotension supported by the appearance of fresh melaena. Recognisable fresh blood in a melaena stool is a sign of massive upper GI bleeding. The patient will need initial resuscitation with IV fluids and blood, close serial observation of the pulse, blood pressure and urine output will be critical, blood loss will have to be documented and central venous cannulation will be required.

Exposing the patient revealed the infected skin abrasion on the lower limb. Any infection in this critically ill patient is potentially important; the wound should be carefully documented and swabbed.

REASSURANCE AND EXPLANATION

The initial assessment indicates that the patient should be forewarned and reassured about the intense activity that will take place in the next day or so. Losing blood from internal

CASE STUDY 5.5   A Heavy-Drinking 55-Year-Old Male With Melaena — cont'd

bleeding is a frightening experience, and initially the patient will be very distressed and will feel out of control. Although pain is not usually a problem, there is likely to be intense thirst (blood loss), nausea and perhaps vomiting.

THE PATIENT'S SUBSEQUENT PROGRESS

The patient was given oxygen via a high-flow mask. Large-bore cannulae were sited in both arms and IV Haemaccel was given — 1 unit over 30 min — while awaiting blood for transfusion. The transfusion technician, the laboratory, and the endoscopy unit were alerted to the potential severity of the problem.

The initial blood tests confirmed marked anaemia (haemoglobin 6.0 g/dL), moderately deranged clotting, and grossly abnormal liver function tests.

Within the first hour, the following procedures were completed:
- Cardiac monitor
- Central line (internal jugular approach)
- Urinary catheter (to monitor the exact urine output)
- Ascitic tap (to exclude infection in the ascitic fluid as the cause of the deterioration)

The initial phase of treatment involved:
- **careful transfusion aiming to maintain a CVP of +5 cmH$_2$O** — patients with liver failure handle excess fluid, particularly saline, badly. However, there is a risk of kidney failure if adequate fluids are not given at an early stage. Despite a careful approach, a subsequent chest film on the patient showed pulmonary oedema.
- **IV vitamin K 10 mg** — this will help, but not totally correct, the abnormal clotting. Specific clotting factors provided as FFP will also be needed. Clotting should only be corrected if there is uncontrolled bleeding as sequential uncorrected clotting tests are the best way to assess the recovery of liver function.
- **IV antibiotics: cefuroxime and metronidazole** — these are administered on the basis of an assumption that infection is already present, or very likely to occur, as a complication. This combination was chosen as most effective against gut organisms that may infect the ascitic fluid or biliary tree. Broad spectrum antibiotics are routinely given at the first suspicion of variceal bleeding.

One hour after admission, the patient had received 2 units of blood, 3 units of FFP and 1 unit of Haemaccel. His CVP had risen to +19 cmH$_2$O, and his chest film (to show the central line) showed pulmonary oedema.

Emergency endoscopy, after treatment of the pulmonary oedema, showed confluent oesophagitis and fresh bleeding from an oesophageal varix. The varix was obliterated with an oesophageal band and as this appeared to control the bleeding the patient was returned to the ward and started on an octreotide infusion at 50 mcg/h.

His observations did not stabilise; his pulse remained high at 115 to 120 beats/min, his SBP stayed below 95 mm Hg and 6 h after admission his CVP dropped to +2 cmH$_2$O and he had a large fresh haematemesis. Repeat endoscopy confirmed further active variceal bleeding and the banding was repeated.

He returned to the ward and overnight his pulse, blood pressure, and CVP stabilised with further blood transfusions and FFP. Hourly urine outputs, however, had dwindled to 10 to 20 mL/h and the patient was difficult to rouse.

His blood results showed worsening kidney function. At mid-morning he had a further very large haematemesis associated with worsening confusion. A Sengstaken balloon was passed as an emergency procedure and he was transferred to the ITU.

At this stage the problems were:
- uncontrolled variceal bleeding
- worsening hepatic failure
- pulmonary oedema
- hepatorenal syndrome (kidney and liver failure in a critically ill patient)

The outlook in this situation is extremely poor.

Acute Jaundice

Jaundice is caused by a buildup of the yellow pigment bilirubin and a breakdown product of haemoglobin and related proteins, which is normally produced and excreted by the liver. Virtually all cases of jaundice on the AMU will be due either to acute liver damage from viral hepatitis (Case Study 5.6) and toxins (usually alcohol) or to obstruction of the bile ducts by gallstones or, less commonly, tumour.

Acute hepatitis presents with flu-like symptoms, joint pains, nausea and discomfort in the right upper abdomen. Most of the symptoms improve with the sudden appearance of jaundice, although the nausea and vomiting may increase. Occasional cases progress to acute liver failure, but for the majority treatment with rest, a light, low-fat diet and alcohol avoidance will lead to a full recovery. Half of the cases of infective hepatitis are due to hepatitis A. This is transmitted by the orofaecal route, but spread to close domestic contacts can be prevented by vaccination. Hepatitis B is less common and tends to be associated with transmission through bodily fluids: transfusion, infected needles, and other high-risk behaviour. Close contacts such as sexual partners also require protective vaccination.

GALLSTONES, ACUTE CHOLECYSTITIS AND ASCENDING CHOLANGITIS

Gallstones usually present with biliary colic—severe upper abdominal pain going through into the back. If they become wedged in the bile ducts, there is a risk of infection, either confined to the gall bladder (acute cholecystitis) or spreading up the bile ducts to the liver (ascending cholangitis; Case Study 5.7). In these situations there is pain, but also signs of sepsis (fever, high white cell count) and, with spreading infection, abnormal liver function tests. Clinical management is focused on assessing the patient's progress and ensuring that while investigations are in progress there is adequate pain relief. An

---

CASE STUDY 5.6 **Acute Jaundice and Malaise in a 60-Year-Old Male**

This male was admitted with a 2-week history of vomiting after meals and a 1-week history of increasing jaundice, dark urine and pale stools. There was no history of pain, gallstones or risk factors for hepatitis (transfusions, travel or at-risk behaviour). He was on no medication and was a light social drinker.

On examination he was fully alert, markedly jaundiced and had a slightly enlarged and tender liver. There were no signs of chronic liver disease.

Blood tests were available from 4 days before and from the day of admission. His bilirubin level had doubled over 4 days but his liver enzymes were falling from markedly high levels (AST from 2800 to 590 IU/L). The albumin and clotting studies (which are the two most important tests of how well the liver cells are working) were normal.

A liver scan showed no abnormality in the liver, no signs of obstruction to the biliary tree, and normal pancreas. A day after admission the tests for glandular fever came back positive. A diagnosis of viral hepatitis due to glandular fever was made.

CASE STUDY 5.7   **A Male With Chest Pain and Chills**

A 75-year-old male was admitted with the sudden onset of prolonged shivering episodes lasting 15 min at a time. This was followed after about 4 h by an attack of retrosternal chest pain associated with nausea. There was a past history of peptic ulcer disease and chronic atrial fibrillation.

On examination he was mildly jaundiced and sweating profusely. His pulse was 85 beats/min in atrial fibrillation and blood pressure normal; the temperature was 38°C. His liver was mildly enlarged and he was tender over the gall bladder.

The liver function tests were abnormal, with a high bilirubin and moderate elevation of the AST (79 IU/L) and alkaline phosphatase (325 IU/L). An urgent ultrasound showed gallstones and a dilated biliary tree.

A diagnosis of infection in the biliary system spreading to the liver (ascending cholangitis) was made and the patient started on IV fluids, ampicillin, and gentamicin.

---

overall deterioration, continuing or worsening pain, and fever that fails to respond to IV antibiotics indicate a need for intervention, either by endoscopic attempts to remove the impacted stones (ERCP with sphincterotomy) or a direct surgical approach.

Acute Abdominal Pain

Abdominal pain is a common complaint on the acute medical ward. Although it is a feature of several medical conditions such as cardiac failure (liver congestion) and acute gastritis, it can also be due to a 'pure' surgical condition such as acute appendicitis or intestinal obstruction in a patient who has been admitted for medical reasons because the diagnosis was not immediately apparent (Fig. 5.5).

CRITICAL CLINICAL TASKS IN ACUTE ABDOMINAL PAIN

Establish the site and pattern of the pain. Midline localised pain is likely to arise from the stomach, duodenum or bowel. Severe pain that radiates into the back suggests either acute pancreatitis (Case Study 5.8), a deep peptic ulcer or an abdominal aortic aneurysm. Right-sided pain may arise from the liver, gall bladder or appendix. Kidney pain starts in the loins and radiates to the front or into the groin. An intra-abdominal catastrophe such as a perforation or a sudden blockage of the blood supply to part of the gut causes severe acute generalised pain from the outset. Pain that waxes and wanes (colic) occurs in acute gastroenteritis but is also seen in obstruction, in which case the pain becomes progressively more severe. If obstruction is suspected, look for evidence of a strangulated hernia—a tender swelling in the groin. Importantly in certain states, notably the elderly, the immunosuppressed, in pregnancy and during chemotherapy, symptoms and signs often do not have 'classical' clinical features.

   Assess the severity of the pain. Patients with severe abdominal pain are often grey, restless and clammy, and may be either lying still not wanting to be moved (acute peritonitis) or doubled up by intestinal colic. Oesophageal and peptic ulcer pain are not

FIGURE 5.5   The common causes of acute abdominal pain.

CASE STUDY 5.8   **Severe Abdominal Pain and Jaundice in a 56-Year-Old Female**

A 56-year-old female was admitted with a 6-month history of intermittent abdominal pains and a 3-week history of jaundice with pale stools. The pain was situated below the rib cage on the right and would be constant for an hour or so before easing off. On the day of admission, the pain was much more severe and prolonged. It also radiated into the back and was associated with vomiting.

On examination she was in pain, mildly jaundiced and looked unwell. There was a low-grade fever, a pulse of 110 beats/min, respiratory rate of 20 breaths/min and a blood pressure of 110/60 mm Hg, with no postural drop. Oxygen saturation was 92%.

She was tender over the gall bladder and there were only scanty bowel sounds.

The abnormal blood tests were as follows: WCC 16.5 ± 10⁹/L, bilirubin 59 mmol/L, AST 182 IU/L, amylase 5727 IU/L.

An urgent abdominal ultrasound showed gallstones and a dilated biliary system.

A diagnosis of gallstone-related pancreatitis was made. The patient was transferred to the surgeons for further management.

---

usually severe unless there are complications such as perforation (Case Study 5.9). Gall bladder pain is generally very severe (Case Study 5.10), as is the pain of acute pancreatitis. Ensure appropriate analgesia is prescribed, including IV opiates if necessary. There is no evidence that providing adequate pain relief masks or delays making the correct diagnosis.

CASE STUDY 5.9 | **Peptic Ulcer Pain**

A 28-year-old male was admitted with 6h of epigastric pain. He gave a long story of similar, less severe pain occurring an hour or so after food or alcohol and relieved by indigestion tablets. He looked well, but had marked epigastric tenderness.

CASE STUDY 5.10 | **Biliary Colic**

A 40-year-old female was admitted with severe constant pain under the right rib margin that radiated into the back. She was restless and in pain, with marked tenderness over the gall bladder area. There was a trace of bile in her urine and she appeared mildly jaundiced. Over the next 24h she developed nausea, vomiting and a fever and was started on IV antibiotics for a diagnosis of presumed acute cholecystitis.

 CRITICAL CLINICAL TASKS IN ACUTE ABDOMINAL PAIN

- Establish the site and pattern of the pain
- Assess the severity of the pain and treat accordingly
- Look for signs of sepsis, shock and bleeding
- Examine for abdominal rigidity and peritonitis
- Prepare for resuscitation

Look for signs of shock and sepsis. Severe abdominal pain with signs of shock—tachycardia, hypotension, and increased respiratory rate—suggests a serious intra-abdominal catastrophe: perforation, acute bowel ischaemia, ruptured aneurysm, acute pancreatitis or intra-abdominal sepsis. A rising pulse rate, increasing pain, falling blood pressure and decreasing hourly urine output suggest an impending intra-abdominal disaster. These patients require urgent resuscitation and medical evaluation, including abdominal films and an immediate surgical opinion.

Examine for abdominal rigidity and peritonitis. The most obvious features of acute peritonitis are localised pain on coughing and board-like abdominal rigidity, accompanied by few, if any, bowel sounds. The patient does not want to move, appears shocked and is usually vomiting. If the condition has been developing over several days, the signs may be less dramatic: abdominal distension, vague tenderness, but a silent abdomen. Common causes of peritonitis are perforation of a peptic ulcer or acute appendicitis. Acute peritonitis may be accompanied by signs of sepsis—hypotension; rapid thready pulse; and cold, mottled extremities.

Prepare for resuscitation. Patients with an acute abdomen, particularly peritonitis, need urgent resuscitation, often in preparation for surgery. The basic requirements are oxygen, IV fluids, nasogastric intubation and urinary catheterisation to ensure an adequate urine output. Once a provisional diagnosis and management plan is in place, the patient must be reassessed to ensure there is adequate pain relief.

IMPORTANT CLINICAL TASKS IN ACUTE ABDOMINAL PAIN

Look at associated clinical features. A review of the reasons for the admission is helpful in evaluating the nature of the pain. Right upper abdominal pain in a patient with heart failure may be due to liver congestion. Pain with jaundice may be due to gallstones. Severe pain developing in a patient with a bleeding ulcer may be due to perforation. Acute pancreatitis is common in alcoholics but can also complicate gallstones and DKA. Note the date of the last menstrual period and ask about vaginal discharge and bleeding. Ruptured ectopic pregnancy and even concealed or unrecognised labour pains are encountered outside the gynaecology wards.

Review the previous history. Review any similar previous pain, particularly if it has been investigated already. Some drugs are commonly associated with upper GI ulcers and erosions: NSAIDs, aspirin and steroids. Old notes are needed urgently, with a particular view to the previous surgical history (Case Study 5.11).

Review the urine test results. Urinary infection is one of the most common causes of abdominal symptoms, either suprapubic discomfort from bladder distension or loin pain from the kidneys. Inspect a urine sample—if it is cloudy and strong-smelling, infection is likely. Send a pregnancy test in a female of childbearing age.

IMPORTANT CLINICAL TASKS IN ACUTE ABDOMINAL PAIN

- Look at associated clinical features
- Review the previous history
- Review the urine test results
- Review the stool chart
- Prepare the patient for further investigations

Review the stool chart. The nature of the patient's bowel actions is of fundamental importance in assessing the cause of abdominal pain. Obstruction is associated with absolute constipation: no motions and no flatus. Colic with diarrhoea suggests colitis, particularly if there is blood in the stool, or gastroenteritis.

It is important to document the exact type of stools that are passed. If the problem includes diarrhoea, the volume and quality of the stool is vital in assessing the fluid replacement needs of the patient. Bloody diarrhoea is a serious problem that has relatively few causes: severe colitis, campylobacter enteritis, and, in the elderly, acute ischaemic colitis. Fresh stool specimens must be sent (*and processed by the laboratory*) urgently.

CASE STUDY 5.11 Renal Pain

A 60-year-old male was admitted with a 4-day history of severe intermittent pain in the right loin, radiating around into his abdomen. For the past 12 h he had a number of sudden 'chills' and had mild urinary frequency. In the past, his left kidney had been removed because of 'infection'. An urgent ultrasound showed a large renal stone wedged in the right ureter and an enlarged and obstructed right kidney. Blood cultures were positive for *Escherichia coli*.

Prepare the patient for further investigations. Basic blood tests are carried out on admission to assess the degree of shock (notably renal function and lactate) and to look for evidence of infection (white cell count and blood cultures). It is vital to obtain an up-to-date ECG to help identify the patient with at-risk cardiac disease. Abdominal and erect chest films identify perforation; abdominal ultrasound and CT will identify other causes such as gallstones, pancreatitis, intra-abdominal abscesses (Case Study 5.12), and abdominal aneurysm.

Acute Diarrhoea: Sources and Courses

INFECTIVE DIARRHOEA

There are six common causes of infective diarrhoea:

- Campylobacter
- Salmonella
- *Escherichia coli*
- Clostridium difficile (due to antibiotics, particularly oral cephalosporins)
- SRSV (small round structured virus or norovirus)
- Rotavirus

The main features are listed in Table 5.3.

Patients are usually admitted to hospital with diarrhoea because of the worries about them maintaining their fluid intake against loss from both the upper and lower GI tract. The secondary problem involves distinguishing between acute infective diarrhoea and the acute inflammatory bowel diseases—ulcerative colitis and Crohn's disease.

Assessment

- History of recent foreign travel
- Ask about other possible cases

CASE STUDY 5.12	Acute Abdominal Catastrophe

CASE 1

Two weeks after a myocardial infarction, an 80-year-old female was admitted to hospital, severely ill with hypotension, tachycardia and acute generalised abdominal pain. Her abdomen was diffusely tender with very few bowel sounds. She remained critically ill despite fluids and antibiotics and underwent emergency laparotomy. The findings were of a gangrenous intestine due to an embolus lodged in the mesenteric artery. The embolus had arisen from the scar at the site of her myocardial infarction.

CASE 2

A 60-year-old female awoke with constant midline upper abdominal pain. During the day, the pain persisted and became more severe. The general practitioner visited and diagnosed constipation. By the evening she was confined to bed with generalised, constant abdominal pain; she had started to shiver and was unable to get warm. On admission to hospital, she was in shock and had marked generalised abdominal tenderness. She was resuscitated with oxygen and IV fluids and transferred to the surgeons. At operation she had a ruptured diverticular abscess of the large bowel, with faecal peritonitis.

TABLE 5.3 ■ **Features of Infective Diarrhoea With Different Causes**

Organism	Food	Incubation (Days)	Main Clinical Features	Complications
Campylobacter	+	5	Bloody diarrhoea	Acute colitis
Salmonella	+	2	Vomiting and diarrhoea	Shock
Escherichia coli (0157:H7)	+	2	Cramps and diarrhoea	HUS
Clostridium difficile	–	10	Acute severe colitis	Acute colitis
SRSV	–	1	Nausea and vomiting	Outbreak
Rotavirus	–	1	Diarrhoea and vomiting	Outbreak

HUS, Haemolytic uraemic syndrome; SRSV, small round structured virus or norovirus.

- Have there been recent doubtful meals/mass catering, etc.?
- History of recent antibiotic therapy

Is This Patient at Special Risk?

- Elderly
- Diabetic
- Immunosuppressed
- Cardiac disease
- Kidney disease

Is there a history of recurrent diarrhoea? A background of recurrent diarrhoea, especially associated with blood and mucus, makes an acute episode of diarrhoea more likely to be due to inflammatory bowel disease than to infection.

Clinical Assessment in Acute Diarrhoea

At all times the ward team should ensure the safety of the patient: ABCDE.

Assess Fluid Loss

- How much is being passed and for how long?
- What has the fluid intake been?
- What have the urine volumes been (approximately)?

Look for Evidence of Shock

- Confusion/drowsiness
- Hypotension
- Oliguria (less than 30 mL/h)
- Evidence of sepsis/fever
- If antibiotic induced, has the original infection resolved?

Diagnosis. Infective diarrhoea is diagnosed from stool cultures, which must be obtained as soon as the patient is admitted to hospital. The organisms are easy to culture and in the case of *Clostridium difficile* the toxin can be identified in the stool.

Clinical Management in Acute Diarrhoea

To protect staff and patients, infection control (following the local guidelines) *must* always be instituted in cases of acute diarrhoea until stool cultures are available (Fig. 5.6). Most cases are self-limiting, provided that attention is paid to correct fluid balance. This

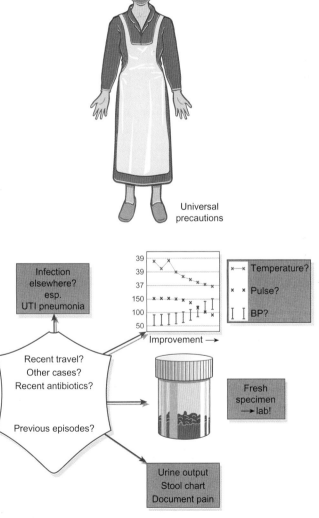

FIGURE 5.6 Acute diarrhoea. *UTI*, Urinary tract infection.

is particularly the case with the viral diarrhoeas: SRSV and rotavirus. Patients who are most at risk are the elderly and frail. The principle of treatment is to correct fluid deficit and keep up with the loss of fluid in the stool and vomit (Case Study 5.13). It follows

---

CASE STUDY 5.13   Salmonella Gastroenteritis

Twenty-four hours after a family celebration, a 75-year-old female developed nausea, short-lived vomiting and acute diarrhoea that persisted for 4 days, culminating in an emergency admission. By this time, she was too weak to stand and complained of persistent mid-abdominal cramps.

INITIAL NURSING ASSESSMENT

ABCDE. The patient was conscious and orientated, complaining of severe thirst and generalised episodic abdominal pains. The respiratory rate was 25 breaths/min, oxygen saturation 90%, pulse rate 120 beats/min and a lying blood pressure of 90/70 mm Hg, decreasing to 70/40 mm Hg on sitting upright. The temperature was raised, at 38.5°C, and the BM stix was normal at 6.0 mmol/L in spite of 4 days of virtual starvation. There were early pressure sores over the buttocks, perianal faecal soiling, and mild bilateral ankle oedema. The patient's abdomen seemed soft but generally tender, with very active bowel sounds.

History. There was no previous history of diarrhoea, recent antibiotic treatment or other significant illnesses. Several other guests at the function had also developed diarrhoea. There had been around eight bowel actions in the past 24 h, but only two or three small amounts of urine had been passed over the previous 4 days.

IMMEDIATE MANAGEMENT

- The assessment was of an elderly unwell female with infective diarrhoea and dehydration, with a marked reduction in urine output, raising the possibility of acute kidney injury. The elevated temperature suggested possible sepsis from the gut or perhaps a urinary infection.
- Oxygen was administered to bring the saturation to 95%.
- Peripheral venous access was not possible and so a central cannula was immediately inserted (intraosseous access was the alternative).
- A urinary catheter was passed to measure an accurate output.
- Rehydration was started, with a combination of isotonic saline and potassium chloride supplements.
- Bloods were taken for full blood count, biochemistry, lactate and culture. An urgent stool specimen was sent directly to the on-call bacteriology technician. The consultant microbiologist was warned of the possibility of a food poisoning outbreak.
- Abdominal x-rays were taken in view of the persistent pain, to exclude complications—severe colitis of any cause can lead to distension and, ultimately, perforation of the large bowel ('toxic dilatation').

PROGRESS

The initial tests confirmed dehydration and kidney injury (urea 54.1 mmol/L, creatinine 504 mmol/L); the sodium and potassium levels were low due to loss of electrolyte in the stool. Oral rehydration was not possible because of nausea and vomiting. Correction of the CVP from −3 to +5 cmH$_2$O over the first 4 h with IV saline brought up the blood pressure. Urine outputs over the first 3 days of admission were 450, 800, and 1500 mL, indicating a return of renal function (this was 'prerenal' rather than established renal failure, as it responded promptly to fluid replacement). After discussion with the consultant microbiologist, the antibiotic ciprofloxacin was administered.

Salmonella enteritidis was isolated from the initial stool specimen and, as usually happens with this infection, the abdominal pain and diarrhoea settled over the first 7 to 10 days of admission.

therefore that the fluid balance and stool charts must be accurate. By its nature, diarrhoea will impair the accurate collection and measurement of urine, but the combined volume of stool and urine in a commode or bedpan can be estimated relatively easily. It is critical to keep a reliable stool chart using the Bristol Scoring System.

Antibiotics are rarely needed unless there are signs of complications:

- Persistent fever with a failure to improve
- Development of severe colitis
- Development of shock
- Signs of infection elsewhere, for example, infected heart valve
- Severe colitis with the risk of haemorrhage, toxic dilatation, and perforation
- HUS (haemolytic uraemic syndrome)

Ciprofloxacin is the drug of choice except for *C. difficile*, for which treatment is usually oral vancomycin or metronidazole.

Clostridium difficile Diarrhoea

The indiscriminate use of antibiotics has led to a large rise in bowel infections due to *C.difficile*. The clinical picture varies from mild diarrhoea to severe colitis with fever, systemic sepsis and death. Certain patients are at a particular risk.

- Age over 65, particularly from nursing or residential homes
- Antibiotics (amoxicillin, co-amoxiclav, erythromycin, cephalosporins) within the past month
- Recent hospitalisation
- Immunocompromised
- Previous *C. difficile* diarrhoea (25% of cases relapse or become re-infected)
- Patients on PPIs (omeprazole, lanzoprazole)

Diagnosis relies on two fresh stool specimens from any patient with mushy or liquid stools being sent urgently to the laboratory with a request for the *C.difficile* toxin. Urine-contaminated faeces can be sent. The result should be available on the same day. Specific treatment is with oral metronidazole and in severe infections oral vancomycin or a new treatment, oral fidaxomicin. In severe cases this will be combined with intravenous fluids and careful attention to nutrition.

The following indicate a potentially severe infection:

- Temperature >38.5
- More than seven episodes of diarrhoea per 24 h
- WCC >15 × 10^9
- A 50% rise in initial creatinine level (developing renal failure)
- Elevated lactate level
- Distended abdomen and no diarrhoea (suggests a toxic megacolon)

Any patient where there is a suspicion of *C. difficile* must be isolated within 2 h of the first loose stool until the stool result is known. The test is in two stages and to diagnose active *C. difficle* infection which needs treatment, both must be positive—the presence of the *bacteria* ("GDH EIA")—meaning the patient must remain isolated—and the presence of its *toxin*—meaning the patient also needs specific treatment.

ENTERIC PRECAUTIONS

C. difficile and its spores contaminate and survive on surfaces such as commodes and bedside equipment and, in a busy ward, are easily spread by staff from one patient to another.

These minimise spread: a single room with an en suite commode, staff wearing gloves and a long sleeved gown who wash their hands with soap and water (not gel) before entering and before leaving (putting their gloves and gowns in a bin within the patient's room), liquid soap and disposable wipes for the patient.

Infective Diarrhoea Versus Acute Ulcerative Colitis

Some cases of severe diarrhoea will be due to acute ulcerative colitis rather than to an infective cause such as *Salmonella* or *Campylobacter*. The history is usually longer, with evidence of previous bowel symptoms. The patients are often more acutely ill with systemic features of anaemia, weight loss and fever associated with copious watery diarrhoea, which is usually bloody, as opposed to the typical green and offensive stool of infection. Some infections, notably, *E.coli* 0157:87, can progress from watery stool to bloody diarrhoea in 24 to 48 h. However the treatment is entirely different—acute ulcerative colitis needs high dose steroids and powerful immunosuppressants.

IMPORTANT CLINICAL TASKS IN ACUTE ULCERATIVE COLITIS

- Reassure the patient and his or her relatives
- Examine the pressure areas and perineum for evidence of damage and initiate protection
- Send stool for culture and *C. difficile* studies
- Explain the management plan
- Ensure the patient understands the significance of the stool and urine output charts
- Involve the dieticians at an early stage
- Avoid prescriptions for opiate analgesics or antidiarrhoeal drugs that can trigger toxic dilatation

---

 CRITICAL CLINICAL TASKS IN ACUTE ULCERATIVE COLITIS

- Look for evidence that the colitis is improving:
  - A falling pulse rate
  - A resolving fever
  - Less frequent diarrhoea
- Look for signs of toxic dilatation of the colon:

- Persistent abdominal pain and tenderness
- Increasing pulse rate
- Increasing daily abdominal girth
- Sudden cessation of diarrhoea
- Look for signs that the colitis is not responding:
  - Persistent fever and tachycardia
  - Persistent severe diarrhoea
  - Continuing or increasing lower GI blood loss
  - No improvement in malaise or abdominal pain

However, the emergency assessment is similar:

- Is there hypovolaemic shock?
- Are there signs of sepsis?
- Is the abdomen tender, silent, board-like or distended (toxic dilatation)?
- What has been the output of stool and urine over the immediate past few days?
- What is the nutritional state (ankle oedema often indicates a low-protein state)?

Medical Conditions Presenting With Gastrointestinal Symptoms

CARDIOVASCULAR DISEASE

Congestion

Hepatic congestion with stretching of the capsule that surrounds the liver leads to right-sided abdominal pain below the ribs, anorexia and nausea. In extreme cardiac failure the liver can fail, with the development of jaundice and grossly abnormal liver function tests.

Ischaemic Bowel

Acute shortage of the blood supply to the gut due to an embolism or to reduced cardiac output after, say, a myocardial infarction can cause acute lower abdominal symptoms: pain and diarrhoea that is often bloody.

Abdominal Aneurysm

Rupture of an aortic aneurysm leads to acute severe abdominal pain and circulatory collapse. Immediate surgical intervention can be life-saving.

Drug-Induced Side Effects

Common GI-related drug side effects are warfarin-induced upper GI bleeding and the clinical features of digoxin toxicity: nausea, vomiting, and anorexia.

Cardiac Cachexia

Extreme anorexia and weight loss are recognised features of advanced cardiac disease, particularly progressive congestive cardiac failure due to chronic valvular disease. This can be sufficient to mimic the development of a GI malignancy, particularly when associated with other gastric symptoms such as abdominal distension (ascites) and the pain from liver congestion.

Respiratory Disease

DIAPHRAGMATIC PLEURISY

The pain from diaphragmatic pleurisy can be referred to the upper abdomen and can be confused with biliary colic or peptic ulceration. The clue is that there are usually associated features of pneumonia (cough, breathlessness and fever), and the pain is much worse on inspiration.

CONGESTION IN COR PULMONALE

Right-sided heart failure in COPD can give rise to hepatic congestion and right upper quadrant pain. In patients with COPD, particularly those who are acutely short of breath, there is often also upper abdominal discomfort, arising from the ribs and diaphragm, that appears to be associated with the extra respiratory effort that these patients have to make.

STEROID-INDUCED SIDE EFFECTS

Patients on long-term oral steroids—chronic asthmatics and those with severe COPD— are prone to gastritis and peptic ulceration. More importantly, as they age these patients are also liable to osteoporotic collapse of their thoracic and lumbar vertebrae. This presents with pain spreading like a girdle from the back around to the front of the abdomen. The pain can be severe and can be confused with an acute abdominal crisis.

Diabetes

DKA can typically present with acute abdominal pain and vomiting. The picture can be very similar to that of acute pancreatitis, with similar biochemical changes in the blood. Interestingly, there is also an increased risk of true acute pancreatitis complicating severe ketoacidosis.

COVID-19 AND THE GASTROINTESTINAL TRACT

Anorexia, nausea, vomiting and diarrhoea are relatively common in acute COVID-19 but are not usually the most significant symptoms and are mostly self-limiting. Specific organ damage, notably hepatitis, pancreatitis and cholecystitis are described but are rare. Liver enzymes are frequently raised on blood tests but this usually a non-specific effect of the acute illness.

Whether it is safe to continue immunosuppressives (eg steroids, infliximab and aza-thioprine) for Crohns Disease and Ulcerative Colitis in the face of COVID-19 is an area of concern. At present the risk of stopping treatment and triggering an exacerbation of a serious inflammatory bowel disease is thought to be greater than a theoretical risk of damping the immune response to the virus.

Further Reading

Gastrointestinal Bleeding

NICE, 2012. Acute Upper Gastrointestinal Bleeding in Over 16s: Management Clinical Guideline. Available from: NICE.org.uk/guidance/cg141.

Stanley, A.J., 2019. Management of acute upper gastrointestinal bleeding. The BMJ;364, l536.

Liver Disease

EASL, 2017. EASL Clinical Practical Guidelines on the management of acute (fulminant) liver failure. Journal of Hepatology 66, 1047–1081.

NICE. Alcohol-use Disorders: Diagnosis and Management of Physical Complications. Available from: www.nice.org.uk/guidance/CG115.

Diarrhoea

Clostridioides difficile infection: antimicrobial prescribing. NICE guideline [NG199]. Published: 23 July 2021. Available from: https://www.nice.org.uk/guidance/NG199.

Ulcerative colitis: management. NICE guideline [NG130]. Available from: https://www.nice.org.uk/guidance/NG130.

Diabetic Complications

Diabetes in the Acute Medical Unit: The General Approach

Diabetes is closely linked with a number of common acute medical conditions. It is a major cause of premature vascular disease involving the heart, brain and kidneys, and therefore diabetes will be encountered in a significant proportion of emergency patients with myocardial infarction, angina, heart failure, stroke and renal insufficiency.

The illnesses to which diabetic individuals are susceptible will, in turn, have an adverse effect on diabetes control. Insulin requirements are increased in most acute medical conditions, and diabetes control can become disrupted. Diabetic patients who are already on insulin may need careful adjustments: those not usually requiring insulin may need to have it introduced. Severe illnesses such as pneumonia or meningitis can even precipitate diabetic ketoacidosis (DKA). The level of short-term diabetes control may alter the longer-term outcomes of an acute illness. High blood sugars are detrimental to the patient's recovery—they must be identified on admission and managed carefully—balancing the benefits of control with the serious risks of hypoglycaemia. Clearly, the acute medical patient who is also diabetic can present some of the most taxing problems in terms of nursing and medical management.

The acute medical unit (AMU) clinician is presented with a dual challenge to manage the primary acute medical problem and to ensure that the patient's diabetes control does not have an adverse effect on the eventual outcome.

Diabetic emergencies, most notably, ketoacidosis and hypoglycaemia, need immediate, expert management. Insulin-dependent diabetes can give rise to dramatic metabolic disturbances due to extreme changes in the blood sugar. The speed and accuracy of the initial assessment of the patient and the treatment in the first 2 to 3 h of admission will have an important bearing on the prognosis. Box 6.1 lists the key points that should be checked in the acute admission of a diabetic patient.

BOX 6.1   Key Points for an Acute Admission of a Diabetic Patient

1. Is the patient hypoglycaemic?
2. Is this a diabetic emergency or an emergency in a patient with diabetes?
3. Confirm the timing of the last insulin/oral hypoglycaemic and the last meal.
4. What is the usual regimen in this patient and how does the patient manage blood sugars that are too high or too low?
5. Critical clinical observations: Glasgow coma score (GCS), pulse, blood pressure, temperature, respiratory rate, oxygen saturation, blood sugar, capillary ketones and urinary ketones.
6. Check the vision.
7. Skin: examine pressure points (heels, soles of the feet, ankles); *remove dressings.*
8. Look for infection: cellulitis (legs and feet)/groins/vaginal discharge?
9. Examine the feet: numb/painful/infected/gangrenous?
10. Urgent venesection for biochemistry, venous bicarbonate, venous pH, etc.

Diabetic individuals are prone to infections: healing is often impaired and extensive soft tissue damage and loss can occur. The feet, in particular, are at risk from acute infection as a result of the combination of diabetic neurological and diabetic vascular damage. Such infections often present as emergencies with spreading infection, uncontrolled diabetes and, in many cases, a lower limb at risk of amputation.

Finally, it is important to take advantage of the opportunities that can arise on the AMU to influence long-term management. In particular, there is an important link between poor compliance and the risk of diabetic complications. A significant proportion of patients with diabetes only seek medical advice when major problems arise. For these patients, their acute admission provides an important chance to look for unrecognised complications and initiate a review of their overall diabetes management.

AIMS OF THIS CHAPTER

- To provide an understanding of normal and abnormal blood sugar control
- To present an overview contrasting type 1 and type 2 diabetes
- To examine the acute medical conditions that are associated with diabetes
- To explain how to control blood sugars in adverse medical situations
- To present the management of diabetic emergencies
- To look at the treatment of infection in the diabetic patient
- To identify opportunities on the AMU to influence longer-term management

Normal Blood Sugar Control and the Nature of Diabetes

The normal blood sugar level is kept within the range of 4–8 mmol/L by a balance between:
- The rate at which glucose is removed from the blood to be used by the muscles
- The rate at which glucose is manufactured by the liver and released into the blood

Insulin is released from the pancreas and *reduces* the blood sugar by:

- Increasing glucose uptake and utilisation by the muscles
- Reducing glucose formation and release by the liver

Normally, the pancreas senses the increase in blood sugar that occurs after food is eaten and secretes a carefully controlled amount of insulin. The insulin lowers the blood sugar and drives metabolism by pushing glucose into the cells, where it is used for energy.

If there is no insulin present, the body behaves as though it is in a state of acute starvation:

- The liver compensates by producing and releasing excessive glucose.
- The muscles stop taking in and using glucose.
- As a result, there is an acute increase in the blood glucose level.

- Fat is burnt as an alternative source of energy to produce fatty acids. These, in turn, form ketones, which are acids. Ketones appear in the blood and the urine.
- The patient becomes acidotic (the blood pH and the bicarbonate—HCO_3 fall). Diabetes occurs in two situations:
- There is a complete failure of insulin production. This is the situation in *type I diabetes*.
- There is a reduction in insulin production and the tissues themselves are resistant to the actions of insulin. This is the situation in *type II diabetes*.

An Overview of Type I and Type II Diabetes

Type I (or 'insulin-dependent' diabetes mellitus [IDDM]) occurs when there is a progressive failure of insulin production.

Type II (or 'non-insulin-dependent' diabetes mellitus [NIDDM]) occurs when there is a combination of two factors:

- The tissues fail to react to insulin.
- The rate of insulin production is reduced.

There are fundamental differences between the two types of diabetes (Table 6.1).

- Type I diabetes
  - There is little or no naturally occurring insulin.
  - Unless supplied with regular carbohydrates and insulin, the patient will become ketotic.
- Type II diabetes
  - There is a relative lack but not a complete absence of insulin.
  - Blood sugars are elevated, but the patient is not usually at risk from DKA unless triggered by severe illness such as acute pancreatitis.

TYPE I DIABETES

Type I diabetes is an autoimmune disease. To develop it, the patient needs to have an inherited tendency that is activated in some way by a viral trigger to switch on a progressive destruction of the body's own ability to produce insulin. Antibodies are produced that are directed against both the insulin hormone and the pancreatic β cells that produce and release insulin. Once 80% of the β cells have been destroyed, insulin concentrations fall to such low levels that the patient develops diabetes.

TABLE 6.1 ■ A Comparison of Type I and Type II Diabetes

	Clinical Onset	Natural Insulin	Risk of Diabetic Ketoacidosis	Obesity	Relative Frequency (%)
Type I	Sudden	Nil	Yes	No	20
Type II	Slow	Low	Rare	80%	80

TYPE II DIABETES

Type II diabetes is a partially inherited, age-related, 'Western' condition that has a strong association with obesity, a poor diet and physical inactivity. Insulin levels are moderately low (the number of pancreatic β cells is reduced by around 20%). More importantly, the patient's tissues are resistant to the action of insulin.

Recent Developments in the Treatment of Diabetes

TYPE I DIABETES

There is increasing emphasis on tight blood sugar control to lessen the risks of long-term complications. To achieve this, there is a wide choice of insulin regimens and insulin injection devices. Many patients are now established on regimens with a basal background of single- or double-dose, long-acting insulin that is fine tuned by thrice-daily, short-acting insulin, regulated according to fingerprick blood sugar profiles. The importance of minimising postprandial increases in blood sugars has been realised and some patients use ultra short-acting insulin (lispro/aspart) with or even just after food to achieve this aim. New analogues such as insulin glargine and detemir are replacing isophane, the traditional basal insulin. Designed to be slowly released from the injection site, these genetically engineered insulins give a more physiological blood sugar profile and represent an important improvement in the management of type I diabetes.

Continuous Subcutaneous Insulin Infusion Pumps (CSII): An increasing number of patients with type 1 diabetes are fitted with CSIIs. These small, battery-driven devices deliver short-acting subcutaneous insulin both as a background basal infusion and, to fine-tune the blood sugars, variable boluses that deal with carbohydrate loads and to correct high glucose levels.

It is *not* an artificial automated pancreas and requires close patient input. Also, because it only administers short-acting insulin, any interruption in delivery can trigger acute DKA or dangerous hyperglycaemia. In acutely ill patients (DKA, unconscious or confused), unless there is immediate and close input from the diabetes specialist team, the pump and infusion device should be completely removed (stored securely) and immediately replaced by an appropriate supply of insulin, for example, a variable rate insulin infusion.

The dietary treatment of type I diabetes remains based on an adequate calorie intake with complex carbohydrates, high fibre and a reduced fat intake.

TYPE II DIABETES

Traditionally, management is based on dietary control with or without oral hypogly-caemics. The aims of dietary treatment in type II diabetes are to reduce the energy intake, correct the blood lipids and reduce the patient's weight. Drug treatment with oral hypoglycaemics acts by stimulating insulin secretion (e.g, glibenclamide and gliclazide), by resensitising the tissues to the action of insulin or by directly reducing the release of glucose by the liver (metformin). An important new class of drugs—sodium–glucose transport protein 2 (SGLT2) inhibitors (EG dapagliflozin) lower blood sugar by increasing the excretion of glucose by the kidneys. As add-on therapy in selected patients, they reduce both cardiovascular and renal complications. Importantly, treatment with SGLT2 inhibitors has been implicated in the development of DKA in acutely ill (particularly in the frail elderly) diabetics in which circumstances they should therefore be withheld.

In time, blood sugar control deteriorates—within 6 years of diagnosis, 25% of patients with type II diabetes will require insulin. The effectiveness of combining twice-daily NPH insulin (isophane) or once-daily insulin glargine or detemir with oral metformin has facilitated a much more active approach to blood sugar management, with the knowledge that this will improve the outlook.

Complications, in particular of vascular origin, are common in type II diabetes. However, there have been major changes in our approach to their prevention. Up to 20% of new cases will have evidence of complications at the time of diagnosis and there is overwhelming evidence that the traditional 'bad companions' of diabetes have a major impact on the frequency with which they occur. Predictably, these are as follows:

- Hypertension
- Hyperglycaemia
- Hyperlipidaemia
- Smoking

Large studies at the end of the 1990s have altered the perception of the importance of addressing these factors in patients with type II diabetes. The evidence indicates that we must take every opportunity to reinforce the need for good diabetic control and the need to reduce the other risk factors, notably, hypertension and smoking. For example:

- Good long-term blood sugar control:
  - Reduces the risk of major diabetic eye disease by a quarter
  - Reduces the risk of early kidney damage by a third
- Lowering abnormally high blood pressure in these patients:
  - Reduces death from long-term complications by a third
  - Reduces the risk of strokes by a third
  - Reduces the risk of serious visual deterioration by a third

This represents a change of emphasis in management. The aim must be to keep the blood sugar and blood pressure in type II diabetes as near normal as possible. The AMU often affords the first opportunity to address these issues, with both new and established diabetes.

Acute Medical Conditions Associated With Diabetes

The presence of widespread arterial damage in many diabetic patients makes them prone to a number of major acute medical problems. The cause of the damage is a combination of direct tissue toxicity from abnormally high sugar levels and the elevated blood lipids that are so common in diabetes. The effect of the damage depends on whether large (e.g., main coronary and cerebral arteries) or small (e.g., skin microcirculation and arteries within the kidney) vessels are predominantly affected (Box 6.2). Unfortunately, in many of the older type II diabetics, there is damage throughout the arterial system, and these people are at risk from ischaemia affecting the coronary, cerebral and renal circulation.

Although there are no fundamental differences between the management of medical conditions in those with and without diabetes, diabetics as a rule fare less well than non-diabetics with the same disease. Thus diabetics with ischaemic heart disease have more widespread and more severe coronary artery disease and if they suffer an infarct they have twice the mortality risk compared with non-diabetics. Complications are common and often remain unrecognised by the patient. Thus a middle-aged patient with type II diabetes may have heart muscle damage that only becomes apparent during other severe illnesses. Similarly, silent diabetic renal disease may lead to hypertension and its complications. It is therefore important that, when a patient with diabetes is admitted with a seemingly unrelated problem such as a urinary infection, the opportunity is taken to make a general assessment: for ischaemic heart disease, for hypertension and for kidney damage.

Tissues become damaged more easily and heal more slowly in diabetes. Immune function is reduced and organ damage is likely, especially where the blood supply is already compromised by diabetic vascular disease. Thus pneumonia is more likely to be complicated by empyema, renal infections may end in abscess formation and pressure sores may progress to osteomyelitis. Opportunistic infections may occur: *Candida* infection of the skin creases and mucous membranes, pseudomonal infections of the ear, and an unusual form of meningitis caused by the organism *Listeria*.

BOX 6.2 ▦ Acute Medical Conditions Resulting From Large Vessel and Small Vessel Disease in Diabetes

Large Vessel Disease	Small Vessel Disease
Stroke	Retinopathy (visual impairment)
Myocardial infarction	Renal failure (proteinuria/hypertension)
Cardiac failure (coronary arteries)	Cardiac failure (heart microcirculation)
Amputation	Foot problems
Sudden death (cardiac)	Sudden death (cardiac)

DIABETIC RENAL DISEASE

One-third of type I and between one-quarter and one-half of type II diabetic patients develop diabetic kidney disease (diabetic nephropathy). Diabetic nephropathy is the main cause of end-stage renal failure in the United Kingdom. Urinary protein loss is often the first indication of renal disease. Normally, we lose less than 30 mg of albumin per 24 h in the urine. An early sign that diabetes is affecting the kidneys is the presence of 'microalbuminuria'—a loss of 30–300 mg per 24 h—which can be detected using a specialised screening test. Once the protein loss exceeds 300 mg per 24 h, however, conventional testing of a random urine sample with Albustix will be positive for protein. It is important to appreciate the significance of finding proteinuria in a diabetic patient on the AMU. It does much more than simply alert us to the possibility of a urinary infection.

- Proteinuria indicates probable renal involvement. (What are the patient's urea and creatinine? Are there any previous records of kidney function in the notes?)
- Proteinuria goes hand in hand with cardiovascular complications and diabetic eye disease.
- Proteinuria is strongly associated with hypertension.
- Switching off the renin–angiotensin–aldosterone system with ACE inhibitors (e.g., lisinopril) or angiotensin II receptor blockade (e.g., irbesartan) slows down the deterioration from microalbuminuria to advanced diabetic nephropathy.

If diabetic renal disease is discovered on the AMU for the first time, the patient must be referred for specialist management so that the risk of further complications can be reduced by:

- Careful blood pressure control
- Treatment with ACE inhibitors and related drugs
- Treatment with the new SGLT2 inhibitors
- Tight diabetic control
- Correction of lipids
- Advice on cessation of smoking

DIABETIC NEUROPATHY

Diabetic nerve damage is very common—it occurs in around one-third of patients with type II diabetes. There are two types of diabetic neuropathy: peripheral neuropathy and autonomic neuropathy. Both are very relevant to the AMU nurse. Peripheral neuropathy causes problems in the feet: numbness, poor skin nutrition and impaired mobility. The patient has no warning of trauma to the feet, so minor abrasions can develop painlessly into infective ulceration. Nerve damage and muscle imbalance lead to foot deformity (claw toes) and pressure damage (calluses and ulcers) over abnormal bony prominences. Elsewhere in the body, nerve damage can lead to neuralgia with severe, recurrent and often undiagnosed pain in the thighs and abdomen.

Autonomic neuropathy leads to abnormal regulation of involuntary muscle activity, notably, in the bladder, in the control of the blood pressure and in gastric emptying. Bladder involvement leads to painless retention, overflow and recurrent urinary infections. Abnormal blood pressure control can lead to severe postural hypotension (decreases in the systolic pressure on standing of more than 20 mm Hg), resulting in dizziness, poor balance and recurrent falls. Acute gastric distension can result in regurgitation and aspiration of the stomach contents—an important cause of death in severely ill diabetics and yet fully preventable by timely nasogastric intubation.

CARDIOVASCULAR DISEASE

Cardiovascular disease is a major problem in diabetes and shortens the life expectancy of the diabetic patient by 5–10 years. Diabetics with ischaemic heart disease have more widespread and more severe coronary artery disease than non-diabetic. The main manifestations of cardiovascular disease are angina, myocardial infarction and heart failure. Due to diabetic neuropathy and an increased pain threshold, angina can present late and myocardial infarcts can be painless. It is not unusual for an infarct to present as a sudden deterioration in diabetic control. The risk of a myocardial infarct is increased in diabetes—by a factor of 2–3 in type II diabetes and by an order of a magnitude in type I diabetes sufficient, for example, to cancel out the protective effect of their sex in a premenopausal diabetic female. There is also increased mortality risk both in hospital and during long-term follow-up. The heart muscle fares badly in these patients and the risk of re-infarction is high. The strong association between diabetes and hypertension also accelerates many of the cardiovascular complications.

CEREBROVASCULAR DISEASE

The vascular damage in diabetes affects both the larger cerebral vessels and the cerebral microcirculation. Patients with diabetes are at two to three times the normal risk of having a stroke. Should they suffer one, the mortality risk is higher and the functional outcome is worse than the equivalent stroke in a non-diabetic. Diabetic cerebrovascular disease presents with typical stroke-like symptoms due to thrombosis or hypertension-related cerebral haemorrhage. It is critically important, however, *not* to misdiagnose a neurological presentation of hypoglycaemia as a stroke. It should be assumed that any change in the conscious level of a diabetic patient has a metabolic cause until proved otherwise.

PERIPHERAL VASCULAR DISEASE

Diabetic peripheral vascular disease presents as an emergency with ischaemic problems in the limbs due either to acute arterial occlusion or to vascular complications in the feet: ulceration, infection and gangrene.

Blood Sugar Control in Adverse Medical Situations

HOW GOOD SHOULD CONTROL BE DURING ACUTE SEVERE ILLNESSES?

Any severe illness will disrupt diabetic control and, in the case of an insulin-dependent patient, may put them at risk of DKA. In the non-insulin-dependent patient, uncontrolled hyperglycaemia can produce a diuresis sufficient to lead to dehydration and hypovolaemia. There is also increasing evidence that elevated blood sugars per se are damaging to some patients, even in the short term. Hyperglycaemia reduces the body's immune function: white cell function, for example, is markedly impaired with blood sugars above 20 mmol/L. This may be of critical importance when the body is trying to deal with acute infection. The target blood sugar for patients who are ill with acute coronary syndrome or stroke is between 6 and 10 mmol/L. In general, however, it is prudent to optimise diabetic control during any acute medical illness, on the assumption that it will avoid the risk of ketoacidosis and may improve the overall outlook.

ASSESSING CONTROL

What are 'osmotic symptoms'? Heavy glycosuria draws water into the urine by osmosis. Osmotic symptoms are, therefore, polyuria and thirst and are a sign either of the onset of diabetes or of diabetes that is out of control. The strength of the osmotic diuresis can lead to dehydration but also to electrolyte loss, most notably, of potassium and sodium.

Laboratory blood sugar versus fingerprick testing. Although the fingerprick blood sugar tests give values that are around 15% less than the laboratory blood sugars, they are an invaluable way to assess diabetic control in the acute, unstable situation. The main problem is the unreliability of the glucose stix at low blood sugar levels. Normally, the glucose stix is used as the initial test in suspected hypoglycaemia, so that immediate action can be taken. Ideally, blood should be drawn simultaneously for checking in the laboratory.

Modern blood glucose meters. Glucose meters and glucose test strips have improved considerably in recent years. At one time they were difficult to use and prone to user error: too little blood on the strip would lead to under-reading; timing had to be to the second; and the technique for wiping blood off the strip was critical. Fortunately, the manufacturers have removed many of the user-dependent problems that led to their unreliability.

Meters such as the Ascensia Control and the Optium Xceed are popular because they are reliable, easy to use and require very small amounts of blood—some do not need calibration (control) and increasingly they also measure blood ketones (e.g., Freestyle Optium Neo). It is critical that the meters are used properly. There must be a Standard Operating Procedure in place, a training programme and a Staff Training Record.

- The new, 'virtually' pain-free, adjustable finger-pricking devices should be used. The lancet should be enclosed in the removable platform of the device, making both sharps injuries and inadvertent re-use impossible.

Good practice in fingerprick testing is outlined in Box 6.3.

In the management of DKA, capillary ketone levels are repeated hourly during the acute phase to assess the success of treatment—defined as a fall in the levels of at least 0.5 mmol/L/h.

Continuous glucose monitors (CGMs) and 'Flash' glucose monitors

Real-time CGMs and Intermittently Scanned ('Flash') monitors are removable glucose sensors that are fitted just under the skin—transmitting data wirelessly to the patient's mobile phone. The ease with which day-to-day blood sugars can now be profiled is revolutionising the control of type 1 diabetes and there is the potential for interfacing glucose results with the output of a continuous subcutaneous insulin infusion pump. Patients with type 1 diabetes should now routinely be offered Real-time or Flash continuous glucose monitoring. A major advantage of this approach is to reduce the fear of hypoglycaemia which can be a significant burden. Carefully selected insulin-dependent type 2 diabetics may also be offered Flash monitoring—especially those who have recurrent hypoglycaemia, where physical or cognitive disability excludes capillary testing or those patients who are dependent on care workers to monitor their blood sugars.

What about urine testing? Urine testing for sugar is unreliable for both the diagnosis and the accurate monitoring of diabetes and has been largely replaced by capillary blood sugar measurement. Normally, glucose spills over from the blood into the

---

BOX 6.3 ■ Good Practice in Fingerprick Testing

- Have you re-read the instructions recently?
- Has your machine been calibrated? Does it measure blood ketones?
- Is the finger warm, dry and clean? Are your hands dry and clean?
- Prick the side, not the pulp, of the fingertips. Use the middle and ring fingers
- Produce a large drop of blood by milking up from the finger base
- Do not let the skin touch the test strip
- Apply the drop to the strip so that it covers the test area—do not smear it on
- Follow the instructions
- If you have to, wipe or blot off the blood as instructed
- Use the meter as instructed
- Do you audit your practice?
- How do your results compare with the laboratory sugars?
- Is your ward's blood glucose monitoring subject to a quality control programme?

urine once the blood sugar is above 11 mmol/L, but the level can vary from as little as 7 mmol/L to as much as 15 mmol/L. Urinary ketones are still used to help identify and help manage DKA − ++ on a Ketostix is roughly equivalent to 3 mmol/L of capillary blood ketones.

What about one high blood sugar on admission? By its nature, the blood sugar in most medical admissions will be a random one rather than fasting. Acute illnesses raise the stress hormones glucagon, adrenaline (epinephrine) and cortisone. Their actions counteract those of insulin. This may lead to a temporary diabetic state or may unmask latent diabetes. This effect can be exacerbated by some of the drugs that are used on the AMU:

- Corticosteroids: especially dexamethasone or high-dose methylprednisolone
- Diuretics

The action that is taken depends on the circumstances and in particular on the health of the patient. A fit type II diabetic can tolerate short-term hyperglycaemia relatively well compared with a patient with an acute illness such as a myocardial infarction. An obese new type II diabetic who has been slaking his increasing thirst with sugary soft drinks may well present with a sugar of 20 mmol/L or more and yet, in the absence of any other complications, this type of patient can often be controlled with dietary advice alone. In contrast, a non-obese patient with marked osmotic symptoms without a high sugar intake will probably need immediate treatment with oral hypoglycaemics or insulin.

Similar considerations apply to type I diabetics. In particular, single injections of insulin to 'bring the sugar down' are usually unhelpful, as they obscure the pattern of diabetic control and are no substitute for planned management of diabetes, taking into account the medical condition and the patient's nutritional needs.

In summary, considerations when planning short-term control include:

- Is there a risk of ketosis? (Urinary and plasma ketone levels)
- Will the blood sugar levels directly influence the medical outcome?
- Are there osmotic symptoms (thirst and polyuria) or dehydration?
- What are the risks and consequences of hypoglycaemia?

What is the importance of capillary and urinary ketones? Checking for urinary ketones and measuring fingerprick capillary ketones are fundamental to identifying patients at risk of (or already suffering from) diabetic ketoacidosis.

There are three types of ketones (also known as ketone bodies):

- Acetoacetic acid
- Acetone
- β-Hydroxybutyrate

Ketones are acidic substances that appear in the blood when there is excessive breakdown of the body's fat stores. They are used by muscles as an important source of energy when glucose is not available, either because of fasting or because there is no insulin available to drive glucose into the muscle cells.

BOX 6.4 ■ Causes of Ketonuria

Starvation (extreme dieting, vomiting)	Small to moderate amounts
Strict dieting in obese type II diabetes	Small to moderate amounts
Diabetic ketoacidosis	Moderate to large amounts

In fasting states and in dietary glucose restriction, the ketone production is insufficient to cause acidosis, and there is only mild or moderate ketonuria. This is in contrast to the situation in severe insulin deficiency, in which there is a large rise in blood ketone levels that can lead to dangerous acidosis (Box 6.4).

Of the three ketones, acetone (which smells like nail varnish remover) is largely excreted in the breath, while acetoacetic acid and β-hydroxybutyrate are excreted in the urine. Urinary ketones can be detected with Ketostix, which is specific for acetoacetic acid. Several blood glucose monitors are now available which will also measure capillary ketone levels, specifically β-hydroxybutyrate. Near-patient testing for capillary ketone levels is replacing urinary ketone measurements for diagnosing and managing DKA.

It is vital for clinicians to appreciate the difference between starvation (or vomiting) ketosis and DKA. This is a particular issue in the anorexic or dieting type II diabetic who shows moderate ketonuria: do you rush in with a DKA regimen, or can you reassure the patient and even congratulate them on sticking so rigidly to their diet? This depends on the clinical picture. In general, ketonuria is much more likely to indicate impending ketoacidosis in the thin type I diabetic than in the obese patient whose diabetes is controlled with oral hypoglycaemics. Moreover, the patient with ketoacidosis is likely to have warning symptoms: thirst, hyperventilation and nausea. The action the clinician would take is also dependent on whether or not there is an acidosis. A diabetic patient with moderate ketonuria may look 'too well' for DKA; measure the capillary ketones and check for acidosis. As a guide:

Capillary Ketone Levels

<0.6 mmol/L	Normal
0.6–1.4 mmol/L	Repeat in 2 h
1.5–2.9 mmol/L	Risk of DKA
>2.9 mmol/L	Probable DKA

A simple venous blood sample for pH and plasma HCO_3 level will reveal if there is a cause for concern: if the pH is less than 7.3 and the bicarbonate level is low (less than 15 mmol/L), there is acidosis, if it is normal, then both nurse and patient can be reassured.

Case Study 6.1 illustrates difficulties with blood sugar control in a type II diabetics. The main problem was steroid-induced hyperglycaemia without ketosis. Metformin is a

---

CASE STUDY 6.1   **Diabetes in Asthma: Steroid-Induced Diabetes and Hypertension?**

A 42-year-old overweight female was admitted with a 3-week history of severe thirst and polyuria. Her blood sugar was 34 mmol/L and there were no ketones in her urine. Her blood pressure was 160/115 mm Hg.

She had chronic asthma controlled by inhaled corticosteroids. For 8 weeks, she had needed high doses of oral steroids 20–30 mg daily to control her worsening symptoms.

Treatment with metformin neither dropped her sugars sufficiently nor did it clear her osmotic symptoms. She was therefore treated with short-term insulin while her asthma was controlled and her oral steroids were withdrawn. She was referred to the respiratory unit for a review of her asthma and control of her blood pressure.

---

commonly prescribed first-line oral hypoglycaemic and tends to be used in obese type II diabetic patients. It was a reasonable choice in this case, although precautions have to be taken when it is used. The main problems concern the risk of lactic acidosis—a life-threatening metabolic disorder. There are a number of situations in which metformin is contraindicated because of this risk, some of which are relevant to the AMU:

- After a myocardial infarction
- In renal failure
- In severe liver disease
- In patients who are shocked or critically ill
- In patients who are more than 80 years old
- In patients who are having IV contrast studies

Recent guidelines for steroid-induced hyperglycaemia prefer once-daily gliclazide to metformin—with up-titration, which in most cases will control the blood sugars.

A blood pressure of 160/115 mm Hg is unacceptable in a diabetic patient since *any* level of hypertension in a diabetic is associated with accelerated vascular and renal disease. Aggressive blood pressure control reduces the risks considerably, and in this patient, a target level of 140/80 mm Hg would be entirely reasonable. It is likely that once oral steroids were withdrawn from this patient, both her hyperglycaemia and her hypertension will settle. Short-term insulin was indicated mainly because of the marked osmotic symptoms.

Case Study 6.2 brings out more difficulties associated with the use of metformin in an elderly diabetic. The main problem here relates to the interaction of an acute medical illness and the patient's oral hypoglycaemic drugs, rather than hyperglycaemia itself. This patient presented a complex problem of acidosis but not ketosis and renal failure (high urea and creatinine). The blood sugar was normal. Metformin has caused lactic acidosis and the two diuretics have combined to produce profound abnormalities in the sodium and potassium levels. Drug side effects are common in elderly patients, and particular care has to be taken in the case of elderly diabetics, who are prone to complicated acute medical problems.

CASE STUDY 6.2	Complication With Metformin in the Elderly: Lactic Acidosis

An 80-year-old male with type II diabetes presented with a 3-week history of vomiting, breathlessness and diminishing mobility. On admission, he was breathless and shivering. His mental test score was 4/10, and his temperature was 37.4°C.

Treatment had been metformin 500 mg tds, spironolactone 100 mg bd, furosemide 80 mg od and gliclazide 160 mg bd.

On admission, test results were as follows:
- BP 150/62 mm Hg
- WCC 21.8 × 10⁹/L
- Potassium 8.6 mmol/L, sodium 120 mmol/L, urea 38.2 mmol/L, creatinine 251 mmol/L, sugar 6.4 mmol/L, bicarbonate 5 mmol/L, lactate 4.6 mmol/L.
- Urine: no glucose and no ketones.

Practical Management of Diabetes in Adverse Circumstances

Several situations are encountered on the AMU in which it would not be appropriate simply to continue with the patient's usual diabetic regimen and in which the management of diabetes becomes an important practical problem:

- Acute medical conditions that destabilise diabetes
- Acute medical conditions in which hyperglycaemia should be avoided
- Diabetic patients who are vomiting or unable to eat and drink normally

Patients with type I diabetes need insulin at all times, whether they are eating or not; the acutely ill medical patient who is also diabetic is at risk from rapidly changing sugar levels and the development of ketoacidosis. In these patients, it is important to ensure good control with as simple a regimen as possible. Whether type II diabetics require the same intensive approach depends on the severity of the medical condition, but in many acute situations due priority has to be given to the diabetic control, in addition to treating the immediate medical problem. The aim in either type is to maintain a reasonable blood sugar without risking hypoglycaemia.

Variable Rate Intravenous Insulin Infusion—VRIII ('Sliding Scale') or GKI? Self-Management of Diabetes in Hospital

To counter the increasing number of errors in the management of IDDM in hospital, appropriate patients should be offered the choice of monitoring their blood sugar and adjusting and administering their own insulin. It requires a written agreement from the patient and does not replace formal documentation of the usual observations and insulin administration. For emergency admissions, factors such as impaired conscious level, DKA or confusion, the need for intravenous insulin precludes self-management.

> **BOX 6.5 ■ Pros and Cons of GKI and a Variable Rate Intravenous Insulin Infusion (VRIII)**
>
> | **GKI** | **VRIII** |
> |---|---|
> | Simple to use | Requires volumetric pump and syringe driver |
> | Risk of water overload | Risk of hypoglycaemia |
> | Insulin + glucose together | Suitable for complex fluid regimens |

Two techniques are used to control diabetes in the sick and unstable patient: the careful use of IV insulin and glucose, either as separate infusions of dextrose and a variable rate of IV insulin—termed a variable rate intravenous insulin infusion (VRIII)—previously called a 'sliding scale'—or with a single infusion (bag) containing glucose, potassium and insulin known as a *GKI* (Box 6.5).

In some hospitals, the VRIII is thought to have several disadvantages compared with the simpler GKI 'single-bag' infusion:

■ The infusions are complicated to administer.
■ The dependence on separate infusions of insulin and glucose increases the risk of inadvertent swings in blood sugar.

The opposing view (and one that is increasingly adopted in many guidelines) is that the advent of sophisticated infusion and syringe pumps has simplified their administration and minimised the risk of error. There are also advantages of having the flexibility of two adjustable infusions, particularly in critical situations in which there is a need for complex fluid regimens. Current guidelines recommend a VRIII in sick type I diabetics who have hyperglycaemia but do not have (or no longer have) ketosis.

The safest approach is to use the regimen that is most familiar to the unit and that has been shown to be trouble-free during its use. Whichever regimen is favoured, the key is the attention to detail in setting up and running the regimen, combined with an appropriate level of monitoring.

Clinicians must appreciate that, whatever their relative advantages and disadvantages, these two techniques do *not* apply to the immediate management of a patient with DKA—in other words, those patients showing:

■ Capillary blood ketones >3 mmol/L/urinary ketones present in moderate to large (>than ++) amounts and
■ Acidosis (low plasma bicarbonate [<15 mmol/L]/pH < 7.3)
■ Sugar levels more than 11 mmol/L

In these patients, the DKA regimen (see later) should be followed.

GLUCOSE INFUSION AND A SLIDING SCALE OF INSULIN (VRIII)

How to manage a diabetic with a variable rate intravenous insulin infusion. A variable rate of insulin (VRIII) is used in unstable patients to match the blood sugar with an appropriate dose of insulin. The insulin must always be administered with a source of glucose (substrate), usually 5% dextrose. The aim of a VRIII is to keep the blood sugar under fairly tight control—in the range of 6–10 mmol/L, while avoiding hypoglycaemia. The indications for a VRIII include an unwell type I diabetic who is not eating or drinking or has recurrent vomiting (not due to DKA) or is severely unwell (e.g., sepsis) and needs good diabetic control.

When using a VRIII:

- Any long-acting basal insulin should be continued at the usual dose and time while on a VRIII.
- Check the capillary blood sugar hourly and the electrolytes at least daily.
- There should be a dependable and constant supply of carbohydrate as IV dextrose to prevent insulin-induced hypoglycaemia.
- The insulin infusion rate should never be zero (unless the patient becomes hypoglycaemic).
- Alter the whole sliding scale if the initial doses do not produce rapid control.
- When discontinuing the infusion, it must be overlapped with the first dose of subcutaneous insulin by an hour.

The glucose infusion. Give 5% dextrose with 40 mmol of KCl at 100 mL/h. If fluids are restricted (e.g., cardiac failure) use 10% dextrose with 20 mmol of KCl (0.3% KCl) at 50 mL/h—omit the potassium if the potassium is more than 5 mmol/L. The potassium should be checked at least 6 hourly.

The insulin infusion. Make up an infusion of neutral insulin solution (Actrapid) 50 units in 50 mL of isotonic saline in a 50-mL syringe and driver. The pump must be alarmed and the lines fitted with safety features to prevent sudden unloading of the insulin into the patient (anti-syphon and anti-back-tracking valves).

Target blood sugar. In sick patients a VRIII should be considered with capillary blood sugars greater than 10 mmol/L. The aim is to achieve capillary blood sugar levels in the range of 6–10 mmol/L. Check the glucose stix hourly while the patient is ill, then reduce to 2–4 hourly once the glucose is stable.

Adjusting the rate of insulin (the sliding scale). Table 6.2 gives three scales relating the insulin rate to the capillary blood sugar: a reduced rate for patients normally on 24 or

TABLE 6.2 ■ Typical Sliding Scales

Capillary Blood Sugar	Reduced Rate (Units/h)	Standard Rate	Increased Rate
<4.0	0	0	0
4.1–8.0	0.5	1	2
8.1–12	1	2	4
12.1–16	2	4	6
16.1–20	3	5	7
20.1–24	4	6	8
>24	6	8	10

fewer units of insulin a day, a standard rate suitable for most patients and an increased rate for patients normally on more than 100 units per day. The scale is reviewed 6 h after starting—if the capillary sugars are above the target range and not falling, the next scale-up is introduced or, if already on the top scale, one is customised. If a patient becomes hypoglycaemic, the VRIII is stopped while the hypo is treated and then restarted, after no more than 20–30 min, stepping down to a lower rate scale.

THE DIGAMI REGIMEN: AN EXAMPLE OF CONTROLLING THE BLOOD SUGAR IN ACUTE ILLNESS

The Diabetes Mellitus, Insulin Glucose Infusion in Acute Myocardial Infarction (DIGAMI) study itself showed a possible survival advantage in keeping sugars within the normal range in patients with acute coronary syndromes who are either known to have diabetes or whose blood sugar at the time of admission is more than 11 mmol/L— findings that may be applicable to other groups such as those with acute stroke (Fig. 6.1). The DIGAMI regimen is an excellent template for the practical approach to the close

FIGURE 6.1 DIGAMI (Diabetes Mellitus, Insulin Glucose Infusion in Acute Myocardial Infarction) regimen: an example of blood sugar control in acute medical illness. *DKA, Diabetic ketoacidosis.*

control of blood sugars in acute severe illness. In contrast to a VRIII, the DIGAMI regimen uses the *trend* in capillary blood sugar to titrate the rate of administration of insulin and may give smoother control.

GLUCOSE, POTASSIUM AND INSULIN

How to manage diabetes with a GKI infusion. The GKI infusion is the preferred way in some units to control blood sugars in a number of situations:

- The recovery period in DKA (i.e., once blood sugars fall below 13 mmol/L)
- Acute, severe illness in a non-ketotic diabetic patient (e.g., sepsis, stroke)
- Post-myocardial infarction hyperglycaemia (once sugars fall below 13 mmol/L)
- Type I diabetics who are nil-by-mouth (e.g., upper gastrointestinal bleeding awaiting endoscopy)

The intravenous infusion

- 500 mL of 10% dextrose and 10 mmol of KCl (omit the KCl if the serum potassium is more than 5 mmol/L)
- Add neutral insulin solution (Actrapid) to the bag according to the blood sugar:

Blood sugar	2.0–7.0 mmol/L	Add 8 units (1 unit/h)
Blood sugar	7.1–11.0 mmol/L	Add 16 units (2 units/h)
Blood sugar	11.1–17.0 mmol/L	Add 32 units (4 units/h)

The doses of insulin may need to be reduced for each range of blood sugars if the patient is sensitive to insulin. Substitute doses of insulin for each range would be 4, 12 and 24 units.

Some types of patients need more insulin than usual:

- The patients with extreme obesity
- Patients on steroid therapy (prednisolone, dexamethasone)
- Patients with cirrhosis
- Patients with previous high insulin doses, for example, >70 units per day

Some patients may need to have the scale 'individualised'. In these situations, it may be necessary to consult with the diabetes team.

Infusion rate. 500 mL every 8 h (approximately 60 mL/h) using an alarmed infusion pump.

Target blood sugar. Aim for blood sugars in the range of 4–12 mmol/L.

Adjustments. Check and record the blood sugar with glucose stix every hour. If it is necessary to change the insulin dose, make up and start a new bag, but do *not* change the infusion rate, which stays constant at 60 mL/h.

Blood sugar more than 17 mmol/L? Stop the dextrose infusion and start isotonic saline (0.9%) at 80 mL/h. Check the capillary blood or urinary ketones and measure the venous bicarbonate. If this is not ketoacidosis, start a low-dose IV infusion of neutral insulin (Actrapid) (see below) at 4 units/h until the sugar falls to less than 17 mmol/L for 2 consecutive hours. Then restart GKI.

Blood sugar less than 2 mmol/L? Stop the GKI and give 10% dextrose 500 mL at 60 mL/h. Check the glucose stix every half hour and restart GKI when the blood sugar increases to 4 mmol/L. If the patient becomes clinically hypoglycaemic, seek urgent medical help and prepare to increase the strength of the dextrose infusion.

Hints on converting from IV infusions to subcutaneous insulin

- Once the patient is stable and able to eat and drink, change to subcutaneous insulin
- Change over in the morning, not at the end of the day
- Plan to give the first subcutaneous injection before breakfast
- If the patient is already on insulin, add 10% to their usual dose for the first few days
- If not previously on insulin, start on 30–40 units of neutral insulin solution (Actrapid) divided into four doses
- Stop the insulin infusion 60 min after the first dose of subcutaneous insulin (IV insulin disappears from the circulation in 5 min)

How good is your subcutaneous insulin injection technique? Insulin should be injected using an 8-mm needle by pinching up the skin and subcutaneous tissue (*not* the muscle) with the thumb and index finger. The injection is given at right angles (perpendicular) to the skin: *make a tent and put the insulin in through the front door.* The fold should be maintained throughout the injection and for 5–10 s afterwards before the needle is removed. During the early hospital stay, the abdomen should be used (for the fastest rate of absorption and onset of action). Only use a specific insulin syringe.

Note: The pinching technique does not apply to the new insulin pens, in which the preferred technique is a vertical injection into the skin.

Managing a case of severe medical problems and hyperglycaemia (Case Study 6.3).

This is the story of acute severe pulmonary oedema with a preceding history of probable recent onset angina. Ischaemic heart disease complicated by a possible myocardial infarction is the most likely primary diagnosis. There is also a problem with diabetes: the patient is on maximum oral hypoglycaemic therapy with two drugs, yet his doctor is still worried about recent blood results.

The patient's vital signs of hypotension, tachycardia and breathlessness are all in keeping with acute pulmonary oedema. However, DKA also can present like this. Although the blood sugar indicates that the patient's diabetes is out of control, the absence of ketones in the urine is reassuring at this stage. It will be important to ensure further urine testing remains negative for ketones and that capillary ketones are less than 0.6 mmol/L. The emergency laboratory blood results will also clarify the situation. The finding of heavy proteinuria without signs or symptoms of infection raises the possibility of diabetic kidney damage, which is characteristically associated with both generalised vascular disease and hypertension.

The investigations confirmed hyperglycaemia without DKA. There is mild renal failure. The GP results are helpful: the renal failure has not developed acutely and the patient's diabetes has not been under good control. The HbA_{1c} measures the amount of haemoglobin that has been linked to glucose in the blood: it has become an important indicator of diabetic control because it reflects the levels of blood sugars that have been occurring over the past 2 or 3 months. The higher the HbA_{1c}, the higher the recent blood sugars. A 'normal' target level of 48 mmol/mol or less in the absence of repeated hypoglycaemic episodes is an indication of good control. In this patient, the level of 97 mmol/mol confirms the suspicion of poor control. Reducing the level from 97 mmol/mol will have a progressive effect on reducing the risk of diabetic complications, particularly neuropathy, retinopathy and nephropathy. The immediate priorities are as follows:

- To clear the pulmonary oedema (symptoms, saturations and respiratory rate)
- To slow the atrial fibrillation (rate from the cardiac monitor)
- To control the blood sugar (hourly glucose stix)

Fluid balance will be critical:

- The patient's heart may not cope with large volumes of fluid.
- There is uncertainty about the patient's renal function.
- The patient may need multiple infusions (e.g., inotropic support or nitrates).

The interventions described in the case study resulted in some improvement in the patient's pulmonary oedema and atrial fibrillation. The main problems were persistent hypotension, with low urine output and continuing hyperglycaemia (but no ketosis). There was uncertainty as to whether or not the patient could be hypovolaemic. High blood sugars like these, particularly if they had been associated with an osmotic diuresis before admission, could have resulted in dehydration.

In summary, the patient in Case Study 6.3 presented with pulmonary oedema due to ischaemic heart disease. These were complications of poorly controlled diabetes, diabetic renal disease and inadequately treated hypertension. His management illustrates how care must be coordinated and prioritised to address both the primary medical problems and the diabetes.

Could We (or Should We) Assess Obesity in the AMU?

At least 75% of all newly diagnosed patients with NIDDM are obese, but this is difficult to quantify in the acutely sick patient. Nonetheless, weight loss of 10 kg in this group will halve their fasting blood sugar, reduce diabetes-related death rates by a third, drop their diastolic blood pressure by 20 mm Hg and cut their cholesterol by 10%.

Patients with a body mass index (weight/height^2) of more than 30 kg/m^2 have significantly increased health risks. Similar considerations apply to waist circumference, which is a lot easier to measure in the acute situation: high risk is associated with waist circumferences greater than 102 cm in males and 88 cm in females.

CASE STUDY 6.3	Severe Breathlessness in a Male With Type II Diabetes

A 55-year-old male was admitted at 4:00 h with a 4-h history of increasing breathlessness associated with chest tightness and copious frothy sputum. He had been a diabetic for 5 years and took a combination of glibenclamide 15 mg once daily and metformin 850 mg twice daily. He was on no other medication. His family gave the additional history that for a month he had complained of chest discomfort on walking from his car to the office. He had also been concerned about his diabetes, his weight was increasing and his GP had not been happy with the results of his recent blood tests.

On admission to the AMU, the patient appeared as a distressed, overweight male, sitting forward on the trolley and fighting for breath. He was clammy, with cold extremities.

His skin, feet and pressure areas were all in good condition; there were no signs of infection.

Initial observations were as follows:
- Pulse 150 beats/min and irregular
- Blood pressure 80/50 mm Hg but difficult to hear
- Temperature 37°C
- Respiratory rate 30 breaths/min
- Oxygen saturation on 35% oxygen: 88%

The patient was conscious and orientated but was too breathless to speak. The finger-prick blood sugar was 28 mmol/L. A small quantity of urine was obtained, which showed large amounts of sugar and protein, but no ketones.

Arterial and venous blood samples were taken. The patient's electrocardiogram (ECG) showed atrial fibrillation at 160 beats/min, with acute ischaemic changes and left ventricular enlargement, but no signs of an actual infarct. A portable chest x-ray confirmed pulmonary oedema. The oxygen was increased to 60%. He was given 80 mg of IV furosemide and a small dose of IV diamorphine. He was started on subcutaneous low-molecular-weight heparin.

By this time his blood tests were back:
- Blood gases

• pH	7.35	Not acidotic
• pO_2	8.0 kPa	Should correct with increased oxygen
• pCO_2	4.0 kPa	Normal (usually low in diabetic ketoacidosis due to hyperventilation)
• Bicarbonate	19 mmol/L	Not acidotic

- Biochemistry

• Sugar	32 mmol/L	High
• Sodium	144 mmol/L	Normal
• Potassium	5.1 mmol/L	Normal
• Urea	28 mmol/L	High
• Creatinine	300 mmol/L	High

- The laboratory computer had some GP results from 6 weeks previously:

• Sugar	19 mmol/L	High
• Urea	24 mmol/L	High
• Creatinine	280 mmol/L	High
• HbA_{1c}	97 mmol/mol	High

To bring the patient's atrial fibrillation under rapid control, IV digoxin 0.75 mg was given in 50 mL of isotonic saline over 2 h. To control the blood sugar, an infusion was started at 6 units of insulin per hour. After careful consideration, a urethral catheter was passed to measure the hourly urine output.

CASE STUDY 6.3	Severe Breathlessness in a Male With Type II Diabetes — cont'd

Two hours later, the patient was less breathless and felt more comfortable. His observations were as follows:

- Pulse — 110 beats/min
- Blood pressure — 85/50 mm Hg
- Respiratory rate — 25 breaths/min
- Oxygen saturation — 95%
- Blood sugar — 25 mmol/L
- Urine output — 20 mL (negative for ketones)

A central line was passed, which showed normal to high central venous pressure (CVP) readings of between 15 and 20 cm H_2O, making it unlikely that the patient was hypovolaemic. He was started on a dobutamine infusion, to improve cardiac function and to increase his blood pressure. His insulin infusion rate was increased to 8 units/h. He was given a further 40 mg dose of IV furosemide.

On this regimen, the blood pressure increased to 110/70 mm Hg and his urine output improved to 70 mL/h. Once the blood sugars had decreased to 11 mmol/L, the infusion was replaced by subcutaneous insulin. The patient continued to improve over the following 24 h.

He was transferred to the care of the diabetic team to look at his cardiac status in more detail and to reassess his long-term diabetic control. Subsequent enquiries confirmed that there had been concerns over previously elevated blood pressures of around 160/110 mm Hg, and that he had been considered for antihypertensive treatment 'if the levels did not settle'.

Management of Acute Diabetic Emergencies

DIABETIC KETOACIDOSIS

A reasonably sized district general hospital can expect to admit around two cases of DKA per month. Most will be of moderate severity, but a few patients will be severely ill. Among this population will be the brittle diabetics with recurrent ketoacidosis and often with a history of poor compliance.

Causes of Diabetic Ketoacidosis (Box 6.6)

Most cases of DKA are precipitated by infection or some form of disruption to the insulin treatment. This is often due to the inappropriate action taken by the patient, or surprisingly, by the in-patient team, at the time of an acute illness: usually stopping or reducing insulin because of problems with maintaining oral intake. An important minority of cases of DKA are the first manifestation of new-onset diabetes. There will also be a number of brittle diabetics with recurrent ketoacidosis—predominantly female, socially disadvantaged and poorly compliant, this group often has associated eating disorders. Recently, an increasing problem of ketoacidosis in type II diabetes is being recognised, particularly in patients of Afro-Caribbean origin. Interestingly, once the episode is over, these patients can return to oral hypoglycaemics or even to dietary treatment alone. Patients on the new SGLT2 inhibitors also appear prone to a form of DKA in which, unusually, the blood sugar can be near normal.

BOX 6.6 ▦ Causes of Diabetic Ketoacidosis

Infection	40%
Disruption of insulin treatment	25%
New onset	15%
Other causes (e.g., infarct, pregnancy)	20%

Underlying Mechanism

In DKA, there is an acute shortage of insulin. As a result, the liver produces and releases excessive amounts of glucose that appear in the blood (*hyperglycaemia*) and that spill over into the urine (*glycosuria*). The heavy glucose load in the urine pulls in water and electrolytes by osmosis, leading to losses of fluid (*dehydration*); loss of potassium (*hypokalaemia*); and loss of sodium (*hyponatraemia*), phosphate and magnesium. Because there is a shortage of insulin, sugar cannot enter the cells and so the body starts to burn adipose tissue (fat stores) as an alternative energy source. The adipose tissue breaks down to free fatty acids, which are in turn converted into ketones by the liver. Some of the ketones are used by muscles for energy and some are excreted in the urine (*urine positive for ketones*). Ketones are acidic substances, so when excess ketones appear in the blood they produce an *acidosis*, indicated by a low pH and bicarbonate level (measured by near-patient testing on venous blood in a blood gas analyser). The ketones can be smelt on the breath and measured in the blood and the urine using modern dual-purpose glucose meters.

The definition of DKA is the presence of all three of:
1. Capillary blood glucose 11 mmol/L or more
2. Capillary blood ketones more than 3 mmol/L (or ++ ketonuria)
3. Venous pH less than 7.3 or bicarbonate less than 15 mmol/L

Severe DKA in which ITU care is required has these features:
- Capillary blood ketones >6 mmol/L pH < 7.1
- HCO_3 <5 mmol/L potassium <3.5 mmol/L
- Sats <92% SBP <90
- Pulse <60 pulse >100
- Drowsy or GCS less than 12

The consequences of DKA are illustrated in Fig. 6.2.

Management

The key to the treatment of DKA should be clear from the above discussion:
- Adequate insulin replacement
- Correction of fluid and electrolyte loss

Acidosis does not usually need correcting, as it responds to the reversal of ketosis by insulin, fluid and electrolyte therapy. Case Study 6.4 describes a case of acute severe DKA.

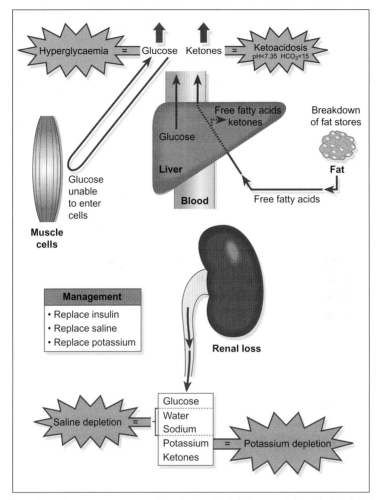

FIGURE 6.2   The consequences of acute insulin deficiency: diabetic ketoacidosis.

Hyperventilation is a sign of acidotic breathing (the body is trying to correct the acidosis by blowing off carbon dioxide). The patient in Case Study 6.4 had not been eating for 2 days and was therefore at risk from ketosis. Missing a single dose of insulin would have been enough to accelerate the onset of ketosis.

The patient had signs of DKA with hypovolaemia (low blood pressure). There were no features of infection or myocardial infarction. In particular, the chest was clear, there was no skin sepsis and there was no renal angle tenderness. There was no sign of meningeal irritation. Abdominal pain and tenderness are common features in DKA and can be due to acute fatty liver infiltration or pancreatitis. The patient was able to protect her airway (GCS above 8).

Hyperkalaemia is common in DKA, but there is usually a rapid fall as soon as fluids and insulin are given and the potassium enters the cells. Normally, we would administer

CASE STUDY 6.4 | Acute Severe Diabetic Ketoacidosis

A female who had been a diabetic for 30 years, now aged 50, was admitted with a 48-h history of anorexia, headache and breathlessness. Her blood sugar the day before admission was 17 mmol/L. Her husband usually administered her insulin, and she had good control, with blood sugars in the range of 3–5 mmol/L on twice daily isophane 9 and 7 units and morning soluble 5 units. After a domestic upset, there was some doubt about whether she had received her insulin on the day of admission to hospital. Her husband came home from work to find her nearly unconscious and hyperventilating. There had been one previous admission with DKA 5 years before.

The ECG showed signs of an acutely raised potassium level. The urine showed large amounts of ketones, protein and sugar. BM stix was 55 mmol/L, capillary blood ketones were 5 mmol/L.

Blood samples, including blood cultures, were sent for analysis, and an immediate injection of calcium gluconate (to provide urgent cardiac protection from the very high potassium) was given intravenously. A central line, nasogastric tube and urethral catheter were passed. A portable chest radiograph was performed.

On examination, the patient was apyrexial, respiration rate was 40/min, pulse was 110 beats/min and blood pressure was 90/60 mm Hg. Oxygen saturations were 99% on air. She was restless and aggressive. Her GCS was 9/15. The examination was otherwise negative, apart from generalised abdominal tenderness. Her breath smelt of ketones.

The following test results came back:

Hb	12.9 g/dL	Normal
WCC	29.7 × 10⁹/L	Very high as is common in diabetic ketoacidosis, even if infection is not present
Glucose	58.7 mmol/L	Very high (DKA *can* occur at sugars as low as 12 mmol/L, but most are >25 mmol/L)
Sodium	127 mmol/L	Low due to sodium lost in the osmotic diuresis
Potassium	8.6 mmol/L	*Very* high; the total body potassium is low, however, and the level will fall rapidly with treatment (known as 'hidden' potassium loss)
Urea	14.2 mmol/L	High due to dehydration
Creatinine	226 mmol/L	High due to dehydration (normal when tested 3 months prior to admission: always check previous notes for pre-existing kidney function)
pH	6.93	Severe acidosis (most patients with DKA will have a pH of 7.0–7.2)
pO₂	21.6 kPa	Good oxygen levels (on oxygen therapy)
pCO₂	1.6 kPa	Low (blown off by hyperventilation)
Bicarbonate	2.0 mmol/L	Low (this increases as the acidosis improves with treatment)

INSULIN THERAPY

A fixed-dose insulin infusion was prepared consisting of 50 mL of 0.9% (normal) saline with 50 units of neutral insulin solution (Actrapid), administered at a rate of 8 units (8 mL) per hour. Her usual basal insulin was continued.

INTRAVENOUS FLUID REPLACEMENT

- 2 L of 0.9% saline were given in the first hour (via an infusion pump).
- 1 L of 0.9% saline was given in the second hour.
- 500 mL/h of 0.9% saline was then given for 4 h.

By 12 h, the patient had improved and her urine was showing moderate amounts of ketones only. A 10% dextrose infusion at 100 mL/h was started in the arm opposite to the saline infusion and the FRIII replaced by a VRIII.

CASE STUDY 6.4   Acute Severe Diabetic Ketoacidosis—cont'd

POTASSIUM REPLACEMENT

- Potassium was added to the infusion at 20 mmol/h once the serum potassium had fallen to less than 5.0 mmol/L

BICARBONATE

- 100 mmol of sodium bicarbonate (600 mL of 1.4% sodium bicarbonate) was given through the central line over 30 min. Bicarbonate is only used in DKA when there is severe acidosis.

MONITORING

- Hourly BM stix and capillary blood ketones were continued until the patient could eat and drink normally.
- Hourly pulse, BP, temperature, respiratory rate, GCS/ACVPU (AVPU plus new-onset confusion) and urine output until the patient was stable (at least 6 h).
- Hourly oxygen saturations and supplementary oxygen to keep the saturations in the range of 94%–98%; 2 hourly potassium, sugar, sodium, urea and bicarbonate until the sugar had fallen to 13 mmol/L.
- A flow diagram was used to show the progress of the blood tests.
- Urinary ketones were checked every 2 h (note that the ketonuria frequently increases initially and may take at least 24 h to clear from the urine).
- Continuous ECG monitor for 24 h (the risk of hyperkalaemia and arrhythmias).

potassium with the second litre of fluid. In this case, however, there were changes on the ECG showing that the high potassium level was putting the heart rhythm at risk. Urgent action was needed to bring the level down. The patient was going to need careful fluid balance—hence the central line and catheter. The nasogastric tube was to prevent aspiration of stomach contents in the event of acute gastric paralysis with distension, a common problem in severe DKA.

The importance of fluid balance in caring the diabetic patient. Clinical staff must be exceptionally careful monitoring the input and output in acutely ill diabetic patients. In DKA and non-ketotic hyperglycaemia, high volumes of fluid are being given to patients who are in a critical state because of fluid depletion amounting to between 4 and 6 L. However, these patients may well have both cardiac and renal problems due to their diabetes and are at risk from fluid overload. This is critical in the first few hours of admission: typically, a patient with severe DKA may not pass urine for the first hour or two of rehydration, but if this persists they may need catheterisation and even a central venous line to ensure that the fluid input is not overly aggressive. Some DKA protocols recommend 2 L of fluid in the first hour, but this would be too fast for the frail, elderly and those with heart disease. Moreover, over-enthusiastic fluid replacement will wash out ketones and lower the blood sugar, but paradoxically lead to a worsening of the acidosis. An example of judicious fluid replacement of, say, a 7 L deficit (severe dehydration) in a frail patient would be as follows:

- 2 L isotonic saline over 4 h
- 1 L isotonic saline over 4 h

- 0.5 L isotonic saline over 8 h
- The remaining 3.5 L over the next 24 h

Careful fluid management is the key to good treatment. The measure of a well-managed acute DKA is an accurate fluid balance chart showing hourly input and output and a flowchart of the capillary blood sugars, insulin infusion rate, capillary ketones, potassium, venous pH and bicarbonate.

What to Avoid While Treatment Is Working

Hypokalaemia. Patients with DKA may start with a high potassium, but the level drops rapidly once the potassium moves back into the cells when insulin is given. Potassium is usually administered as a pre-mixed bag of saline containing 40 mmol/potassium per litre of saline. Adjustments to the rate of potassium replacement can be made according to the 2-hourly potassium results. An example of the way to adjust the potassium supplements is shown in Table 6.3.

Hypoglycaemia. Start 10% glucose once the sugar falls to less than 14 mmol/L.

Fluid overload. The overall fluid deficit will be between 4 and 6 L. In a sick diabetic patient, it is wise to use a central line and monitor the CVP. Any infusion should be controlled with a volumetric pump.

Aspiration. Care of the patient with altered consciousness. Empty the stomach contents with a nasogastric tube if necessary.

Intracerebral oedema. This grave complication is unusual and tends to occur in those patients younger than 20 years old. It usually occurs during the first 24 h after initial apparent metabolic and clinical improvement. There is a sudden deterioration in the conscious level (fall in the GCS) with neurological signs such as severe headache, neck stiffness, fitting and bilateral upgoing plantars. It may be seen with over-enthusiastic fluid replacement (in these cases the blood appears diluted and the sodium level falls below normal, e.g., to 120 mmol/L) or it can simply occur for no obvious reason in a severe DKA. Diagnosis is by CT scan (and excluding meningitis or stroke) and treatment aims to reduce the raised intracranial pressure with mannitol (100 mL of 20% mannitol over 20 min) and dexamethasone.

A management protocol for DKA

Adequate fluid replacement is the most important early intervention: Intravenous fluids correct dehydration, wash out the ketones and correct the electrolyte levels in the

TABLE 6.3 ■ Adjustment of Potassium Level With Supplements

Serum Potassium (mmol/L)	Potassium Added to Each Litre of Saline
<3.5	Senior advice
3.5–5.5	40 (mmol)
>5.5 or anuric	Nil

blood. Large volumes are required but caution is necessary in the elderly, those with renal or heart failure and in young adolescents.

Weight-based *fixed-rate* **insulin infusion (FRIII)**: From the outset, Actrapid insulin is infused intravenously at a fixed rate of 0.1 unit/kg/h. Thus a 70 kg patient requires 7 units/h. Regardless of weight, the rate should not exceed 15 units/h. No initial bolus is necessary. Once the capillary glucose falls below 14 mmol/L consider reducing the FRIII to 0.05 units kg/h.

Patients already on basal analogue or basal human insulin should have this continued at their normal dose and time. A patient's own insulin pump and its infusion set should be removed entirely and stored securely (for later interrogation).

Bedside testing to drive successful management (Table 6.4): Management is based on hourly near-patient testing (handheld glucose/ketone meters and ward blood gas machines) of the capillary blood glucose and ketone levels, venous (not arterial) bicarbonate and pH, and electrolytes (notably the potassium level). These are the markers of successful treatment—with the biochemical targets over the first 6 h of:

- Increasing the bicarbonate level at 3 mmol/L/h
- Reducing the blood sugar at 3 mmol/L/h
- Reducing the capillary blood ketones at 0.5 mmol/L/h
- Maintaining the potassium at 4.0 to 5.5 mmol/L

Resolution of DKA is recognised by:

- Blood sugar less than 14 mmol/L
- Capillary blood ketones less than 0.6 mmol/L

Paradoxically, large volumes of saline initially reduce the level of (HCO3)—rendering it an unreliable indicator of resolution.

A saline arm and a glucose arm: Once the blood sugar falls below 14 mmol/L the patient needs glucose on which the insulin can work—as a 10% solution running in parallel to the saline and insulin infusions and preferably given in the opposite arm.

Four stages in management:

0 to 60 min: Immediately start insulin and restore the fluids.

60 min to 6 h: Make IV fluid adjustments and confirm that the treatment targets are on course.

6 to 12 h: Continue FRIII and start glucose infusion using the opposite arm.

12 h and beyond: Confirm resolution of DKA and change to a VRIII or switch to subcutaneous insulin.

TABLE 6.4 ■ **Blood Sugar and the Rates of IV Insulin and Dextrose**

Blood Sugar	Insulin (units/h)	10% Dextrose (mL/h)
14	6	Nil
9–13.9	3	100
9	2	200

The DKA Treatment Regime

0 to 60 Min: FRIII and Initial Fluid Replacement

Prepare 50 units of Actrapid insulin or Humulin S in 50 mL of 0.9% saline and infuse intravenously at 0.1 units/kg/h (FRIII). Administer any usual long-acting insulin (e.g., Glargine, Detemir or Degludec) at their normal dose and time.

Restore the circulating volume: if the SBP is less than 90, give 500 mL of 0.9% saline over 15 min and repeat if the SBP stays below 90. Once the SBP is above 90 (or if it had not initially been that low) give 1 L of 0.9% saline over an hour. The insulin and saline should, if possible, be given in opposite arms.

60 Min to 6 H: Hitting Biochemical Targets and Avoiding Hypoglycaemia

Check glucose, capillary blood ketones and urinary ketones hourly, check venous blood gases and potassium at 60 min, 2, 4 and 6 h. Continue fluid replacement—usually starting potassium with the second litre of fluid. One litre of 0.9% saline with 40 mmol of potassium chloride over 2 h, 1 L of 0.9% saline with 40 mmol of potassium chloride over 2 h, 1 L of 0.9% saline with 40 mmol of potassium chloride over 4 h.

Check biochemical targets are being met—see above. If they are not—check the lines, the pump and the amount of insulin left in the syringe. Consider increasing the FRIII in increments of 1 unit/h.

When the capillary glucose falls below 14 mmol/L, start 10% glucose IV at 125 mL/h in parallel to the IV saline and potassium (in the opposite arm). Consider reducing the FRIII to 0.05 U/kg/h.

6 to 12 H: Monitor the Biochemistry, Avoid Fluid Overload and Avoid Hypoglycaemia

Maintain fluids with:

1 L of 0.9% saline with 40 mmol of potassium chloride over 4 h and 1 L of 0.9% saline with 40 mmol of potassium chloride over 6 h.

The urine output by now should be at least 0.5 mL/kg/h.

Continue hourly measurements of glucose and ketones with venous blood gases for pH, bicarbonate and potassium at 6 and 12 h. The FRIII is likely to be needed for at least 6 h before the DKA resolves. When the capillary glucose falls below 14 mmol/L start 10% glucose IV at 125 mL/h in parallel to the IV saline and potassium. To avoid hypoglycaemia, consider reducing the FRIII to 0.05 U/kg/h.

12 to 24 H: VRIII or 'Usual' Insulin

Check for DKA resolution: if the blood ketones are less than 0.6 mmol/L, the pH > 7.3 and the patient can eat and drink, switch to a subcutaneous insulin regimen. Do not stop the intravenous insulin until 30 min after the first dose of subcutaneous insulin. If the patients cannot eat or drink or if they need IV insulin because of severe sepsis or other acute illness, start a VRIII as described above.

Restarting Insulin and Insulin-Naive Patients

Restart a previous basal/bolus subcutaneous regimen by giving the first bolus dose at mealtime followed 30 min later by a discontinuation of the intravenous insulin infusion. The long-acting basal insulin should have been continued at the normal dose and timing throughout the DKA treatment. In new diabetics, the required total daily dose of insulin will be around 0.5× their weight in kg—giving half the dose as a long-acting analogue with the evening meal and the other half as rapid-acting insulin divided equally and given before breakfast, lunch and the evening meal. In the very obese, the daily requirement may be increased to 0.75× their weight.

DKA With a Normal Blood Sugar

Some patients (e.g., partial correction of DKA at home or patients using SGLT2 inhibitors) present with DKA but with normal sugars. In these, saline is given as normal but an insulin FRIII (at 0.05 U/kg/h) with a 10% dextrose infusion (125 mL/h) is also started at the same time.

General Care

Ensure intravenous fluids are started immediately, if necessary involving ITU outreach to secure venous access.

- Catheterise if no urine has been passed within 3 h or if there is hypotension.
- Insert a nasogastric tube if the conscious level is disturbed (GCS less than 8).
- Administer broad-spectrum antibiotics if sepsis is suspected (e.g., co-amoxiclav and cephalexin).
- Administer a prophylactic dose low-molecular-weight heparin as there are risk factors for venous thromboembolic disease (Box 6.7).

 CRITICAL CLINICAL OBSERVATIONS IN DKA

- Is the airway safe?
- Oxygen saturation and respiratory rate
- Blood sugar and capillary blood ketones
- Blood pressure
- Pulse (ECG)

BOX 6.7 ■ Indications for Anticoagulation in Diabetic Ketoacidosis (DKA)

- No contraindication
- Severe DKA
- Previous thromboembolism
- Hyperosmolar
- 'Phlebitic' legs

IMPORTANT CLINICAL OBSERVATIONS IN DKA

- Glasgow coma score/ACVPU
- Temperature
- Test for urinary ketones
- Examine for signs of infection

Caring for the Patient With Diabetic Ketoacidosis

The first 4–5 h are critical in the care of the patient with ketoacidosis. The ward team will be caring for a very sick, distressed and possibly confused patient going through a period of intense clinical activity. The staff will be combining the technical expertise necessary to administer a complex treatment regimen and the skills required to meet the personal needs of a patient who is vulnerable, feels dreadful and is probably terrified for their life.

Critical Clinical Tasks in Diabetic Ketoacidosis

Ensure that the initial infusions are correctly prescribed and administered. It is vital that there is absolutely no delay in initiating the saline and insulin infusions. The protocol must be followed and the correct amounts of fluid given during the first critical few hours. Particular attention must be paid to the potassium supplements and the subsequent blood levels.

Monitor the patient's progress. The hourly observations should chart: a falling pulse, rising blood pressure and increasing urine output as dehydration is corrected. If there is confusion or impairment of the conscious level, the GCS will improve. As acidosis resolves, the respiratory rate will fall and symptoms will improve.

CRITICAL CLINICAL TASKS IN DKA

- Ensure that the initial infusions are correctly prescribed and administered
- Monitor the patient's progress
- Address the patient's physical needs
- Provide reassurance and support
- Initiate plans to prevent this from happening to the patient again
- Refer to the diabetes specialist team
- Do a pregnancy test in patients of childbearing age
- Remove and store securely any insulin pump and its connections

Address the patient's physical needs. If the patient is unconscious, the priority is the nursing care of coma. The patient may be in discomfort and possibly in pain. If this is severe, a judgement will be made about the need for effective analgesics. The patient should adopt a comfortable position in bed and due attention should be paid to the pressure sites, *in particular to the heels*. Mouth care will be important because hyperventilation and dehydration will dry out the oral mucosa. There will be nausea, so sucking ice may be preferable to oral fluids. During the first few hours of admission, there will be numerous medical and nursing interventions performed, so the patient's physical comfort will need to be continually reassessed.

Provide reassurance and support. Initially, the patient may feel frightened and powerless. Patients with long-standing diabetes may be worried about relinquishing control to nurses and medical staff who are not part of the usual diabetic team. These fears will need to be addressed and the patient reassured about the temporary need for intensive insulin and fluid therapy. If there is disorientation or confusion, the patient will need support and explanation as the situation improves.

Initiate plans to prevent this from happening to the patient again. If your communication and assessment have been effective, why this has happened should be clear. Involve the diabetes specialist nurse at an early stage and make sure that when the patient is transferred from the AMU it is to the care of a diabetes team.

Referral to the Diabetes Specialist team. All patients with DKA (and those admitted with hypoglycaemia) must be referred on admission to the Diabetes Specialist Team who should see the patient within 24 h of referral.

Reassurance for Patients With Diabetic Ketoacidosis

- Your nausea and vomiting will stop as the drips start to work.
- You are breathing quickly to blow off the toxic ketones.
- Your breathlessness will improve as your diabetes is brought under control.
- The nasal tube is to stop your stomach from overfilling with air.
- You are getting all the insulin and nutrition that you need in the drips.
- Try not to panic on the oxygen mask—you need it to boost your oxygen levels.
- Your appetite will return as soon as the diabetes comes under control again.
- All the blood tests and close monitoring are needed for the first few hours only.
- You can take over blood testing and insulin treatment once you feel well enough.
- We are giving you powerful antibiotics to cover any possible infections.
- Your heart is fine: the monitor is simply telling us its rate and rhythm.

Answering Relatives' Questions in Diabetic Ketoacidosis

The patient's relatives will be extremely concerned and frightened by the way in which the diabetes appears to have suddenly become a threat to the patient's life. They will need to be reassured.

Should we have acted sooner? Examine the relatives' understanding of diabetes. To what extent are they involved in the patient's diabetic care? If the DKA has been precipitated by an intercurrent infection, are they aware of the problems of acute illness in the diabetic? What warning signs did they act on to seek help, and were these appropriate?

What else could we have done? Are there areas where they would like more information? The relatives may be frightened by the idea of diabetes, injections, adjusting insulin and so forth. In these circumstances, the diabetes specialist nurse will have an important educational and supportive role and will need to be involved.

What will happen next? You can reassure the relatives that the vast majority of patients with DKA make a complete recovery. There are, however, complications that can occur and the management will have to be particularly intensive for the first 6 h or so. There will be a lot of clinical activity during this time and it is usually helpful to put some constraints on the number of visitors during this period.

Clinical details from the relatives. The relatives may also be an important source of urgent clinical information, particularly if the patient is too unwell or confused to give a full history. The relatives can provide important clinical details of the illness and the usual level of diabetic control. The description of the symptoms and how they progressed will help determine the nature of any precipitating infection. Was there headache and fever to suggest meningitis; dysuria and renal tract pain to suggest urinary sepsis; or diarrhoea and vomiting to suggest gastroenteritis? What evidence do the relatives have concerning the usual level of diabetic control and the degree of cooperation and compliance with treatment? Is there a blood sugar diary card to look at? What is the usual insulin regimen? When was it last administered and when did the patient last eat or drink? On a general note: is there a history of heavy alcohol intake (which can have an impact on diabetic control) and are there any allergies, particularly to antibiotics?

The Importance of Patients' and Relatives' Education in Diabetes

The patient in Case Study 6.5 is typical of a diabetic who is uncertain what to do when acutely unwell. There were clear warning signs from his osmotic symptoms that his diabetic control was deteriorating. His acute abdominal symptoms were either gastroenteritis or the first indications of DKA. He should have sought urgent help when he first found urinary ketones, or preferably when he had the combination of vomiting and an inability to keep up with his fluids. Before he was discharged from the AMU, the patient and his mother were given a clear explanation of what had happened and what action they could take in the future.

CASE STUDY 6.5	Diabetic Ketoacidosis—No Advice on What to Do on Sick Days

A 17-year-old boy with a year's history of type I diabetes gave a 2-week history of tiredness, polyuria and high BM stix. He did not seek help or adjust his insulin. Two days before admission to hospital, he developed diarrhoea and continued to vomit all day. He continued his insulin but was unable to take any fluids. By the evening, his urine showed ketones, but he waited a further 12 h before asking for help. On admission, he was dry and hypotensive. There were large amounts of ketones in his urine. Test results: blood sugar 28.5 mmol/L, creatinine 112 mmol/L, urea 8.5 mmol/L, pH was 7.29, bicarbonate was low at 12 mmol/L. He improved rapidly with IV fluids and insulin.

Information for Diabetics: What to Do on Days When You Are Sick

- The main problems occur with gastroenteritis and infections.
- When you are ill you may need *more* short-acting insulin than normal.
- Your blood sugar can rise even if you cannot eat your normal diet.
- While you are ill, check your blood sugar between 2 and 4 hourly. Your target blood sugar should be around 10 mmol/L.
- Check your urine (Ketostix) or blood (Optium B Ketone test and Xceed Meter) for ketones between 2 and 4 hourly. Depending on the levels:
  - Trace (<1.5 mmol/L)—increase fluids, consider a small increase in background insulin.
  - Moderate to Large (>1.5 mmol/L)—increase fluids. Give 10% or 20% of the total daily dose of insulin as extra insulin injections every 2 h. Check blood glucose and ketones every 2 h.
- Adjust your insulin only if you are confident in doing so. If you have persistent vomiting or you cannot control your blood sugar or ketone levels, seek urgent help. *Never stop your insulin.*
- Keep your carbohydrate intake up with milk and sugar, snacks, ice cream and high-sugar soft drinks.
- Aim to drink 4–6 pints (3.6–5.4 L) of sugar-free liquid per day.
- If the breathing becomes rapid, the vomiting persists and there is drowsiness, you, the patient or your relatives, *must* seek urgent medical attention.

Hyperosmolar Non-Ketotic Diabetic Coma

This relatively rare complication is seen in elderly type II diabetic patients and has a 50% mortality rate. The patients present extremely unwell, with very high sugars (>30 mmol/L) and impaired conscious levels, but without ketoacidosis (blood ketones <3 mmol/L, HCO_3 >15). They are usually profoundly dehydrated due to osmotic fluid loss. The history usually involves a precipitating illness—an infection in 80% of cases—with vomiting and thirst that has often been relieved by high volumes of very sugary drinks. The diagnosis is made from the clinical setting and the finding of a high blood osmolality (over-concentrated blood). The osmolality can be calculated by a simple formula using standard blood results: Osmolality = 2 × (plasma sodium + potassium) + urea + glucose.

The normal osmolality is 275–295 mOsmol/kg; in a hyperosmolar non-ketotic diabetic coma, the level is greater than 320 mOsmol/kg.

Management includes central venous pressure monitoring, nasogastric intubation to prevent aspiration and the same saline regimen used to treat DKA. Caution is needed, however, as these patients are often frail with renal and cardiac problems.

Potassium replacement follows the same principles for their use in DKA.

Insulin is given as a fixed rate intravenous infusion at 0.05 units/kg/h (half the rate of DKA) with a 10% dextrose infusion run at 125 mL/h in parallel and is either started once the glucose level stops falling (importantly, it is only started when the glucose falls below 14 mmol) with fluid replacement alone or immediately if there are ketones present (urine > ++ or blood >1 mmol/L). Biochemistry and fluid balance should be corrected more slowly than is done in DKA—up to 72 h. Osmolality is checked hourly to assess progress but should not fall at more than 5 mOsmol/kg/h.

Hypoglycaemia

The possibility of hypoglycaemia must always be the first consideration when faced with an acute neurological or behavioural disturbance, whether the patient is diabetic or not. It is a major danger for patients who are on insulin.

SYMPTOMS

The symptoms of hypoglycaemia present acutely and progress rapidly as the blood sugar drops. For example, mild symptoms of headache, slight mood changes, excessive sweating of the face and hands or subtle changes in behaviour occur as sugars fall to 3 mmol/L. Blood sugars less than 4 in in-patient diabetics should be corrected ('make four the floor'). As the sugar decreases, adrenaline (epinephrine) is released, which produces the classic warning signs: sweating, irritability, tremors, palpitations and intense hunger. There may be double vision, aggression and poor cooperation. With severe hypoglycaemia, at sugar levels of 1 to 2 mmol/L, there may be epileptic fits, confusion, stroke-like symptoms and coma. Untreated, severe hypoglycaemia can result in irreversible damage. In prolonged hypoglycaemia, death may occur, but this is a rare occurrence and tends to be associated with deliberate overdosing of either insulin or oral hypoglycaemics.

CAUSES

Hypoglycaemia is most common in type I diabetes as a result of mismatches of insulin, carbohydrate intake and carbohydrate utilisation. Many type I diabetics now tend to aim for low/normal blood sugars using three or four times daily short-acting insulin. Although these intensive regimens reduce the incidence of long-term complications, they can put the patients at an increased risk of hypoglycaemia. Missed meals, excessive unplanned exercise and (particularly the morning after) an alcoholic binge can all lead to acute hypoglycaemia. Interestingly, islet cell function partially recovers when new diabetics are first started on insulin. This is a temporary effect that lasts only a few months, but the extra natural insulin puts new diabetics at risk from hypoglycaemia during this 'honeymoon period'.

Prolonged hypoglycaemia can occur in patients with type II diabetes if they are taking oral hypoglycaemics combined with insulin. It is a particular problem in the elderly if they are inappropriately given long-acting hypoglycaemics such as glibenclamide or chlorpropamide, if they eat poorly and, particularly if they abuse alcohol or have renal failure.

In-patient hypoglycaemia can occur as a result of insulin prescribing errors, for example confusing the insulin name (e.g., Humalog Mix 25) with the dose. There is a particular risk of confusing the two intravenous insulin preparations:

50 U Actrapid in 50 mL saline is used for VRIII and FRIII.

10 U Actrapid and 50 mL 50% glucose are used for emergency treatment of hyperkalaemia.

HYPOGLYCAEMIC UNAWARENESS

In some diabetics, there are no warning signs of hypoglycaemia on which they can take action—a condition termed hypoglycaemic unawareness. These patients can pass rapidly through a stage of confusion to hypoglycaemic coma. Hypoglycaemic unawareness is seen mainly in diabetics who have frequent hypoglycaemic attacks. These appear to blunt the usual symptoms of impending hypoglycaemia. Even one hypoglycaemic episode will blunt the awareness of a second episode for 24 h or more, so these patients are in a vicious circle. Diabetic autonomic neuropathy will also reduce the body's normal warning response to hypoglycaemia. Therefore if there is a history of recurrent and potentially dangerous hypoglycaemia, the patient needs an urgent referral for a detailed assessment of their diabetes, in particular, to exclude hypoglycaemic unawareness. Fortunately, awareness can be restored if further hypoglycaemic episodes are avoided.

MANAGEMENT

Hypoglycaemia is the ultimate medical emergency: the presentation is dramatic, the benefits of treatment are immediate and, most importantly, to miss or to delay treatment is a disaster. Permanent neurological damage from hypoglycaemia, although rare, can be devastating. If you suspect hypoglycaemia, check the glucose stix and, if possible, send a laboratory glucose for later confirmation. Stop any IV insulin infusion until normal blood sugars have been restored. As intravenous insulin stops working within about 5 min, it must be restarted within 20 min of correcting the hypoglycaemia.

If the patient is in a coma, your priority is to ensure the patient's safety with regard to the airway, breathing and circulation. If the patient is conscious and cooperative and you diagnose hypoglycaemia (glucose < 4 mmol/L), you should give 20 g of quick-acting carbohydrate as:

- 200 mL of pure fruit juice.
- Six glucose tablets.

TABLE 6.5 ■ Constitution of Glucose Solutions

Glucose Solution (%)	25 g Glucose in
50	50 mL (now seldom used in hypoglycaemia)
20	125 mL
10	250 mL

- Repeat this step if the blood glucose remains less than 4 mmol/L after 15 min. Give no more than three of these steps. Consider IV glucose or glucagon if still hypoglycaemic. Once recovered, give a long-acting carbohydrate (two biscuits or 200 mL milk or the next meal).
- Review but do not omit any insulin that is due.

If the patient is uncooperative but able to swallow, squeeze two tubes of a glucose gel between the cheeks and the gums and massage the cheek to help absorption.

Intravenous glucose. A large-bore cannula will be needed if there is an impaired conscious level, as IV glucose will be needed (Table 6.5). Give 200 mL of 10% or 100 mL of 20% glucose over 15 min. Check the glucose stix 10 min after treatment has been given. The infused doses can be repeated. Hypoglycaemia due to oral hypoglycaemics can be prolonged, as some of the drugs have a long course of action. These patients will need careful monitoring for recurrence and may need a 10% infusion of glucose continued at 100 mL/h for a number of hours.

Intramuscular glucagon. If you cannot get immediate venous access, then glucagon can be used. Glucagon is a naturally occurring hormone that has the exact opposite effect of insulin. Give 1 mg of glucagon intramuscularly. It acts more slowly than glucose (in a coma, consciousness returns in 10–15 min). Glucagon also causes nausea and vomiting and is not very effective in patients who are starved or who have consumed excessive alcohol. After glucagon, the amount of long-acting carbohydrate given after recovery is double that suggested above.

ALWAYS SEEK THE CAUSE FOR HYPOGLYCAEMIA

Case Study 6.6 illustrates why it is important to find out the cause of the hypoglycaemia. Cortisone, like adrenaline (epinephrine) and glucagon, is a stress hormone that is released in response to hypoglycaemia to try and correct the body's blood sugar. Addison's disease, like diabetes, is another autoimmune disease in which the body produces antibodies against the adrenal gland, the source of cortisone. This patient's natural ability to correct hypoglycaemia was impaired due to his lack of cortisone. Addison's disease and diabetes share a similar mechanism and are known to occur together, in the same patient. This case illustrates the need to follow up any case of hypoglycaemia to establish the exact reason for its occurrence.

CASE STUDY 6.6   **Failure to Recover From Hypoglycaemia**

A 35-year-old diabetic was admitted with severe hypoglycaemia. He had been seen by his parents the evening before and had then been found in a confused and barely rousable state in the morning. He had been a diabetic for a year and was quite depressed about its implications for the future. He remained confused and hypoglycaemic for several days, despite high-dose IV glucose. Initial suspicions that he had taken an insulin overdose could not be substantiated. He was discharged home after eventual recovery but was admitted a day later with further hypoglycaemia.

Further investigations revealed that he had also developed Addison's disease. He responded well to cortisone therapy and his hypoglycaemia resolved.

TABLE 6.6 ■ A Guide to Infusions and Additives in Diabetes

Infusion/Additive	Route	Indications/Uses	Risks
Isotonic saline[a]	Peripheral line	Dehydration diabetic ketoacidosis	LVF (fluid overload)
Hypotonic saline	Peripheral line	Hyperosmolar (high sodium)	Overdilution (watch sodium)
5% Glucose[b]	Peripheral line	GKI	Overdilution if given >24 h
10% Glucose	Large bore	GKI/hypoglycaemia	Hyperglycaemia
20% Glucose	Central/large bore	Hypoglycaemia	
50% Glucose	Central/large bore	Hypoglycaemia	
KCl solution (2 mmol/mL)	Mix *thoroughly* in saline or glucose	Potassium depletion	Potassium overload
Sodium bicarbonate 1.26% (600 mL gives 100 mmol of bicarbonate)	Central line	Severe acidosis (pH < 6.9)	Extravasation
		Severe hyperkalemia (protective action)	Sodium overload (LVF)

LVF, Left ventricular failure.
[a]Also known as normal saline, 0.9% sodium chloride and physiological saline.
[b]Also known as dextrose.

In managing all these diabetic emergencies, it is important to be familiar with the various IV infusions (Table 6.6).

Infective Complications in Diabetes: The Acute Diabetic Foot

Acute infections involving the lower limbs and feet are a common cause of emergency admission in the diabetic patient. The feet are extremely vulnerable in diabetes due to the combination of vascular damage, peripheral nerve damage and the patient's inherent susceptibility to infection. Half of those with type II diabetes who are older than

60 years have established peripheral nerve damage. This leads to two major problems in the feet:

- Loss of sensation
- Muscle imbalance, with resulting foot deformity

If the feet are numb, minor trauma goes unheeded, so that simple abrasions progress to ulceration and infection. Deformity of the feet, and in particular clawing of the toes, puts areas over the soles of the feet at risk from the effects of abnormal pressure loading. Calluses form over the metatarsal heads, which are the main pressure points; these break down and become ulcerated.

As a result of diabetic vascular disease, the blood supply to the tissues is poor: they heal badly and may ulcerate, particularly around the ankles. Infections do not clear and may progress proximally from localised involvement of the feet to the rest of the leg. Ultimately, the tissues may die, with the development of wet or dry gangrene.

ASSESSMENT OF THE DIABETIC FOOT

The severely infected foot that brings the diabetic patient in as an emergency will characteristically have cellulitis spreading from an area of ulceration. The likely sequence is that a trivial abrasion starts silently and progresses to ulceration. By the time the patient needs admission, the ulcer will have become infected and the whole foot may be at risk. Diabetes may be out of control and if the patient is septic (i.e., the infection has spread into the bloodstream), they may also be ketoacidotic.

It is important to recognise that in some patients, particularly the elderly and socially disadvantaged, the acutely infected foot is only part of a picture of generalised self-neglect (Box 6.8 and Fig. 6.3).

BOX 6.8 ■ Self-Neglect in the Elderly Diabetic Patient

- Poor vision
- Poor mobility
- Poor motivation
- Multiple medical problems
- Poor skin: sores, excoriation and abrasions
- Hypertension and hyperglycaemia
- Advanced diabetic feet, calluses and foot ulcers
- Obesity
- Superficial candida infection in skin creases, between the toes, and in the groin
- Uncut nails with infected nail beds
- Neglected dentition
- Old and dirty dressings/bandages
- Heavy nicotine staining

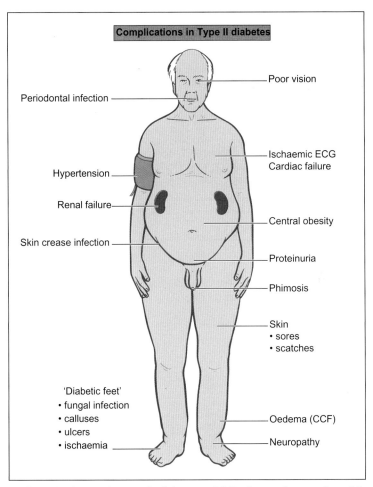

Complications in Type II diabetes

- Poor vision
- Periodontal infection
- Ischaemic ECG
- Cardiac failure
- Hypertension
- Renal failure
- Central obesity
- Skin crease infection
- Proteinuria
- Phimosis
- Skin
  - sores
  - scatches
- 'Diabetic feet'
  - fungal infection
  - calluses
  - ulcers
  - ischaemia
- Oedema (CCF)
- Neuropathy

FIGURE 6.3 Complications of type II diabetes. *CCF*, Congestive cardiac failure; *ECG*, electrocardiogram.

A reasonable idea of the degree of vascular and nerve damage can be obtained from the patient's history (Box 6.9). Diabetic vascular disease is indicated by a history of exertional calf pain progressing to severe rest pain in the legs and feet, a history of previous bypass procedures and/or amputation of some of the toes. Diabetic nerve damage is suggested by a history of unpleasant burning, pins and needles or diffuse pain in the feet, all of which are worse at night. The feet feel numb, and there may be a previous history of painless damage from ill-fitting shoes or minor trauma. If the ankle is damaged the whole foot can appear hot, red and swollen—a situation easily confused with an acute infection but one in which, in contrast to cellulitis, the skin is usually intact.

BOX 6.9 ■ Indications of Ischaemic and Neuropathic Feet in Diabetes

Ischaemic feet

- History of exertional calf pain and resting foot pain
- Previous lower limb bypass procedures
- Cold, poorly nourished feet, with shiny red skin
- Areas of gangrene/necrosis

Neuropathic Feet

- Burning and tingling feet, particularly at night
- Numb to the touch
- Warm feet
- Calluses over pressure points
- Ulcers over pressure points
- Foot deformity (clawed toes)

HOW TO LOOK AT THE FEET

- Remove all old dressings on the lower limbs.
- Ask the patient if their feet are numb—can the patient feel you touching their feet? Ideally use a customised monofilament, which buckles when a slight pressure (10 g) is applied to it, to test sensation over the balls of the feet.
- What colour is the skin?
  - Red, shiny and hairless skin indicates poor nutrition (ischaemia).
  - Are there any black areas?
  - Are the feet blue and cold, suggesting arterial insufficiency?
  - Are they warm and wet (oedema)? This can indicate nerve damage.
- Have any foot or leg pulses been found?
  - There may be elements of both arterial and nerve damage.
- Look at the nails and between the toes (maceration and fungal infection).
- Are the feet a normal shape?
  - Clawed toes indicate small muscle damage and make the feet vulnerable to pressure damage, with callus formation over weight-bearing areas.
  - A deformed ankle may indicate painless joint damage (Charcot joint).
- Are there any breaks in the skin or ulcer formation? If there are ulcers:
  - How deep are they? (Superficial or penetrating) 'Probe to bone' is a test for osteomyelitis in which a thin sterile rod is introduced through the ulcer to feel for grittiness or solid bone, indicating the depth of penetration.
  - How big are they? (Foot ulcers with an area of more than 2 cm^2 often involve the bone.)
  - Do they look infected (red, exuding pus and smelling) or are they simply chronic pressure ulcers?

- Is there any cellulitis: tender, red, raised areas around breaks in the skin?
  - The foot may be hot and there may be an obvious collection of pus beneath the skin. There may be a strong odour, suggesting a gram-negative infection. Sometimes gas can be felt as bubbling (crepitus) within the tissues.
- There may be areas of wet or dry gangrene. The distinction is important (Box 6.10).

Signs of Worsening and Spreading Infection

- The foot becomes increasingly hot, swollen and painful.
- The patient looks ill.
- The skin goes purple and red or black blisters appear.
- There is an increase in:
  - Pulse
  - Temperature
  - Blood sugar and blood ketones
  - White cell count
  - Respiration rate (acidotic breathing)
- The infection spreads into the leg.

Box 6.11 summarises the important points to check for in the acute diabetic foot.

MANAGEMENT

In the first 24 to 48 h, the priorities in managing the acute diabetic foot are to:
- Control the diabetes
- Treat infection

BOX 6.10 ▦ Distinction Between Wet and Dry Gangrene

Wet Gangrene	Dry Gangrene
Swollen	Hard
Moist	Dry
Blistering	Demarcation of blackened tissue
In a large portion of the foot	In toes and toe ends
Early debridement/amputation	Early angiograms/revascularisation?

BOX 6.11 ▦ Checklist for the Acute Diabetic Foot

- Is the foot chronically damaged or is there an acute problem?
- Are any skin breaks superficial or penetrating and deep?
- Is there any cellulitis?
- Are the ulcers clean and punched out or secondarily infected?
- What is the dominant problem: nerve damage, arterial disease or both?
- Is the patient becoming ketoacidotic?

- Provide adequate pain relief
- Salvage the limb if there is critical ischaemia
- Prevent the worsening of any pressure damage
- Urgently involve the multidisciplinary diabetic foot care team

The infection is identified by taking deep swabs/wound debris from any ulcers and sets of blood cultures. If there is severe local or spreading infection, broad-spectrum antibiotics are used, for example, IV Tazocin and clindamycin. If Methicillin-resistant *Staphylococcus aureus* is suspected, IV vancomycin and teicoplanin are also used. These will be modified once the results of cultures are known. If the ulcers are deep, the feet are x-rayed to identify any spread of the infection to the underlying bone.

If the foot deteriorates or there is wet gangrene, there must be an immediate surgical opinion regarding the need for debridement. Critical (limb-threatening) ischaemia should be suspected if there is a history of severe rest pain, signs of ischaemic ulceration and areas of gangrene. The surgeons must see these patients urgently with a view to immediate angiography and a limb-salvaging procedure (e.g., bypass or angioplasty).

Pressure damage to the heels is a major hazard in these patients, and appropriate protective action is necessary. The position in which the patient is nursed is important because if the feet are dependent they will become oedematous, and if they are elevated, a poor blood supply will become even worse. Decisions on longer-term and preventative actions and the choice of appropriate dressings, wound management and pressure off-loading lower limb appliances can be left to be made later by the diabetes foot care team.

The key points in emergency treatment and management of the acute diabetic foot are presented in Box 6.12.

BOX 6.12 ■ Emergency Treatment and Management of the Diabetic Foot

Emergency Treatment
- Control the diabetes
- Treat sepsis
- Exclude limb-threatening ischaemia

Managing the Infected Foot
- Urgent referral to the Diabetes Foot Care Team
- Control diabetes
- Neuropathic/vascular or both?
- Look at the pressure points
- Avoid pressure damage to heels
- Assess the extent and depth of any ulceration
- Deep swabs and blood cultures
- Intravenous antibiotics for cellulitis/treat sepsis urgently
- Urgent vascular surgical opinion?
- Improve any local oedema (avoid elevation in ischaemia)

Excellent Diabetic Care

- Ward protocols for the emergency management of DKA and hypoglycaemia
- Protocol for the use of variable and fixed-rate intravenous insulin infusions
- Management protocol for the acute diabetic foot and acute limb ischaemia
- Planned protocol reviews and updates
- Review of the significance of finding glycosuria, proteinuria and ketonuria
- Appropriate and timely access to the diabetes specialist teams
- A system to review techniques for measuring blood sugars, near-patient testing using venous blood gases and injecting insulin
- A system to calibrate and maintain the blood glucose and blood ketone meters
- An audit of the management of diabetic patient on the AMU
- Educational resources for staff, patients and relatives

Further Reading

NICE guideline [NG17]. Type 1 diabetes in adults: diagnosis and management. Published: 26 August 2015 Last updated: 17 August 2022. https://www.nice.org.uk/guidance/NG17.

NICE. (2015). Diabetic foot problems: prevention, management. NICE Guideline. https://www.nice.org.uk/guidance/ng19.

Series of current Joint British Diabetes Societies documents on DKA, HONK, Hypoglycaemia, VRIII. http://www.diabetologists-abcd.org.uk/JBDS/JBDS.htm.

Thromboembolic Disease

Introduction

Almost a tenth of acute medical admissions were with either a provisional diagnosis of deep vein thrombosis (DVT) or a possible pulmonary embolus (PE). Owing to the unreliability of the clinical signs and the anxiety of missing a dangerous clot, these patients had usually been admitted and treated with IV heparin infusions until tests confirmed or refuted the diagnosis.

The situation has changed for three reasons:

- Rapid and reliable screening tests are now available for venous thromboembolism (VTE).
- Simplified anticoagulation with once-daily subcutaneous low-molecular-weight heparin (LMWH) has replaced the heparin infusion (and itself is now being replaced by the new direct-acting oral anticoagulants [DOACs]).
- The introduction of ambulatory care units.

There are two important clinical issues:

- Differentiating between the various causes of a red, swollen and painful leg: venous thrombosis, cellulitis, varicose eczema and arterial insufficiency
- Remembering to consider the possibility of pulmonary emboli in any ill and breathless patient—particularly where there is pleuritic chest pain and pre-existing lung disease—notably, chronic obstructive pulmonary disease (COPD) and lung cancer

The overriding consideration in these situations is that a missed diagnosis of venous thromboembolic disease carries with it the potential of a preventable death from a massive pulmonary embolus. It should be remembered that post-mortem studies have shown that 10% of hospital deaths are due to pulmonary emboli; most of them were unrecognised.

The Nature of the Disease

THROMBOSIS AND THROMBOEMBOLISATION

Mechanisms

Thrombosis refers to the process in which a mass of clot forms inside an artery or a vein. It consists of a dense network of fibrin, in which there are trapped variable proportions of red cells and platelets. Thrombosis blocks the vessel and impairs blood flow. Arterial thrombosis leads to ischaemic tissue damage (myocardial infarction, stroke and peripheral vascular disease), whereas in venous thrombosis the consequences are due to back pressure and local swelling (oedema). If the clot disintegrates, parts of it can break off, producing emboli that travel onward—in venous thrombosis through the veins to the lungs (pulmonary embolus) and in arterial thrombosis through the arteries to major organs such as the brain (cerebral embolus), limbs (peripheral embolus), kidneys (renal infarction) and intestine (acute bowel ischaemia).

The trigger for thrombosis depends on whether it occurs in an artery or a vein.

- In the arteries, local damage to the vessel wall, usually in the form of a ruptured atheromatous plaque, initiates thrombosis by the release and activation of clotting factors and the adhesion of platelet clumps to the damaged surface.
- In the veins, there are three factors that contribute to abnormal clotting and increase the risk of venous thromboembolic disease (DVT and PE):
  - Stagnation of the blood flow

- Damage to the vein wall
- Abnormalities of the clotting mechanism

Stagnation of the blood flow. Stagnation within the veins is the most important factor in initiating venous thrombosis. Calf muscles act as a venous pump, returning blood to the heart. Failure of the calf pump due to enforced immobility (e.g., post-operative bed rest, plaster cast, paralysed limb) leads to venous stasis. This is a particular problem in the elderly, the obese and those with varicose veins: in these patients, even 3 or 4 days of immobility can be critical.

Damage to the vein wall. Thrombosis is triggered by the activation of clotting mechanisms that occur when there is damage to the vein wall—indeed, this is the normal mechanism for preventing bleeding at the sites of trauma. Typical situations that lead to vein damage are pressure injuries to the calf from the operating theatre table and the deterioration that occurs in the veins as a result of recurrent venous thrombosis.

Abnormalities of the clotting mechanism. Several inherited and acquired abnormalities of the clotting mechanisms increase the risk of venous thromboembolic disease (Box 7.1). The most common acquired abnormalities are those associated with the oral contraceptive pill, hormone replacement therapy (HRT), pregnancy and the presence of malignant disease.

Inherited clotting abnormalities (thrombophilias) are increasingly recognised as underlying the cause of recurrent DVTs, particularly in younger patients and in those with a positive family history. The most important of several inherited coagulation abnormalities, known as Factor V Leiden, is present in 5% of the population and increases the risk of thrombosis by 10 times the normal rate. One in five patients with their first DVT is positive for Factor V Leiden. Recent estimates suggest up to half of all patients who present with a venous thromboembolic episode, either DVT or pulmonary embolus, may have a single or multiple inherited abnormalities of their clotting. In these individuals, each episode can be triggered by trivial external events such as minor surgery or immobility. In the future, increasing attention will be paid to identifying these inherited risk factors.

Multiple risk factors. In most situations in which the chances of a venous thrombosis are high, there are multiple risk factors. Thus in major orthopaedic procedures on the leg, there is vein damage and immobility; in pregnancy there is abnormal clotting and stagnation of blood due to intra-abdominal mechanical effects; and in prolonged air travel, there is immobility, often associated with a degree of dehydration. The

---

BOX 7.1 ■ Examples of Inherited Thrombophilia

- Antithrombin deficiency
- Protein C deficiency
- Antiphospholipid syndrome
- Protein S deficiency
- Factor V Leiden

combination of the oral contraceptive pill and the presence of Factor V Leiden increases the risk of a DVT 30-fold.

Major risk factors. In a patient with suspicious symptoms, the presence of these *major* risk factors (those that increase the risk by 5–20 times normal) makes the diagnosis of a PE much more likely:

- Recent surgery (hip and knee replacement, major abdominal and pelvic surgery)
- Decreased mobility (institutional care, prolonged hospital stay)
- Malignancy
- Lower limb problems (post-phlebitic limb, varicose veins)
- Pregnancy (not the pill), especially in the third trimester and post-delivery/caesarian
- Previous DVT/PE

Superficial Thrombophlebitis

Thrombophlebitis is a painful inflammation of the superficial veins. Classically it is seen in infected venous cannulae, but it also commonly occurs in patients with varicose veins. The clinical picture is of palpable and very tender cords of thrombosed and inflamed veins, with the overlying skin appearing reddened or bruised. Thrombophlebitis is not in itself dangerous: it does not progress to, but may accompany, DVT. The management is based on removing any cause (e.g., an IV cannula) and treating the symptoms. Importantly, recurrent unexplained phlebitis is found in patients with unrecognised malignant disease, particularly adenocarcinomas of the gastrointestinal (GI) tract and lung.

Deep Vein Thrombosis

DVT is a more serious problem because of the risk of fatal pulmonary embolus. Most DVTs start in the deep veins of the calf, termed the distal veins, where they cause local pain and swelling.

Although calf vein thromboses do not themselves give rise to emboli, one in five subsequently extends up the leg to involve the proximal veins in the thigh and pelvis—*popliteal and iliofemoral thrombosis*. The risk of a pulmonary embolus from a proximal vein thrombosis is very high, around 50%, and some will be fatal. A significant proportion of the survivors, around one in five, will develop a post-phlebitic syndrome in the affected leg, with chronic swelling, varicose veins, skin pigmentation, recurrent thrombosis and venous ulceration.

The management is based on preventing the progression of the thrombotic process through immediate anticoagulation, followed by maintenance of anticoagulants in the medium to long term to lower the risk of recurrence. The aim of treatment is to stabilise the situation. Anticoagulants (unlike fibrinolytics such as alteplase) do not dissolve established clots but are given to:

- Prevent extension
- Reduce the chances of embolisation
- Lower the risk of recurrence

Pulmonary Thromboembolism

Most pulmonary emboli (90%) arise from the proximal veins in the thigh and pelvis. Depending on their size, emboli that travel to the lung either become wedged in the main pulmonary arteries, where they block the outflow of blood from the right side of the heart or pass onward to become trapped in the lung peripheries. The former, termed massive pulmonary emboli, produce a disastrous decrease in cardiac output, leading to sudden death or acute hypotensive collapse. The right side of the heart may become acutely decompensated as it tries to squeeze blood through obstructed pulmonary vessels—leading to further cardiovascular instability. Right heart strain can be seen as right ventricular enlargement on the CTPA, echocardiogram (ECHO) and elevated cardiac biomarkers on the blood tests.

The smaller emboli in the periphery of the lungs produce wedge-shaped areas of lung damage (producing breathlessness and haemoptysis) and give rise to overlying pleurisy (acute chest pain and fever; Fig. 7.1).

Massive pulmonary emboli can move or start to break up either naturally or during the course of cardiopulmonary resuscitation. Thrombolytic drugs such as alteplase can help to dissolve the embolus and are used in unstable patients with hypotension. Concurrent treatment with heparin (usually as an intravenous infusion) will prevent

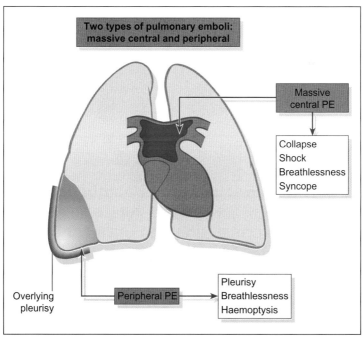

FIGURE 7.1   The two types of pulmonary emboli (PE): massive central and peripheral.

further emboli, and as most patients who survive the first embolus can die from a recurrence within the first few hours, it is important to start treatment urgently.

The management of smaller peripheral emboli is based on preventing further and possibly bigger emboli by giving appropriate immediate and long-term anticoagulation.

Reducing the Risk of Venous Thromboembolism

There is a significant risk that the admission of a patient with an acute medical illness will be complicated by a DVT and/or pulmonary embolus. This risk should be assessed in every patient, and if it is significant, preventative measures—either drugs (LMWH or fondaparinux as, due to the bleeding risk, DOACs are not recommended as prophylaxis in acute medical patients) or mechanical measures (anti-embolism stockings, intermittent pneumatic compression or foot impulse devices)—should be considered. Risk factors for complications such as current active GI bleeding or potential bleeding into the brain or spinal cord (e.g., recent acute stroke or the need for a lumbar puncture) may make mechanical techniques preferable to drug treatment.

Significant risk of VTE in an acute medical admission is defined as:

- Decreased mobility anticipated for 3 or more days or one or more of the following risk factors:
  - Age >60 years
  - Obesity (body mass index >30 kg/m^2)
  - Medical comorbidities (diabetes, congestive cardiac failure [CCF], COPD, chronic arthritis, etc.)
  - Dehydration
  - Active malignancy
  - Phlebitic lower limbs
  - Previous or significant close family history of VTE
  - Pregnant with an associated risk factor (e.g., age >35 years, hyperemesis, ovarian hyperstimulation)
  - HRT or oral contraceptive

Tests to Identify Venous Thromboembolic Disease
DIAGNOSTIC APPROACH: THE TWO-LEVEL PULMONARY EMBOLISM WELLS SCORE: LIKELY OR UNLIKELY

Pulmonary emboli can be ruled out, without additional tests, in a significant number of patients based on their age (less than 50 years); heart rate (less than 100 beats/min); saturations (more than 94%) and no swollen leg, no haemoptysis and no recent surgery or trauma.

For the remainder, confirmatory tests are chosen according to the likelihood of a pulmonary embolus based on the clinical features and the presence of major risk factors.

The two-level Wells PE score (TABLE 7.1) is used to score the probability of a pulmonary embolus. If the score makes a PE **likely** (>4 points), the patient has an immediate CTPA and, if positive, immediate anticoagulation. Immediate interim anticoagulation should be given if the CTPA is likely to be delayed. If the CTPA is negative and a DVT is suspected, the patient should have a proximal leg-vein ultrasound to look for the source of a clot. If this is negative, then there must be an alternative diagnosis.

If the two-level Wells score makes a PE **unlikely** (≤4 points), the patient has a D-dimer test. If it is positive, the patient has an immediate CTPA and, if this confirms a PE, immediate anticoagulation. Immediate interim anticoagulation should be given if the CTPA is likely delayed. If the CTPA or the D-dimers are negative, there must be an alternative diagnosis.

Several tests are available to identify venous thromboembolic disease:

CTPA. The investigation of possible pulmonary emboli has been revolutionised by the introduction of the CTPA. It is superior to both the isotope lung scan and the conventional angiogram. The CTPA also identifies right ventricular enlargement (strain on the right side of the heart). A negative CTPA rules out a significant pulmonary embolus and often gives additional information on alternative causes of the patient's symptoms.

Isotope lung scan. Lung scans are easy to perform and, when used in conjunction with clinical details, are useful in the diagnosis of pulmonary emboli. Although positive scans are also seen in other conditions and must be interpreted with care, a normal scan result is very helpful, as it rules out the possibility of a pulmonary embolus. Lung scans are used if the patient is allergic to contrast media, if the renal function is poor or if radiation exposure has to be minimised.

D-dimer measurements. D-dimers are fragments of dissolving blood clots that can be identified from a blood sample whenever a thromboembolic process is underway. A positive test is also seen after surgery, in infections, after myocardial infarction and in malignant disease: a positive D-dimer test is not therefore in itself diagnostic. D-dimer tests are most useful for ruling out thromboembolism when the initial clinical assessment

TABLE 7.1 ■ **Two-Level Pulmonary Embolism (PE) Wells Score**

Clinical feature	Score
Leg swelling and pain palpating deep veins suggesting a deep vein thrombosis (DVT)	3
An alternative diagnosis is less likely than a PE	3
Pulse greater than 100 beats/min	1.5
Immobilisation for more than 3 days or surgery within 4 weeks	1.5
Previous DVT/PE	1.5
Haemoptysis	1
Malignancy (active treatment, within 6 months or palliative)	1
Clinical probability	
PE likely	>4
PE unlikely	≤4

suggests a low suspicion of the diagnosis. For example, a patient who is breathless may have a major risk factor such as recent hip surgery but also has other likely causes of breathlessness such as COPD: in this situation, a negative D-dimer means there is another cause for the breathlessness. When the clinical suspicion is high, D-dimers are not helpful because a negative result under these circumstances is not reliable enough to rule out the diagnosis (an example would be a patient who is breathless, with no alternative explanation, plus a major risk factor for pulmonary embolus).

Lower limb compression ultrasound. This looks at the compressibility of the vein with an ultrasound probe and also examines venous blood flow using colour Doppler. Compression ultrasound is accurate for thigh vein thrombosis but not for thrombosis in the pelvis or calf. It is also unreliable at picking up recurrent thrombotic episodes. Despite these drawbacks, ultrasound is a simple, rapid and very effective diagnostic tool, particularly when combined with clinical assessment and initial screening by the measurement of D-dimers. If a DVT is thought likely (based on clinical assessment in the form of a scoring system and an elevated D-dimer) but a compression scan is negative, the scan should be repeated in 7 days in case a calf vein thrombosis (not dangerous) has extended above the knee to involve the thigh veins (dangerous).

Contrast venogram and pulmonary angiogram. The venogram examines the veins of the legs and pelvis and the inferior vena cava and was considered to be the 'gold standard' for the identification of venous thrombosis. An invasive test and unpleasant for the patient, its use is confined to difficult cases, particularly those in which active intervention with a vena cava filter is under consideration. The pulmonary angiogram has largely been replaced by the CTPA.

Cardiac biomarkers. If the emboli are big enough to strain the right side of the heart, the cardiac biomarkers NT-proBNP and troponin are released into the circulation. In any patient, the combination of elevated cardiac biomarkers and CT (or ECHO) evidence of acute right heart strain is a warning that outpatient management of the pulmonary embolus would not be safe.

Management of Pulmonary Thromboembolism

The following case studies are used to illustrate the management of pulmonary thromboembolism (Case Studies 7.1–7.4). The classic features of a pulmonary embolus are listed in Box 7.2.

There are two problems with the patient in Case Study 7.3—the management of recalcitrant pulmonary emboli and the problem of assessing her swollen leg. The assessment of a painful calf in a patient with diabetes needs care because the diagnostic possibilities include:

- Cellulitis
- Critical limb ischaemia
- DVT

CASE STUDY 7.1   Acute Massive Pulmonary Emboli

A 35-year-old female was admitted to the hospital after having collapsed at home. She had arisen to go to the toilet and collapsed with a loss of consciousness for a few seconds. She recovered but remained clammy and confused with a thready pulse and felt very breathless. The day before, she had complained of a slight pain in the left calf. She was taking a third-generation combined oral contraceptive pill; she was obese and a smoker. She also had chronic bilateral varicose veins. Three months earlier, she had been admitted with swelling and tenderness of the left calf coming on after exercise, but after equivocal tests she had been discharged without anticoagulation.

On examination, her pulse was 110 beats/min, blood pressure 104/78 mm Hg and oxygen saturations 100% on 6 L/min oxygen. Respiratory rate was 20 breaths/min. The right calf diameter measured 42 cm and the left 46 cm (similar readings to the previous admission). An urgent CTPA showed multiple pulmonary emboli. Seven hours after admission, she collapsed again while walking to the toilet, but on this occasion, there was a cardiorespiratory arrest. Despite prolonged resuscitation and the use of alteplase, she remained in electromechanical dissociation (EMD) and did not survive.

CASE STUDY 7.2   Emboli Treated With Alteplase

CASE 1

A 54-year-old female was admitted with a 1-week history of right upper abdominal pain radiating to her back and right shoulder and worse on lying or on deep inspiration. She had become breathless over 2 days.

On admission, the patient had a respiratory rate of 16 breaths/min, pulse of 80 beats/min and normal blood pressure. The arterial oxygen level was reduced to 88% on air, and the chest film showed changes at both lung bases. A provisional diagnosis of diaphragmatic pleurisy due to pulmonary emboli was made, and LMWH was started.

On the second day, the oxygen saturations fell to 76% on air and the pulse had increased to 110 beats/min. Examination and ECG showed increasing strain on the right side of the heart. On the third day, there was a sudden attack of near syncope and breathlessness while standing associated with further drops in oxygen saturation and a blood pressure of 90/60 mm Hg. The oxygen saturation remained low at 85% despite high-flow oxygen.

The CTPA showed multiple pulmonary emboli. She was thrombolysed with IV alteplase. LMWH was changed to an intravenous heparin infusion. Her condition improved, with a fall in the pulse rate and an increase in oxygen saturation and blood pressure.

A subsequent compression ultrasound showed an extensive right-sided proximal DVT.

CASE 2

A 64-year-old female was admitted with a 5-day history of severe progressive breathlessness and exertional faintness. Two years earlier, extensive investigations for unexplained breathlessness concluded that the diagnosis was hyperventilation.

In her past history, there had been extensive plastic surgery on the left calf. On admission, she was obese with bilateral ankle oedema. She was having episodic attacks of breathlessness and pain. Oxygen saturations were dropping to 70% on air. An urgent lung scan showed multiple pulmonary emboli. She was treated with an IV heparin infusion and alteplase but remained very ill. Combined pulmonary angiogram and venogram showed multiple emboli originating from a left iliac vein thrombosis. A permanent inferior vena cava filter was inserted by the radiologist to lie in the vena cava just below the renal veins. This prevented further emboli, and she slowly recovered.

At review a year later, she remained well, with much-improved exercise tolerance and significant weight loss. She was on lifelong warfarin.

CASE STUDY 7.3   Moderate Pulmonary Emboli

A 67-year-old female was admitted to the hospital with a 1-week history of breathlessness on minimal exertion and 2 days of left-sided pleurisy. She had been immobile for a month with back pain, and for 2 days the left leg had been swollen. She had been on tamoxifen for 4 years after a mastectomy for breast cancer and had insulin-dependent diabetes.

The lung scan showed multiple emboli; she was given LMWH, and because of increasing breathlessness she was also given alteplase (current guidelines suggest that alteplase should **only** be used in acute massive emboli with hypotension or shock).

CASE STUDY 7.4   Two Cases of Acute Pleurisy—Embolus or Infection?

CASE 1

A 50-year-old male was admitted with a 48-h history of very severe right-sided pleurisy, breathlessness and haemoptysis. There was no history of calf pain and no other risk factors. He was sweaty but apyrexial, with a pulse of 110 beats/min, respiratory rate of 20 breaths/min, and shallow painful breathing. Oxygen saturation was 90% on air. He was in extreme pain and very anxious. His legs were normal and he was of a slim build. There was fresh haemoptysis. Chest film showed shadowing at the bases of both lungs. His white cell count was normal. He was given IV opiate analgesia, immediate oxygen and subcutaneous LMWH 12,000 units subcutaneously (175 units/kg). An urgent CTPA showed multiple peripheral pulmonary emboli.

CASE 2

A 45-year-old overweight male was admitted with haemoptysis and severe right-sided pleurisy. He had a week's history of flu-like symptoms culminating in a wheezy-sounding productive cough. For 48h, his sputum had been green but then became blood-stained and then brown. His legs were normal, and there were no risk factors apart from obesity. His pulse was 100 beats/min, temperature 38.5°C and saturation 97% on air. There was a brassy-sounding painful cough and brown mucopurulent sputum. His calves were normal. Chest film was normal, and the white cell count was elevated at 15,000 × 10⁹/L. He was started on antibiotics and analgesics (NSAIDs). A lung scan was requested as a precaution and was reported to be normal.

BOX 7.2 ■ Classic Features of a Pulmonary Embolus

- Pleuritic chest pain
- Breathlessness
- Respiratory rate >20 breaths/min
- Haemoptysis

In cellulitis, there is a clear upper limit of demarcation to a swollen red limb. In critical ischaemia due to arterial insufficiency, the leg can be red and swollen, particularly if the patient has been sitting with the leg in a dependent position. Importantly, the limb will be cool, probably pulseless, and lose its colour when it is elevated.

- Differentiating between an acute chest infection with pleurisy and a PE can be difficult. Key symptoms are chest pain, breathlessness and syncope.
- Pulmonary emboli can arise from silent DVT.
- Oxygen saturations (on air) are commonly below 92% (but can be normal).
- For all pulmonary emboli, the 3-month mortality rate is 15%, but patients who do particularly badly are:
  - Those with a severe acute pulmonary embolus
  - The elderly
  - Those with COPD
  - Those with CCF
  - Those who have an underlying malignancy

CRITICAL CLINICAL TASKS IN A SEVERE ACUTE PULMONARY EMBOLUS

ABCDE: Immediate resuscitation. If the patient has collapsed with a cardiac arrest, cardiopulmonary resuscitation is started without delay. A massive embolus can present with a cardiac arrest, typically in the form of EMD (an ECG rhythm trace but no palpable pulse or blood pressure). Alternatively, patients can present with severe shock—confusion, reduced conscious level, hypotension (systolic blood pressure < 90 mm Hg), desaturation (<90%) and cold clammy extremities—that look very much like sepsis. An urgent bedside cardiac ECHO will confirm acute right-sided heart strain.

Ensure adequate oxygenation. A major embolus cuts off the circulation to the lung, so the patient becomes acutely cyanosed. Immediate high-flow oxygen with a reservoir mask is indicated to correct this. Intubation and ventilation may be needed in extreme cases.

CRITICAL CLINICAL TASKS IN ACUTE PULMONARY EMBOLUS

- ABCDE: immediate resuscitation
- Ensure adequate oxygenation
- Provide adequate circulation

Provide adequate circulation. There is an immediate decrease in cardiac output due to interruption of the circulation by the clot. The blood pressure falls dramatically even though the heart may continue to beat strongly. To help the heart by maximising venous return, the patient must be kept flat with the legs raised. A persistently low blood pressure is an indication for IV fluids. *However*, a safe fluid challenge would be no more than 500 mL of 0.9% saline over 30 min, as the right side of the heart is already under strain and may not cope with a large volume load.

If these measures do not restore the blood pressure, then inotropic support is needed; the options are noradrenaline (norepinephrine), dopamine, dobutamine and adrenaline (epinephrine). Drugs such as glyceryl trinitrate or furosemide are contraindicated, as they will reduce an already dangerously low blood pressure.

IMPORTANT CLINICAL TASKS IN ACUTE PULMONARY EMBOLUS

Relieve the patient's symptoms. Chest pain, breathlessness and severe anxiety, the dominant symptoms in a major pulmonary embolus, respond to IV opiates: morphine or diamorphine. These patients are often terrified by the sudden onset and will need constant reassurance. Unlike acute left ventricular failure (which in other respects gives a very similar picture to a major pulmonary embolus), the patient's breathlessness is not relieved by sitting up—these patients are most comfortable lying flat.

Assess the response to treatment. While resuscitation continues, the pulse, blood pressure and oxygen saturation need to be measured every few minutes. Persistent hypotension and tachycardia, despite efforts to restore the circulation, suggest that the clot has not shifted and that it continues to obstruct the circulation to the lung. Repeated urgent blood gas measurements will be needed during the initial phase.

> **IMPORTANT CLINICAL TASKS IN ACUTE PULMONARY EMBOLUS**
> - Relieve the patient's symptoms
> - Assess the response to treatment
> - Anticipate the need for urgent heparin therapy or thrombolysis
> - Prepare the patient for further procedures

Anticipate the need for urgent heparin therapy or thrombolysis. If the initial management is successful and while the patient's condition stabilises, IV heparin is given as a 5000 to 10,000 unit loading dose followed by an infusion at 18 U/kg/h to prevent further and possibly fatal emboli. The choice lies between IV heparin as an initial bolus, then infusion, and subcutaneous LMWH. Heparin prevents further clotting and allows the body's natural enzymes to disperse existing clots. In patients who remain hypotensive and ill, the thrombolytic recombinant tissue plasminogen activator (rt-PA) (alteplase) can be used in parallel to help break up the emboli more rapidly. The recommended treatment is a 10 mg IV bolus over 2 min followed by 90 mg over 2 h. In a cardiac arrest from a proven PE, a 50-mg bolus can be used.

Prepare the patient for further procedures. Further tests will be needed to confirm the diagnosis, usually a CTPA or, less commonly, a pulmonary angiogram. A pulmonary angiogram is primarily diagnostic, but it can help the patient directly if the catheter is used to dislodge the clot or put thrombolytic drugs directly into the pulmonary vessels where the embolus is lodged. In extreme cases, if thrombolysis has been unsuccessful and the patient remains collapsed, emergency surgery and clot removal can salvage an apparently hopeless situation.

If, despite adequate anticoagulation, recurrent emboli arisie from residual clots in the deep veins, filter devices can be placed in the inferior vena cava. These are effective in preventing further emboli and are usually well tolerated.

NB: Prompt heparinisation and subsequent anticoagulation for 3 to 6 months reduce the risk of recurrent thromboembolic events and fatal pulmonary emboli by 90%.

PULMONARY EMBOLISM IN PREGNANCY

The main cause of pregnancy-related death in the developed world is PE—the risk is greatest in the third trimester and post-caesarian section. In an uncomplicated pregnancy, symptoms such as breathlessness, chest discomfort and ankle swelling are common, and D-dimers can be elevated. There are also concerns about exposing the mother and foetus to unnecessary radiation. During the first two trimesters, a CTPA probably exposes the foetus to less radiation than a nuclear medicine perfusion scan—during the third trimester, they are about equal. Exposure levels from both tests (60–130 µGy), however, are well below those that could be harmful (50,000 µGy). The implications of a missed diagnosis are so grave that the most helpful test has to be selected—this will usually be a CTPA. The "YEARS" decision tool minimises the number of unnecessary scans and is widely used. The tool uses three items from the Wells criteria: (1) clinical signs of a DVT, (2) haemoptysis and (3) pulmonary embolus being the most likely diagnosis, and two cut-off points for the D-dimer result. If no items are present, a D-dimer level of less than 1000 ng/mL excludes a pulmonary embolus, and if one or more items are present, a D-dimer level of less than 500 ng/mL excludes an embolus.

Pregnancy does not influence emergency treatment, but subsequent prevention is based on daily LMWH as warfarin can harm foetal development, and there is insufficient safety data on DOACs.

ANSWERING RELATIVES' QUESTIONS IN PULMONARY EMBOLISM

Why did the patient collapse? A blood clot became dislodged from a thrombosis in the leg and travelled to the lungs, where it became trapped, preventing blood from leaving the heart and reaching the lungs. In effect, circulation of the blood stopped at that point.

What are the risks of a pulmonary embolus? The risk of death in a pulmonary embolus is about 5% (reduced from 30% by treatment).

Is it the clot that is being coughed up? No. The blood-stained sputum is from lung tissue that has been starved of oxygen because the clot has cut off its blood supply.

What happens to the clot? It will break up and dissolve through the body's natural anticoagulants, helped by the treatment the patient is receiving from us. Anticoagulant tablets and heparin prevent the clot from spreading, whereas rt-PA (alteplase) actually melts any clot. However, we only use alteplase in very ill patients as it can cause dangerous bleeding.

What are the risks of further emboli now that the patient is on heparin? They are very low indeed (although not reduced to zero). The heparin will be followed by a variable time on anticoagulant tablets to reduce the risk even further.

Caring for the Patient With a Suspected Deep Vein Thrombosis

The history and examination are unreliable in the diagnosis of venous thrombosis. Seventy per cent of patients who are initially thought to have a DVT will prove to have an alternative diagnosis. Conversely, patients can present with a major pulmonary embolus that has arisen from a completely silent DVT.

There is a high cost for missing a proximal (iliofemoral as opposed to calf vein) DVT: a 50% chance of a further episode and a 10% chance of a fatal PE within 3 months. The emphasis is therefore on using the combination of key clinical features and further investigations to ensure that the number missed is kept to a minimum.

CLINICAL ASSESSMENT OF A POSSIBLE DEEP VEIN THROMBOSIS

Risk factors from the patient's history. The major risk factors are as follows:
- Lower limb immobility
- Major surgery within the previous 12 weeks
- More than two first-degree relatives with a history of DVTs
- Active cancer within the previous 6 months
- Recently bedridden for more than 3 days

Lower limb immobility. After a stroke, a paralysed lower limb often develops chronic ankle oedema, so the diagnosis of a DVT can be difficult, particularly if there is a problem with communication. The risks are similar if a lower limb is immobilised in a full-length plaster cast.

Surgery within the previous 12 weeks. Venous thrombosis is especially common after hip and knee replacements and can occur 4 to 6 weeks after surgery. Diagnosis can be difficult because of swelling and discomfort due to the surgery itself, but investigations need to be pursued because 20% of patients undergoing a major lower limb joint replacement will develop a DVT despite prophylactic subcutaneous heparin in the immediate post-operative period.

Cancer. Active malignant disease within the previous 6 months increases the risk of DVT. Malignancy, particularly in the lung, prostate and pancreas, can also present as unexplained, often recurrent, venous thrombosis.

Positive family history. There is increasing recognition of the importance of a positive history of venous thromboembolic disease in first-degree relatives. The inherited thrombophilias are passed on to half of the offspring, as they are all inherited as autosomal dominant characteristics.

Other Important Features in the History

Previous DVT/PE. A previous thromboembolic episode is a major risk factor. The recurrence rate at 5 years is 25%; it is particularly high if there are residual associated risk factors such as malignant disease or immobility.

Obesity. Obesity is an important risk factor for both DVT and cellulitis. Commonly, obese middle-aged and elderly medical patients have chronically swollen and oedematous ankles, with areas of pigmentation, old healed varicose ulceration and discrete cellulitic-looking areas. These legs can be difficult to assess, in particular, to differentiate between acute and long-standing changes.

Smoking and hypertension. Heavy smoking and hypertension both increase the risk of thromboembolic disease, particularly in middle-aged overweight females.

Examination of the legs. There are three important signs of venous thrombosis in the legs (Fig. 7.2):

- Local tenderness of the calf or thigh
- Swelling of the calf and thigh
- Unilateral calf swelling (>3 cm at 10 cm below the tibial tuberosity)

Three additional signs may be present:

- Ankle oedema
- Unilateral dilated veins
- Calf redness

There is increasing interest in using procedures that combine the results of clinical assessment in the form of a scoring system with the results of a screening test procedure such as the D-dimer tests to determine the next step: immediate discharge, immediate anticoagulation or further investigation with D-dimer measurement and proximal vein ultrasound (Box 7.3; Fig. 7.3).

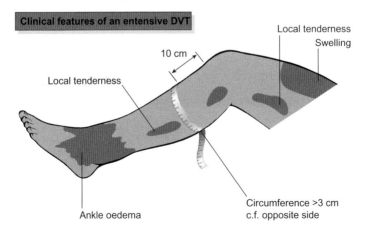

FIGURE 7.2   Clinical features of an extensive deep vein thrombosis (DVT).

BOX 7.3 ■ Scoring of the Probability of a Deep Vein Thrombosis (DVT) From Clinical Features[a]

Clinical Feature	Score
Active cancer (within the previous 6 months)	1
Paralysis or plaster cast immobilising the whole lower limb	1
Bed rest for more than 3 days or major surgery within 3 months	1
Localised tenderness along the deep veins	1
Whole leg swollen	1
Unilateral calf swelling of more than 3 cm	1
Unilateral pitting oedema	1
Distended superficial veins	1
Previous DVT	1
More or as likely alternative diagnosis	−2
DVT unlikely	<1
DVT likely	>2

[a]*Reprinted with permission from Elsevier (The Lancet, 1997, 350, 1795–1798).*

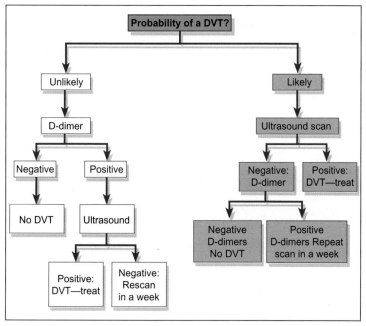

FIGURE 7.3 How probability scores can be utilised to diagnose deep vein thrombosis (DVT).

The Two-Level Deep Vein Thrombosis Wells Score: Likely and Unlikely

A modified Wells score (see Box 7.3) is used to score the patient's DVT as *likely* or *unlikely*. If it is *unlikely* and the D-dimer is negative, a DVT can be ruled out—if the D-dimer is positive, a proximal leg compression ultrasound is carried out to exclude a DVT. If a DVT is *likely*, the definitive test, compression ultrasound, is performed. Only if this is negative, a D-dimer is performed, which, if elevated (suggesting a calf vein clot undetectable by ultrasound), leads to a follow-up scan in 7 days to exclude extension of the clot into the thigh.

OTHER CAUSES OF ACUTE CALF PAIN

Pain arising from the knee joint. Mechanical pain from the knee is suggested by a sudden onset during twisting, turning or crouching. The joint may be swollen, stiff and tender. The history is particularly important in the rupture of a Baker cyst, as the signs in the leg can be identical to those found in a DVT (Fig. 7.4).

Muscle tears, ruptured Achilles tendon. The history is all-important. Torn muscle fibres usually occur during exertion and may be associated with local bruising around the heel and side of the foot. Patients on long-term oral steroids are prone to rupture of the Achilles tendon, which may occur with surprisingly little effort—even using the stairs.

Sciatica. There is a clear relationship in the history of lifting or sudden straining, with the pain commonly radiating from the spine down the back of the leg. With the patient lying on his back, the pain can be triggered by lifting the affected leg straight up in the air.

FIGURE 7.4   Differential diagnosis of a deep vein thrombosis (DVT).

OTHER CAUSES OF A SWOLLEN PAINFUL LEG

Acutely swollen red legs: illustrative cases. The following case studies illustrate possible diagnoses for acutely swollen red legs (Case Studies 7.5–7.7).

CASE STUDY 7.5   Deep Vein Thrombosis

Three weeks after a routine right hip replacement, a 55-year-old female was admitted with an increasingly swollen and painful right leg. There had been mild post-operative swelling, but this had spread from the calf to the thigh. On examination, the leg was swollen, oedematous, shiny and warm to the touch, both above and below the knee. The surgical wound was clean and well healed.

A diagnosis of iliofemoral thrombosis was made, and the patient was started on tinzaparin 175 U/kg subcutaneously once daily.
- The risk of a postarthroplasty DVT persists for up to 6 weeks.
- Half of the patients will have had a silent pulmonary embolus by the time the DVT presents.

CASE STUDY 7.6   Cellulitis

An obese 75-year-old male gave a 10-day history of an increasingly painful and swollen right leg. Initially, the foot was red and extremely tender, but 3 days before admission, the redness spread to involve the whole lower leg. He felt ill and shivery.

On examination, the pulse was 110 beats/min and the temperature was 38°C. The right calf and foot were hot, shiny, swollen and very tender. There was a deep purple/red discolouration of the lower leg, with a sudden line of demarcation 3 in (7.5 cm) below the knee. There were some tender red streaks at the back of the calf, spreading upward toward the buttocks. There was no obvious skin wound, but the spaces between the toes were soggy and inflamed. A diagnosis of acute cellulitis was made, with a site of entry presumed to be the infected web spaces. Intravenous benzylpenicillin 1.2 g qds and flucloxacillin 1 g qds were started, and the leg was elevated and rested. The web spaces were treated with antifungal agents. Prophylactic tinzaparin 3500 units daily was given in view of the risks of a subsequent DVT.

CASE STUDY 7.7   Varicose (Gravitational) Eczema

An 80-year-old male was admitted with bilateral, red, swollen legs and immobility. His legs had been troubling him for years: he had chronic varicose veins, a previous leg ulcer that had eventually healed and intermittent ankle swelling. His main complaint was of skin irritation and itching in the legs. He also noticed that both legs would 'break out' and discharge fluid.

On examination, he looked well and was apyrexial. The lower legs were very discoloured by brown pigmentation, surrounded by red and inflamed areas. The skin was crusty, flaking and covered in scratch marks up to the knees. There were also multiple small raised blisters, some of which were discharging fluid. The white cell count and blood cultures were negative.

A diagnosis of acute varicose eczema rather than cellulitis was made, and after dermatological advice, the legs were cleaned with twice daily 1:10,000 potassium permanganate astringent solution and started on high-potency local steroid cream to the skin.

Cellulitis

Major risk factors for cellulitis are as follows:

- Chronic lymphoedema of the leg (chronic brawny non-pitting oedema)
- An obvious portal of entry such as a skin wound
- Obesity
- Previous leg ulcer

Necrotising fasciitis. *NB*: If the pain from a 'cellulitic' leg is extreme, worsening and seemingly out of proportion to the changes in the leg, it is important to consider the possibility of necrotising fasciitis, a deep, rapidly spreading soft tissue infection.

The main features of necrotising fasciitis are as follows:

- Extreme pain and localised numbness
- Skin blisters and bullae
- Necrotic skin
- Hypotension
- White cell count $>15.4 \times 10^9$/L and sodium <135 mmol/L
- History of IV drug abuse

Necrotising fasciitis requires urgent surgical assessment with a view to extensive debridement if the patient is to survive.

Varicose eczema. Cellulitis can be confused with varicose eczema:

- In both conditions, the legs are red and inflamed.
- Crusting and scaling are seen only in varicose eczema.
- The skin is shiny and smooth in cellulitis.
- If there is doubt, start IV antibiotics and seek dermatologic help.

Management of a Deep Vein Thrombosis

AIM: To Prevent Extension of the Thrombosis and Prevent Embolisation

- Identify risk factors before starting therapy
- Baseline full blood count, clotting screen, biochemistry, liver function tests, consider thrombophilia screen
- Obtain an accurate weight to determine the dose of LMWH
- Identify any possible contraindications to anticoagulation therapy
- If thromboembolism is scored as *unlikely* but with positive D-dimers and there is no contraindication start anti-coagulation immediately, to be followed by confirmation of the diagnosis (compression vein ultra-sound)
- If scored as *likely*, start immediate anticoagulation and confirm with a proximal venous compression ultrasound. If the scan is negative measure the D-dimers and if positive repeat the scan in a week to ensure that a calf vein thrombosis (not seen on a compression ultra-sound) has not spread in to the thigh.
  - To anti-coagulate: give an immediate DOAC, either apixaban or rivaroxaban. Alternatively give five days of subcutaneous LMWH eg tinzaparin 175.0 units/kg.

For the patients on LMWH give 10 mg oral warfarin loading dose on the same day the heparin is started, continue heparin for five days or until the INR is two or above for two consecutive days.

- Subsequent warfarin doses can be predicted using the standard flexible induction dose regimen, which should be available on the ward (DOACS do not need blood test monitoring)
- Raise the leg and, in extensive symptomatic thrombosis, apply class II elastic stockings
- If there is extensive swelling: immobilise for 48 h to allow swelling to reduce, then mobilise in stockings
- Watch for ischaemia
  - loss of sensation
  - pain
  - seek urgent medical assessment if ischaemia is suspected in a swollen leg
- When resting: in bed with leg elevated, not down
- Discharge with or without class II thigh-length hosiery and sleep with foot of bed raised
- Daily walks
- Encourage weight loss
- There is a 6% risk of venous ulceration and chronic disability

Box 7.4 summarises the key points in mobilisation of a DVT patient in the first 24 h.

CRITICAL CLINICAL TASKS IN A SUSPECTED DVT

In a suspected thromboembolic event, give the first dose of heparin immediately. Once investigations are under way, the patient may be off the ward for some time during the critical first few hours. The safest course of action is, in the absence of an obvious contraindication, to give the first dose of subcutaneous heparin as soon as the initial assessment is completed.

BOX 7.4 ■ Bed Rest or Mobilisation in the First 24 h?

- Elevate and rest a tense, swollen leg due to iliofemoral thrombosis
- Do not elevate a leg that may be ischaemic (be wary of the patient with diabetes)
- Rest a leg affected by acute cellulitis
- Mobilise an uncomplicated DVT within the limits of patient comfort
- Do not allow any patient with a swollen leg to sit with the legs dependent. If the leg is elevated or subjected to pressure dressings, watch for ischaemia:
  - Increasing pain
  - Increasing discolouration or pallor of the feet
  - Numbness, loss of sensation
  - Loss or absence of the pulses

CRITICAL CLINICAL TASKS IN SUSPECTED DEEP VEIN THROMBOSIS

- Give the first dose of heparin immediately
- Ensure there is adequate pain relief
- Be vigilant for acute ischaemia

Ensure there is adequate pain relief. A severely swollen leg will cause intense pain. Non-steroidal anti-inflammatory drugs and aspirin are unsafe once warfarin has been started, and paracetamol may not be adequate. Oral dihydrocodeine or tramadol may be sufficient, but in extreme pain subcutaneous morphine 10 mg 2–4 hourly may be needed.

Be vigilant for acute ischaemia. Any acutely oedematous leg is at risk from ischaemia as a result of increased soft tissue pressure compromising the circulation to the legs. *Persistent or increasing pain* is the main warning feature, but there may simply be colour change or loss of feeling in the leg.

IMPORTANT CLINICAL TASKS IN A SUSPECTED DEEP VEIN THROMBOSIS

Care of pressure areas. The heels and sides of the feet are particularly vulnerable in cases of acutely swollen legs. Inspect these areas regularly, use pressure-relieving strategies and encourage early mobilisation. Oedematous legs are prone to superficial skin infections, particularly if pre-existing foot hygiene is poor.

Reassure the patient. The prospect of a clot breaking off and travelling to the lungs terrifies most patients. They will want to know about mobilisation (to be encouraged once any severe swelling has resolved), about what exactly happens to the clot in the leg and when the swelling will disappear.

IMPORTANT CLINICAL TASKS IN A SUSPECTED DEEP VEIN THROMBOSIS

- Care of the pressure areas
- Reassure the patient
- Document all current regular and intermittent medication
- Document the target INR (usually 2.5)
- Ensure a warfarin loading schedule is followed by the prescribing doctors

Document all current regular and intermittent medication. Potential drug interactions will become important once anticoagulation is established.

Document the target INR (usually 2.5). It is important to oversee the anticoagulant therapy, particularly as the patient may be on and off the ward in the first 24 h having tests, and there may be a delay, with associated uncertainty, before all the tests come back to the ward. This can lead to a delay in anticoagulation or failures in communication among the staff.

Ensure a warfarin loading schedule is followed by the prescribing doctors.
Table 7.2 details the warfarin loading schedule, depending on INR.

ANSWERING RELATIVES' QUESTIONS IN DEEP VEIN THROMBOSIS

Why did the thrombosis occur? There are three reasons that may be important: stagnation
of the blood in the leg veins, damage to the walls of the veins that may have triggered it
and an abnormality in the blood itself that can make it more liable to clot.

Is it because of the family history? It is increasingly recognised that, in many patients
(especially those with recurrent episodes or unexplained DVT in young people), there is
an inherited tendency that could also be present in close family members. Sometimes it
becomes necessary to screen family members because some of these abnormalities can
be passed on.

Was it the result of bad post-operative nursing? Even with preventative measures
(LMWH, etc.), there remains a significant risk after any surgery, particularly complex
surgery and major joint replacements.

Does the warfarin continue for life? It depends on the circumstances: for example, if a
second DVT is treated with warfarin for 6 months, the recurrence rate is 20%, compared
with 2% if the warfarin is continued for life.

What about the contraceptive pill, pregnancy and HRT? The risk is increased in all three
situations, but particularly in pregnancy. Even so, the overall figures are still low in absolute terms: of 100,000 women on a third-generation pill for a year, only 25 will suffer a
thromboembolic event (Table 7.3).

TABLE 7.2 ■ Warfarin loading

Day	INR	Warfarin
1	<1.4	10 mg
2	<1.8	10 mg
	1.8	1.0 mg
	>1.8	0.5 mg

TABLE 7.3 ■ Risk of a Thromboembolic Event Among Contraceptive Pill Users

	Rate per 100,000 Females per Year
Normal non-pregnant	5
Second-generation combined pill	15
Third-generation combined pill	25
Pregnant	60

Excellent Care for Thromboembolic Disease

- Staff awareness of the critical issues in thromboembolic disease
  - difficulties in diagnosis
  - the importance of immediate treatment
  - preventable mortality and morbidity
  - immediate access to investigation results (e.g., CTPA)
- Staff training in cardiopulmonary resuscitation
- Guidelines for suspected DVT
  - documentation of risk factors
  - use of a clinical scoring system
  - immediate treatment in suspected DVT
- Access to screening tests: D-dimers/ultrasound/lung scanning
- Anticoagulation guidelines
  - the use of LMWH
  - warfarin guidelines
  - a system for writing up anticoagulation prescriptions
  - managing over-anticoagulation
  - familiarisation with DOACs
- Patient information
  - anticoagulation handbook
  - information leaflets
- Clinical audit
  - initial documentation
  - delay to first dose of heparin
  - event monitoring (e.g., sudden collapse from unrecognised PE)
- Access to ambulatory management
  - Risk stratification to identify low-risk patients
  - Trained nurse – led Ambulatory DVT/PE team

The risk of thromboembolism with HRT is lower than that with second-generation oral contraceptives.

Will it happen again? Even with warfarin therapy, there is a risk of recurrence after it is stopped. The rate is around 20% over the subsequent five years but will be less if there was an obvious trigger such as a hip replacement.

What are the risks of warfarin? Standard treatment with warfarin carries an annual risk of haemorrhage of 7% and death of 0.2%.

Why is the leg still so swollen – will it ever go down completely? Thrombosis damages the valves in the veins that are necessary for the efficient return of blood from the legs to the heart. The leg may remain swollen for some time, and sometimes it may never return to normal. The situation can be helped by regular exercise, the use of support stockings and avoiding sitting with dependent legs.

ANTICOAGULATION THERAPY

Intravenous heparin. Heparin increases the effect of the naturally occurring anticoagulant called antithrombin. There is a wide variation in the response to IV heparin, so that the treatment needs careful monitoring, using the APPT in order to individualise the dose. Inadequate initial therapy is associated with a much worse outcome. The aim is to anticoagulate to 1.5–2.5 times the control APPT. Intravenous heparin is continued for at least 4 days and should overlap with warfarin treatment until the INR is in the therapeutic range of 2.0–3.0 for at least 2 days.

Many audits have shown a tendency to undertreat patients with heparin, particularly in the first critical 24 h: this problem can be minimised by the use of a heparin protocol.

The main role of intravenous heparin is in patients with severe renal impairment, those with a high risk of bleeding and those with a PE and haemodynamic instability who may need additional measures.

Subcutaneous low-molecular-weight heparin. LMWH has replaced the heparin infusion in most situations because it is as effective in treating both DVT and pulmonary embolus. Its simplicity raises the prospect of outpatient treatment.

In contrast to conventional heparin, LMWH:

- can be given once daily
- has a consistent action in every patient that is determined solely by the patient's weight
- can be given as a fixed-dose subcutaneous injection
- does not require laboratory monitoring
- is not safe in severe renal insufficiency (eGFR < 30 mL/min/1.73 m^2)

LMWH is given for at least 5 days while warfarin is introduced, until the INR is within the therapeutic range (2.5–3.0) for two consecutive days.

Doses (using tinzaparin as an example)
Prophylaxis
Low-risk surgery. 3500 units of tinzaparin 2 h pre-op and once daily for 7 days post-op.

High-risk surgery/high-risk medical condition, e.g., severe diabetic ketoacidosis. 50 units/kg 12 h pre-op and once daily for 7 days.

Treatment of thromboembolic event. 175 units/kg of tinzaparin once daily.

- *Weigh the patient*
  - 100 kg = 18,000 units/day
  - 80 kg = 14,000 units/day
  - 55 kg = 10,000 units/day
- *Check renal function*: If eGFR is less than 30, consider intravenous heparin infusion or enoxaparin

Reversing heparin

- **Excessive bleeding on heparin usually responds to stopping the heparin and, if necessary, transfusion. Intravenous protamine sulfate will neutralise heparin at a dose of 1 mg per 100 units given slowly over 10 min, but it only partially reverses LMWH and no more than 40 mg should be given at any one injection. Treatment can be repeated hourly. FFP is not indicated for heparin overdosage.**

Warfarin therapy. Warfarin interferes with vitamin K metabolism and ensures that the naturally occurring clotting factors are manufactured by the liver in an inactive form. Warfarin prolongs the prothrombin time and is monitored by using the INR, a standardised form of the prothrombin time that should be kept in the range of 2.0–3.0, with a target of 2.5 unless there are exceptional circumstances such as recurrent thromboembolic events despite warfarin treatment. Daily INR measurements are necessary in the initial stages of anticoagulation, and the adjusted warfarin dose must be given at the same time each day.

Over-anticoagulation. The most common causes for over-anticoagulation are:

- drug interactions
- errors with warfarin therapy
- the development of cardiac failure
- deterioration in liver function

Many drugs increase the effect of warfarin: those most commonly implicated are broad-spectrum antibiotics. Progressive cardiac failure, particularly in the elderly, is often associated with a sudden deterioration in anticoagulant control – INR values of 10 or more are not uncommon. Liver disease itself prolongs the prothrombin time, so clearly its development would have a major effect on the patient who is also taking warfarin.

Once the INR increases above 5.0 there is a risk of bleeding. However, provided that there is no major blood loss, INR values in the range 4–8 can be managed by discontinuing warfarin treatment until the INR falls. If the INR is greater than 8, warfarin should be stopped and if there are additional risks for bleeding (e.g., over 70 years old, previous bleeding, nose bleeds) a small dose (0.5–2.5 mg *orally* of the IV preparation) of vitamin K should be given. This will partially reverse the effects of the warfarin.

In serious or life-threatening bleeding anticoagulation must be reversed urgently. Intravenous vitamin K – 2 mg will normalise the INR within 6 h while intravenous Prothrombin Complex Concentrate (25–50 units/kg depending on the INR) works immediately. Fresh frozen plasma (FFP) is the alternative to PCC but carries a risk of transfusion reaction and has a slower onset of action. The clotting factors restored by PCC and FFP only last a few hours so IV Vitamin K must be given at the same time.

Direct action oral anti-coagulants: dabigatran, rivaroxaban, apixaban and edoxaban

DOACs (previously known as NOACs), a new class of oral anticoagulants, have revolutionized the management of pulmonary thrombo-embolic disease. Unlike warfarin, which blocks a number of Vitamin K – dependent clotting factors, these drugs act on single sites ('direct') and importantly:

- no INR monitoring and dose adjustment is required
- their onset of action is rapid
- apixaban and rivaroxaban do not need initial LMWH cover
  - Rivaroxaban dose: 15 mg bd for three weeks then 20 mg once daily
  - Apixaban dose 10 mg bd for one week then 5 mg bd
- they carry less risk than warfarin of major bleeding

However, warfarin retains an important role, particularly in patients who have renal failure or are severely overweight or who have liver disease. Significantly, unlike warfarin, DOACs cannot be easily reversed.

Reversal of DOACS

The increased use of DOACS has led to a rise in the number of life-threatening bleeding.

Praxbind, is an artificial antibody, which binds to and inactivates dabigatran.

Ondexxya blocks rivaroxaban and apixaban. These drugs have limited availability and may also increase the risk of triggering thrombosis - their use is therefore confined to life saving treatment and where specialist advice is available.

OUTPATIENT MANAGEMENT OF VENOUS THROMBOEMBOLIC DISEASE

Increasingly patients with an uncomplicated DVT or a pulmonary embolus are being assessed for possible management in an ambulatory care setting. Up to half of all patients with a pulmonary embolus may be suitable for this approach, but a set of strict exclusion criteria have to be applied. The Simplified Pulmonary Embolism Severity Index (sPESI) identifies low risk patients, who if social circumstances permit, may be suitable for ambulatory care. The index is also an *aide memoir* for emphasizing which in-patients may have an adverse outcome.

The simplified Pulmonary Embolism Severity Index

sPESI criteria	Points
Age >80 years	1
History of cancer	1
Chronic cardiopulmonary disease	1
Systolic blood pressure <100 mmHg	1
Heart rate ≥110 b.p.m.	1
Arterial oxygen saturation <90%	1

Only if the sSPESI scores 0 points consider ambulatory care

The new DOACs, apixaban and rivaroxaban, are particularly suited to ambulatory management since they are used in a single-drug regime without the need for initial heparin or blood tests with dose adjustments.

COVID-19 and Thromboembolic Disease

Patients with COVID-19 are at particular risk of thrombotic events. For example, patients with COVID-19 in the intensive therapy unit have a one in five chance of a pulmonary embolism, and any thrombotic event is associated with a significantly increased risk of death. Current recommendations are that severe COVID-19 cases should receive standard-dose prophylactic subcutaneous LMWH. Moderately severe cases should be considered for full therapeutic subcutaneous LMWH, which should be continued until the patient comes off oxygen. A proven thrombotic event should be treated with apixaban or rivaroxaban unless patient instability or reduced conscious level precludes oral medication, in which case LMWH should be used.

Further Reading

British Thoracic Society, 2018. Guidelines for the outpatient management of pulmonary embolism. https://www.brit-thoracic.org.uk/standards-of-care/guidelines/.
NICE, 2023. Venous thromboembolic diseases: diagnosis, management, thrombophilia testing, clinical guideline 2020. https://www.nice.org.uk/guidance/NG158.

CHAPTER 8

Deliberate Self-Harm, Alcohol and Substance Use Disorders

Deliberate Self-Harm

GENERAL PRINCIPLES

Each day an acute admitting ward in an average-sized district general hospital will take in two to three patients with deliberate self-harm. The pressures on medical and nursing time, combined with the problems of finding sufficient beds, often mean that this group of patients is granted a low priority. Although mortality rates are very low, most patients will be discharged without an adequate psychosocial assessment and without any care plan or follow-up. This is not acceptable because:

- This is a vulnerable population.
- Self-harm is invariably associated with considerable emotional distress.
- With correct management, the long- and short-term outcomes can be improved.
- The contribution of personal culpability for an illness does not influence the management in other areas of health—alcoholic liver disease, lung cancer, chronic obstructive pulmonary disease, HIV—and should not in deliberate self-harm.
- The problem is getting larger: the numbers admitted with deliberate self-harm have increased by 50% in 10 years.

Principles of Treatment

- Appropriate emergency management to ensure the safety of the patient.
- Granting the same care, respect and privacy as any other patient.
- Proper psychosocial assessment.
- Identification of patients at risk from further self-harm.
- Where possible, the patient should be given the choice of a male or female member of staff for the assessment process.
- Identification of safeguarding issues (domestic abuse, violence, exploitation).

Who Commits Suicide?

There are 5000 suicides per year in England and Wales: 45% by violent methods, mainly jumping from heights, strangulation and drowning; and 35% by drug overdose, predominantly antidepressants and paracetamol. Interestingly, the rates in both sexes are falling throughout the age range. Numerous factors are said to contribute to this: higher employment rates, recent initiatives to counteract self-harm and reduction in carbon monoxide levels in exhausts. There is still concern, however, over rates in young males, which, compared with two decades ago, are particularly high. Young males are reluctant to acknowledge emotional distress and the need to address it.

WHO IS AT A PARTICULARLY HIGH RISK OF SUICIDE?

It is important to be aware of the vulnerable groups because they will be encountered in the acute medical wards as a result of self-harm or because of their high rates of poor overall physical health.

- Recent acute psychiatric illness, particularly during the first week after discharge.
- Schizophrenia, especially in patients who are poorly compliant or lost to follow-up.
- History of drug and alcohol use disorder.
- Any patient who says that they are feeling suicidal, especially if accompanied by feelings of hopelessness.
- Patients living in social isolation with no family support.
- Several previous episodes of deliberate self-harm (25% of successful suicides have tried before within the past year).
- A single episode of deliberate self-harm carries a 1 in 20 rate of suicide within 10 years.
- Those involved with the legal system, most notably prisoners.

Which Type of Patients Are Admitted With Deliberate Self-Harm?

The admission rate for deliberate self-harm is 300 per 100,000 of the population per year and is increasing, particularly among males aged 15 to 24 years.

- The average age is 30 years.
- Forty per cent will have taken a previous overdose.
- Twenty per cent will take a further overdose within a year, particularly those:
  - Who have a history of alcohol and substance use disorder.
  - Who discharge themselves before the initial assessment has been completed.
  - Who have had several previous episodes.
- Social deprivation and social isolation are common.

- Up to 10% will have a serious psychiatric disorder, commonly depression.
- There is a strong link with a history of epilepsy, particularly in males.
- There is often a history of early parental death or separation.
- A quarter will have been in contact with the psychiatric services.
- Common triggers are major domestic arguments or a recent separation.

THE EMBARRASSED AND IMPULSIVE

- The spur of the moment
- Often triggered by a row and alcohol
- Not necessarily a trivial amount, often paracetamol
- Low risk of recurrence or future suicide

THE SERIOUS ATTEMPT

- A planned event
- Carried out alone and in secret
- No attempt to get help
- Suicide note
- Admits to the intended outcome
- Even 'trivial' overdoses may represent a determined attempt at suicide

THE RECURRENT ATTENDER

- Severe personality disorder
- History of drug and alcohol use disorder
- History of violence and criminal convictions
- High risk of eventual success

THE HIGH-RISK SELF-HARM

- Older
- Male
- Isolated
- Unemployed/retired
- Alcohol dependence
- Poor general health
- Violent method used
- Repeated attempts over a short time frame
- Suicide note
- Mental illness in the past 12 months—especially involving an admission

Why Do Patients Deliberately Harm Themselves?

- **To gain temporary respite**—'I just wanted to get some sleep/escape/to get away for a while'
- **As a cry for help**—'I didn't know what to do next/where to go/who to turn to'
- **As a signal of distress**—'Nobody listened/I just couldn't explain what was happening to me'
- **Communicating anger/eliciting guilt/influencing others**
  - 'I did it on the spur of the moment in front of them all'
  - 'This will show her/him what it's been like for me'
- **To end their lives**—'There's no point in any of it any more'

TWO HIGH-RISK PATIENTS

Case Studies 8.1 and 8.2 illustrate different types of self-harm cases.

From Case Study 8.1, it is clear that:

- The history needed unearthing.
- This patient had a long, unrecognised history involving a major psychosis: probably schizophrenia.

The male in Case Study 8.2 is at very high risk:

- Elderly male
- Violent method of self-harm

CASE STUDY 8.1   Overdose

A 40-year-old male was admitted with an overdose of one of the newer less toxic antidepressants.

He complained of feeling generally upset and lonely but denied significant past illnesses. He was single and lived alone, visiting his father at weekends. He presented as an outwardly cheerful, middle-class articulate male who could not really account for the overdose. Nothing else was noted in the medical or nursing notes.

On subsequent very close questioning, he admitted to previous problems with depression and recalled having electroconvulsive therapy (ECT) in his 20s after a period when he thought he was going mad. He had been treated with antipsychotics at that time. There was a history of progressive social isolation, with only occasional visits away from his bedsit to visit his father.

CASE STUDY 8.2   Violent Self-Harm

A 75-year-old male with severe ischaemic heart disease, cardiac failure and persistent hypotension was admitted because of self-harm.

He had become increasingly frustrated and angry with an unexplained pain in his lower abdomen, which had been thoroughly investigated. He was feeling low and had been sleeping badly. He went into the kitchen, took the scissors and made multiple superficial incisions across his upper abdomen to 'relieve the blood congestion'. On admission, he was tearful and frustrated but embarrassed to have caused so much trouble.

- Features of depression
- Failing physical health

In this age group, deliberate self-harm is commonly triggered by disability, social isolation, chronic pain and untreated depression. It is important to recognise the symptoms of depression in the elderly:

- Anorexia and weight loss
- Constipation
- Change in sleep
- A pattern of mood swings, especially early morning depression
- Physical and mental slowing
- Suicidal ideas

Because the highest rates of suicide are seen in elderly males, it is important to ensure that they receive an urgent psychosocial assessment.

Caring for the Patient With Self-Harm

Acute Medical Assessment Units should have Internet access to TOXBASE, the UK database of the National Poisons Information Service. This provides detailed descriptions of the management of individual clinical problems.

CRITICAL CLINICAL TASKS IN DELIBERATE SELF-HARM

Care of the Unconscious Patient: ABCDE and NEWS2

- Is the airway patent and protected? Remove food and vomit from the mouth.
- Consider an oropharyngeal or a nasopharyngeal airway.
- Place the patient's head down in the recovery position to prevent aspiration.
- Assess the patient's breathing: measure the respiratory rate.
- Document the pulse and blood pressure.
- Measure and correct oxygen saturation.
- Is the patient hypothermic? This is common with barbiturates and phenothiazines. Use a space blanket to warm the patient.
- Is the patient hypoglycaemic?
- Measure the Glasgow Coma Score (GCS): if less than 8, the airway is at risk.
- Expose the patient:
  - As with any unconscious patient, look assiduously for any evidence to suggest a head injury—bruising or bogginess over the scalp and bleeding from the nose or ears.
  - Skin blisters are common after overdoses, especially over the fingers, knees, shoulders and hips. Extensive blistering may occur over areas on which the patient has been lying, for example, the lateral aspect of the feet. Bullae should not be punctured—de-roof them once they have burst and cover them with a nonadherent dressing.

- Look for and document any areas of swelling and bruising, particularly in areas exposed to pressure in unconscious patients: underlying tissue damage may lead to complications, for example, muscle breakdown (rhabdomyolysis), leading to kidney failure and acute limb ischaemia. Muscle damage is common in overdoses of ecstasy, theophyllines and opiates. Paralysis of a limb (wrist or foot drop) can also occur and is caused by nerve palsies due to the local effects of pressure.
- Examine for signs of self-injury (wrists) and of substance use disorder (needle tracks, abscesses).
- Site an IV cannula.
- Place on an electrocardiogram (ECG) monitor and arrange for a standard 12-lead ECG.
- Monitor the oxygen saturations.
- Consider a nasogastric tube if the patient is vomiting and may need activated charcoal.
- Correct hypotension by nursing the patient head down and consider a fluid challenge.

 CRITICAL CLINICAL TASKS IN SELF-HARM

- Institute the care of the unconscious patient: ABCDE
- Take appropriate blood and urine tests
- Consider gut decontamination

Take Appropriate Blood and Urine Tests

- Take blood for measurement of the following:
  - Glucose
  - Alcohol
  - Paracetamol
  - Aspirin
  - Liver function tests
  - Clotting profile, particularly the INR (internal normalised ratio)
  - Special levels, for example, theophylline
- Urine—retain for toxicology screen:
  - Opiates
  - Cocaine
  - Amphetamines
  - Ecstasy
  - Hallucinogens

Assuming, after the initial assessment, that the patient does not need to be transferred to the high-dependency unit (HDU), steps should be taken to decontaminate the gut.

ACTIVATED CHARCOAL

Single dose. A single oral dose of 50 g activated charcoal enhances the elimination of several drugs and is used when anything more than a trivial amount has been taken (accepting the unreliability of the history in this group of patients). It is most effective when given within an hour of the overdose.

It is most useful in:

- Paracetamol
- Tricyclic antidepressants
- Aspirin
- Theophylline
- Phenytoin
- Carbamazepine
- Digoxin

It is of no value in poisoning with:

- Iron tablets
- Lithium
- Methanol
- Antifreeze

Multiple doses of activated charcoal (MDAC): 50 g immediately and 50 g every 4 h are given for life-threatening poisoning with:

- Slow-release theophyllines
- Carbamazepine
- Digoxin
- Phenobarbitone

To avoid the risk of aspiration, the airway must be secure before charcoal is used; it may be necessary to administer MDAC via a nasogastric tube.

Repeated vomiting reduces the effectiveness of charcoal treatment, so antiemetics such as IV cyclizine 50 mg 4 hourly or IV ondansetron may be indicated.

Decontamination of the gut

Gastric lavage. Gastric lavage is no longer indicated as routine in self-poisoning. Occasionally it is used:

- Within the first hour of ingestion (particularly with iron tablets or lithium).
- If the airway is secure.
- If a potentially life-threatening overdose has been taken.

Experimental and new treatments. Recent advances in the treatment of self-poisoning include a new antidote for methanol and antifreeze poisoning: fomepizole. Whole-bowel irrigation with polyethylene glycol is sometimes used for serious overdoses of enteric-coated drugs, iron-containing compounds or sustained-release preparations. Severe digoxin toxicity can be treated with a synthetic digoxin specific antibody.

IMPORTANT CLINICAL TASKS IN DELIBERATE SELF-HARM

Ensure that all the relevant information is available. If the patient is unable to give a reliable history but there is a strong suspicion of self-harm:

- What is available to the patient?
    - The patient's usual medication, including insulin
    - Other tablets and medications at home
    - Illicit and recreational drugs
- Is there evidence of self-poisoning?
    - Empty bottles, blister packs, foil wrappers
    - Has alcohol been involved?
- Is there a suicide note?

Other information from the patient or relatives. The key pieces of information needed in the patient's history are listed in Box 8.1.

IMPORTANT CLINICAL TASKS IN SELF-HARM

- Ensure that all the relevant information is available.
- Provide a suitable and safe environment in which to recover consciousness.

Confidentiality. When dealing with the patient's family, the clinical needs to know the nature and timing of the overdose must be balanced against the patient's right to confidentiality. There may be sensitive matters that the patient would not want to disclose to a third party. Common issues in this area include extramarital relationships, serious difficulties at work, unwanted pregnancy and conflict over child custody.

RELEVANT MEDICAL HISTORY

- Heart disease (tricyclics trigger arrhythmias)
- Liver disease (paracetamol increases the risk of liver damage)
- Alcohol use disorder (liver damage and a marker for high suicidal intent)
- Chronic disability (increases the likelihood of significant depression)

BOX 8.1 ■ History

The history must include the following:
- Mental state
- Past psychiatric history
- Previous self-harm
- Alcohol use
- An assessment of suicidal intent

PSYCHOSOCIAL HISTORY

- The sequence of events that triggered the overdose
- Psychiatric history, especially of depressive illness
- Domestic situation and family support:
  - Marital status
  - Who else lives in the home
  - Names and ages of children and who is caring for them
  - Recent bereavements, anniversaries of deaths
  - Has the patient got a social worker/community psychiatric nurse?
- Previous self-harm
- Are there any vulnerable children/possible abuse? This requires urgent attention.
- Job and financial worries
- Alcohol or drug use disorder
- Evidence of domestic violence—it is acceptable to ask directly about possible abuse by a partner.
- Recent childbirth
- Sexual orientation and sex identity—gay and bisexual males have a 10-fold increased rate of self-poisoning compared with the general population.
- Is there still suicidal intent?

Provide a Suitable and Safe Environment in Which to Recover Consciousness

- Physical safety is ensured by the use of the recovery position combined with appropriate monitoring of the conscious level and vital signs.
- It is important to maintain a calm, competent and non-judgemental approach. You are dealing with a very vulnerable group with low self-esteem, high stress levels, guilt about 'wasting everybody's time' and perhaps just extreme embarrassment.
- Respect the patient's privacy. Try to encourage staff on the consultant's round to discuss the patient's personal details somewhere other than the foot of the bed.
- Organise appropriate communication with the mental health liaison nurse or social services, who can provide effective help.
- Listen to the patient. Try to understand why the patient took the overdose at that particular time and with what intent. Avoid too many direct questions; rather, facilitate the conversation, for example, 'You must have been upset by that' or 'Things seem to have become too much for you'.
- Recent guidelines on self-harm assessment have moved away from a simple measurement of risk (low, moderate and high) to a needs-based assessment that then informs a multiagency care plan.

Case Study 8.3 illustrates the importance of reacting appropriately to the results of nursing observations:

- The combination of carbamazepine and diazepam produced a prolonged period of sedation.
- The patient's initial aggression overshadowed the later fall in conscious level.
- The clinical observations were not acted on with sufficient urgency.
- The falling GCS and the increasing respiratory rate should have alerted the clinical team to the impending need for ventilation. These patients are better nursed in the HDU.

Case Study 8.4 shows that assessment has to be performed with care, if necessary, by conforming to a checklist of high-risk factors. However, a checklist cannot replace sympathetic listening. Furthermore, simply asking if the patient 'feels suicidal' is often enough to identify risk, for example, 'What are your feelings about living and dying?' When time is at a premium, there are *two key questions* that are known to be an accurate prediction of genuine depression:

CASE STUDY 8.3   Deliberate Self-Harm and Progressive Deterioration in Conscious Level

A 20-year-old male with financial problems lost his job and, on impulse, took 30 of his father's carbamazepine tablets (a total of 12 g), without any alcohol.

On arrival in the Accident and Emergency Department (AED), at 1:30, he was agitated and very aggressive and refused oral charcoal. He was given 15 mg of rectal diazepam and admitted.

At 3:00 a.m., his GCS was noted to be 3/15. He remained in the medical ward.

By 4:30 a.m. he became aggressive again and was given a further dose of 10 mg diazepam. He had improved by 9:30 a.m. but deteriorated again by 9:15 p.m. the following evening:

- Oxygen saturation 80%
- Low pO_2 (8.0 kPa)
- Pulse 120 beats/min

He was given high-flow oxygen and observed.

By 5:00 a.m., his GCS had fallen to 7/15. Oxygen saturations were 86% on high-flow oxygen. His respiratory rate was 20 breaths/min.

Over the next 3 h, his GCS dropped to 6/15. His respiratory rate increased to 50 breaths/min and his pulse to 120 beats/min. He was deemed unable to protect his airway and transferred to ITU for ventilation. X-ray showed aspiration pneumonia.

After 4 days on a ventilator, he made a full recovery.

CASE STUDY 8.4   A Previous Concealed Episode of Deliberate Self-Harm

A 49-year-old female was admitted to hospital with a significant overdose of amitriptyline. She had left a suicide note to her son and had only been found at home by luck. She made a good recovery and did not appear depressed on the ward. However, on further questioning, she admitted that, 2 weeks before admission, she had taken 30 nitrazepam tablets but had not told anyone about it, and her husband had not been aware of her depression.

She was considered to be at high suicidal risk and admitted as an informal patient for further psychiatric assessment.

During the past month, have you often been bothered by:

1. Feeling down/depressed or hopeless?
2. Having little interest or pleasure in doing things?

A major advance in the management of self-harm has been the ready access to Liaison Psychiatry—firstly, to perform rapid psychosocial assessments (ideally within an hour of admission) and secondly, to advise on the challenging issues of consent, capacity and confidentiality.

The Patient Who Refuses Treatment

This is one of the most difficult areas of clinical practice, even for the most experienced medical and nursing staff. There are a number of common scenarios:

- A patient is admitted from casualty but refuses to stay in the ward.
- A recovering patient refuses to wait to see a psychiatrist.
- A patient absconds from the ward.
- A patient is intoxicated and abusive and refuses to cooperate.
- A patient is cooperative but will not see a psychiatrist.
- A patient refuses specific medical treatment for the overdose.
- A patient with acute alcohol withdrawal discharges himself.

In all such cases, a balance must be struck between *the duty of care* that we owe to our patients and *respect for their autonomy*, which is based on their competence *at the time* to make a decision. Patients can only be treated without their consent if they are not competent to make a decision and the proposed treatment is justified by the seriousness of the situation. Treating a patient against their wishes is done within the framework of the 1983 Mental Health Act when the treatment is of a psychiatric disease (e.g., an acute psychotic episode) and within the 2005 Mental Capacity Act when brain function and reasoning (competency) are affected by a physical illness (e.g., acute delirium or intoxication) that requires treatment.

Within the decision-making process, there are two components to this competency:

- Understanding and retaining the details of the proposed treatment—its benefits, risks and the consequences of turning it down.
- Having the ability to weigh up the alternatives when coming to a decision.

It is important to understand that it is the *ability of the patient to participate in the decision-making process* and *not* the *quality* of the decision, that is important. A competent patient can refuse treatment even if the decision seems irrational, abnormal or lacking common sense and, perhaps, may even result in the patient's death.

An assessment of competency (or *capacity*, as it is termed legally) will, in difficult cases, require the expertise of senior medical staff, although it is clear that in most acute situations, the combination of emotional distress and the effects of drugs or alcohol makes it fairly obvious when a patient is not competent to make such important decisions. The patient's capacity and how it has been assessed must be carefully documented in the records.

In extreme emergencies where capacity appears impaired but there is insufficient time for it to be formally assessed, treatment to 'save life and limb' can be given against the patient's wishes under what is termed, in England and Wales, *Common Law*.

The Mental Health Act can be used in medical wards to detain and, in some situations, treat a patient against their wishes. The Mental Health Act will allow treatment for a mental health problem but would not allow treatment of, for example, an overdose unless it is a symptom or consequence of the person's mental disorder. However, this would only apply in exceptional circumstances: the laws are complex, they rely on careful psychiatric assessment and the laws themselves vary within the United Kingdom. In England and Wales, Section 5(2) of the Mental Health Act (1983) can be invoked to detain a medical inpatient against their will for an emergency period of 72 h. Certain criteria must be met:

- The capacity to make a decision should be impaired because of a psychiatric disorder.
- In the case of an overdose, the law allows life-saving treatment to be administered against the patient's wishes if the act of deliberate self-harm was itself a direct consequence of a psychiatric disorder.
- The Mental Health Act can also be used to detain a patient with a mental disorder against their will if the patient is a danger to themselves or to others.

Using the Mental Health Act is not ideal: it takes time and organisation, and for an emergency section on the medical ward, the consultant physician has to be there in person. By their nature, these acute problems arise at extremely unsocial hours—usually at 2:00 a.m. or 3:00.

The skill in dealing with such patients is to try and prevent the situation from arising by:

- Avoiding confrontation.
- Maintaining a supportive and non-judgemental approach.
- Establishing a good relationship with the patient.
- Using persuasion and negotiation rather than coercion or bullying.
- Avoiding predictions of the time when a drip comes down/when a psychiatrist visits/of discharge.
- Involving relatives, within the confines of patient confidentiality.

In difficult situations, these principles should be followed:

- Act reasonably and in the best interest of the patient.
- Involve senior nursing and medical staff at an early stage.
- Give the patient options should they change their mind.
- Document events and outcomes in detail.
- Use common sense.

If patients abscond or discharge themselves, it is important to consider *who* needs to be informed and *when* would be the most appropriate time to do it:

- The next of kin
- The general practitioner
- Social services
- Community psychiatric services
- The health visitor (if children are involved)
- The police
- The probation officer

Case Studies 8.5 and 8.6 illustrate the kinds of difficulties that may occur in cases of self-harm.

Specific Overdoses

Three types of drugs make up 85% of the overdoses: of these, paracetamol and antidepressants are particularly toxic.

- Paracetamol, 45%
- Benzodiazepines, 20%
- Antidepressants, 20%

CASE STUDY 8.5	Substance Use Disorder, Deliberate Self-Harm and Absconding

A 25-year-old known heroin user was admitted to hospital with an overdose of diazepam and slashed wrists, soon after leaving prison. He was described by the police as a violent male and had struck his wife because of suspicion that she had been unfaithful. On admission, he was conscious but had slurred speech and was drowsy.

Soon after admission, in the middle of the night, he walked out of the ward taking his drip and drip stand with him, to stay with his friends near the hospital. The police were informed and persuaded him to return. By 3:00 a.m., he was threatening to walk out again, saying that he was going to kill himself.

What were the options?

- **Let him go again.** He exhibited several high-risk features for suicide: substance use disorder, male, etc.
- **Detain him under Common Law.** He is under the influence of a diazepam overdose and is probably not competent to make decisions. He is a danger to himself.
- **Section 5(2) of the Mental Health Act.** There is no mental illness immediately obvious.
- **Persuasion.** After a long talk with a senior doctor, he calmed down. It transpired he was virtually illiterate, was depressed about his hopeless employment prospects and had been denied access to his children because of his behaviour. His marriage looked unlikely to survive the effect of his prison sentence. He was referred for some form of problem-solving therapy.
- **Negotiation.** Typically for this type of situation, the problem of smoking on the ward became a major issue. Agreeing to let the patient find an acceptable place to smoke can defuse tension and also form the basis of negotiation to try and encourage the patient to stay on a voluntary basis.

CASE STUDY 8.6	Detention Under the Mental Health Act

A 40-year-old male was admitted to the hospital having taken a trivial amount of nitrazepam. He had cut his left arm (to 'let out the badness'). He was hearing voices that were telling him to kill himself, and he was demanding to leave hospital. He was pacing the room and wringing his hands in agitation, saying he just wanted to be left in peace to go home and die.

He had previously had ECT and had been on various psychotropic drugs.

In the early hours, he continued in his efforts to leave the ward, and there were practical problems in obtaining psychiatric help. The security staff were called and the consultant physician came in. After evaluating the situation, the consultant signed Form 12 (Section 5(2)) which, after being received by the manager of the mental health services, detained the patient against his will for 72 h to allow a psychiatric assessment to be made. A mental health nurse was seconded to look after the patient until the morning, when he was transferred to the mental health unit.

Benzodiazepines

Benzodiazepines, unless taken as part of a more toxic cocktail, depress the conscious level but not sufficiently to put respiration at risk unless the patient also aspirates. Management is based on maintaining respiration and keeping a secure airway. The specific antagonist, IV flumazenil, reverses benzodiazepine coma immediately, but the drug has potential problems:

- The effects of a single-dose wear off after 2 h.
- If tricyclic antidepressants may also have been taken, flumazenil is contraindicated: the surge in excitability associated with sudden benzodiazepine reversal may trigger a life-threatening tricyclic-induced cardiac arrhythmia.
- The sudden reversal of benzodiazepine coma may trigger acute agitation—this will need careful management.

Paracetamol Poisoning

Paracetamol poisoning is common and dangerous. There are 70,000 cases per year in the United Kingdom, and of these 200 will die due to liver damage—paracetamol remains the most common cause of acute liver failure.

How does it cause liver damage? Paracetamol is handled by the liver through two biochemical pathways. After a normal-sized dose, 90% is converted to harmless by-products, but 10% is converted by the p450 enzyme system to a highly active and toxic compound, NAPQI. NAPQI is deactivated in the body by glutathione.

In overdosage, the first pathway is swamped and large quantities of paracetamol are sent down the p450 route to produce NAPQI. Glutathione stores are eventually exhausted in mopping up excessive NAPQI. Once this happens, NAPQI starts to destroy the liver.

These simple biochemical pathways explain three important facts:

- Chronic alcoholics and malnourished patients have low glutathione levels and are therefore particularly susceptible to paracetamol toxicity.

- *N-acetylcysteine (Parvolex)* and methionine, which replenish glutathione stores, will act as effective antidotes in paracetamol poisoning.
- Drugs that increase p450 levels (anticonvulsant therapy, antituberculous (anti-TB) treatment, St. Johns Wort) send more of the paracetamol down the 'toxic route' and increase the toxicity of paracetamol.

How much is a significant overdose? It is important to express the dose of paracetamol that has been taken in mg/kg body weight. If the patient weighs more than 110 kg, use 110 kg as the body weight to avoid underestimating the toxic dose. Liver damage is unlikely at less than 75 mg/kg (approx. 12 tablets in an average-sized adult). However, 150 mg/kg (24 tablets) is likely to cause severe liver toxicity.

- In susceptible patients—the malnourished (especially patients with HIV, cystic fibrosis and eating disorders) or patients with alcohol use disorder–half of this amount can be dangerous.
- Liver toxicity may occur even if the tablets are ingested over the course of several hours.
- You cannot rely on the patient's story for the quantity or timing of the overdose.
- Patients will often have taken combination tablets (e.g., dextropropoxyphene and paracetamol) or a cocktail of drugs and alcohol that may each need treatment in their own right.

CLINICAL PICTURE OF SEVERE PARACETAMOL TOXICITY

0 to 24 h

- Minimal immediate symptoms
- Mild nausea and vomiting within a few hours
- Liver function tests are normal in the first 12 h, abnormal by 18 h

48 to 72 h

- Right upper abdominal pain with continued vomiting
- Liver tenderness
- Progressively deranged liver function tests (LFTs: alanine transaminase and aspartate transaminase levels >1000 IU/L indicate severe damage)
- Prolonged prothrombin time
- Loin pain, haematuria, proteinuria and deteriorating kidney function

Days 3 and 4

- Maximum liver damage on the fourth day
- Jaundice
- Increasing confusion with grade 3/4 hepatic encephalopathy

IMMEDIATE MANAGEMENT

- It is critical to establish the exact timing of the overdose. Focus on the history:
  - Time tablets purchased
  - Time tablets swallowed
  - Time help arrived
  - Could the overdose have been staggered over several hours?
- What else was taken?
  - Alcohol?
  - Antidepressants?
  - Aspirin/codeine?
- Is this a susceptible patient?
  - Eating disorder, HIV, cystic fibrosis or malnourished
  - Chronic alcoholic
  - Epileptic medication/anti-TB drugs
  - Underweight (toxic dose [150 mg/kg] in a 50-kg patient is 15 tablets)
  - Consider activated charcoal
    - Overdose taken within an hour, particularly if more than 150 mg/kg ingested
    - Methionine is not going to be used (charcoal inactivates methionine)
- Take blood for measurement of paracetamol levels (if overdose was taken within an hour or so of admission, wait 4 h before testing, but if more than 24 tablets were taken, still consider immediate antidote). Determine baseline LFTs and clotting, particularly if there is a substantial overdose or uncertain timing.
- Start *N-acetylcysteine (Parvolex)* treatment if indicated. Repeat LFTs and prothrombin time at the end of the infusion (20 h).

LATE PRESENTATION (8–24 H) OR STAGGERED INGESTION OVER SEVERAL HOURS

The situation is urgent because any delay progressively reduces the effectiveness of *N*-acetylcysteine (Parvolex) and patients who present late tend to have more serious overdoses. If more than 150 mg/kg or 12 g have been taken, it is safest to start treatment while awaiting the blood results. The following factors are considered:

- History (toxic dose of >150 mg/kg per day)
- Symptoms (abdominal pain and vomiting)
- Blood levels (of limited value in staggered overdoses)
- Prothrombin time
- LFTs and creatinine
- Blood gases

The use of *N*-acetylcysteine (Parvolex) at times in excess of 24 h is uncertain, but it should be given if the prothrombin time, creatinine or liver enzymes are abnormal or if the blood gases show an acidosis.

WHO GETS IV *N*-ACETYLCYSTEINE (PARVOLEX) OR METHIONINE?

A single paracetamol blood level measured at 4 h or more after the overdose will predict who is at risk from liver damage. Blood levels from earlier than 4 h are of no value in assessing the risk of liver damage. The graph of the blood levels of paracetamol against time since the overdose is used to determine who needs the antidote (Fig. 8.1). The timing of the overdose is therefore critical to the management of the patient.

- The graph only applies to tablets taken as a single dose over a 1-h time period: overdoses stretching over hours or days (staggered overdose) should be treated regardless of the blood levels.
- When in any doubt, *treat and treat without delay.*
- For example:
  - Within 24 h of an overdose exceeding 150 mg/kg, start treating while awaiting blood levels.
  - For more than 24 h, treat if the patient is jaundiced, has a tender liver or has abnormal LFTs/clotting.

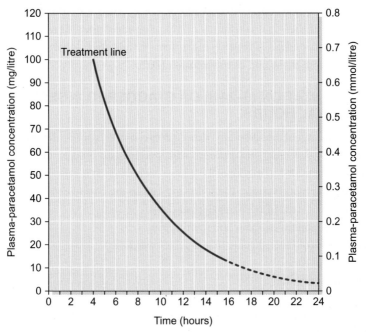

FIGURE 8.1 The use of plasma paracetamol levels in the decision to use *N*-acetylcysteine (Parvolex).

N-Acetylcysteine (Parvolex) and methionine are most effective if given within 12 h of the overdose, but Parvolex works up to 24 h and possibly longer. It is the treatment of choice in the acute medical unit, but methionine is useful in particular situations:

- The patient refuses a drip.
- The patient insists on leaving hospital but would take methionine with them.

N-acetylcysteine (Parvolex). The patient must be weighed so that the correct dose can be given:

- 150 mg/kg in 200 mL of 5% dextrose over 1 h
- 50 mg/kg in 500 mL of 5% dextrose over 4 h
- 100 mg/kg in 1000 mL of 5% dextrose over 16 h

Double-check that the correct dose of N-acetylcysteine (Parvolex) *is drawn up: for patients over 110 kg, the dose is based on a maximum weight of 110 kg.*

In cases of severe overdosage, the infusion will be used beyond 24 h (at a rate of 150 mg/kg per 24 h) until the prothrombin time decreases to less than 20 s. If there is severe liver damage, the patient must be kept very well hydrated, and broad-spectrum antibiotics such as IV cefuroxime should be given.

There is a 1 in 20 risk of a rash/wheeze/itching or some other generalised reaction within an hour of starting *N*-acetylcysteine (Parvolex). The infusion should be stopped for 60 min while the reaction settles before restarting at 50 mg/kg over 4 h. If the reaction is severe, IV antihistamines and hydrocortisone should be given.

Oral methionine. Methionine is an alternative to *N*-acetylcysteine (Parvolex) and is easier to give—the dose is 2.5 g immediately and 2.5 g every 4 h for three further doses. However,

- Patients are frequently vomiting at the time it needs to be given.
- It is only helpful within 10 to 12 h of the overdose.
- It is inactivated by oral charcoal.

When to discharge. Patients should be discharged only:

- After psychosocial assessment.
- After completion of *N-acetylcysteine (Parvolex)*, provided that the liver enzymes, creatinine and prothrombin time are normal.
- If there are no symptoms.

There is a poor prognosis 24 h after the overdose, and a Liver Unit must be consulted if:

- Prothrombin time is more than 75 s (clotting must not be corrected as serial measurements determine the likelihood of recovery)
- Arterial pH <7.3.
- Creatinine is > 300 mmol/L.
- Arterial lactate > 3 to 3.5 mmol/L.
- Hepatic encephalopathy (grade III–IV).

Clear instructions, as outlined in Box 8.2, should be given to the patients who discharge themselves.

BOX 8.2 ■ Clear Written Instructions to Patients Who Go Home or Self-Discharge After Paracetamol Overdose

- Return if there is:
  - Abdominal pain
  - Persistent vomiting
  - Confusion
- Consider oral methionine

Antidepressant Overdose

There are two important types of antidepressants used in deliberate self-harm:
- The older tricyclic antidepressants (e.g., dothiepin, amitriptyline, protriptyline):
  - These are dangerous and cause coma, convulsions and cardiac arrhythmias.
  - Dothiepin is the most dangerous, particularly as it is available in 75 mg tablet strength.
- The new generation of antidepressants (selective serotonin reuptake (SSRI) inhibitors)
  - Drugs such as fluoxetine, while safer than tricyclics, can cause 'serotonin syndrome'—acute confusion, fever, muscular rigidity and twitching. The syndrome can progress to marked blood pressure and pulse instability, melted muscles (rhabdomyolysis), convulsions, kidney failure and grossly abnormal clotting.

MANAGEMENT

Patients initially show features of atropine-like poisoning, with a dry mouth, blurred vision and dilated pupils. In severe toxicity, for example, more than 750 mg of a tricyclic drug, the patient becomes increasingly drowsy over a period of 4 h or so. A dose of 2 g or more produces severe toxicity that lasts several hours.

The tricyclic overdose provides the classic example of patients who 'were fine' in the AED but then deteriorated at a frightening rate when they reached the ward—often doing so in the critical interval between the initial clinical assessment and when they were seen by the junior doctor.

The main dangers include:
- **Respiratory depression**. The GCS, respiratory rate and oxygen saturation (National Early Warning Score 2 [NEWS2]) should be monitored hourly in these patients, more often if they are showing any signs of toxicity. Blood gases are checked: tricyclic poisoning can cause a dangerous acidosis that needs correction with IV sodium bicarbonate.
- **Cardiac arrhythmias**. Patients must be monitored and cared for near the nursing station. The first sign of trouble may be a cardiac arrest in ventricular fibrillation. A standard ECG recording may show warning signs of cardiac toxicity

(the QRS complexes are slurred to more than the width of four small squares). Arrhythmias can be abolished with IV sodium bicarbonate (50 mL of 8.4%) which can be given prophylactically if there are warning ECG changes or hypotension—conventional antiarrhythmic drugs can make the situation worse by depressing cardiac function.

- **Convulsions.** These are treated with IV diazepam or lorazepam.

Patients remain at risk for at least 12 h after admission and are prone to arrhythmias if they mobilise prematurely. Dothiepin, in particular, has been associated with a significant number of in-hospital deaths.

IMMEDIATE MANAGEMENT OF TRICYCLIC AND SSRI OVERDOSES

Gastric lavage? There is little point in lavage unless large amounts of the drug have been taken within the hour. Indeed, by pushing the tablets further down the gut, lavage may increase absorption.

Single-dose activated charcoal. A single dose of 50 g of activated charcoal reduces absorption if given within an hour of ingestion. If there are signs of significant drug toxicity, a further dose can be given at 2 h.

Carbon Monoxide Poisoning

BASIC MECHANISMS

Carbon monoxide is odourless, colourless and extremely dangerous. It binds to and poisons circulating haemoglobin, preventing it from taking up, or releasing, oxygen. As a consequence, patients suffer hypoxic damage to the heart and central nervous system.

The gas has two important sources:

- Incomplete combustion of carboniferous domestic fuel (gas, coke, coal, wood) associated with faulty installations or accidental fires.
- Car exhaust fumes (catalytic converters reduce the amount of carbon monoxide).

CLINICAL PICTURE

Acute exposure. Headache, nausea and dizziness progressing to collapse and loss of consciousness. In severe poisoning with coma, there may be skin blistering and pressure-induced muscle damage (rhabdomyolysis). The limbs are spastic and there may be acute heart damage, pulmonary oedema or increased intracranial pressure.

Subacute exposure. Slower onset of nausea, vomiting, headaches and drowsiness. The clinical picture can mimic flu or gastroenteritis—a source of confusion. As with gastroenteritis, a whole household can be affected if exposed to the same source.

ASSESSMENT AND MANAGEMENT

- ABCDE: care of the patient with an impaired conscious level:
  - Airway management.
  - Assess cardiac function, monitor the heart rhythm and measure troponins.
  - Monitor oxygen saturations.
  - Monitor blood gases and venous blood for carboxyhaemoglobin (COHb) levels. Severe toxicity is associated with COHb levels greater than 20% (heavy smokers reach levels of 8%–10%).
- Give immediate high-concentration oxygen—100% oxygen is indicated for significant toxicity. This will need to be delivered via a tightly fitting mask with an inflated face seal (seek anaesthetists' advice, as the standard nonrebreathing masks are inadequate).
- Consider *hyperbaric oxygen* (oxygen given in a specialist unit at 2.4 times normal atmospheric pressure), especially in cases of:
  - Pregnancy
  - COHb more than 20%
  - Signs of neurological dysfunction
- If it is accidental domestic exposure, the local environmental health department should be involved to assess the safety of the house.

Alcohol Use Disorder

PROBLEMS OF ALCOHOL IN THE ACUTE MEDICAL UNIT

Estimates suggest that around 20% of acute medical admissions are directly or indirectly the result of alcohol use disorder (Fig. 8.2). Acute alcohol intoxication is potentially dangerous in terms of respiratory depression and aspiration and must be managed carefully. It is equally important to recognise chronic alcohol dependence—those patients who, while they would not necessarily concede to being 'alcoholic', have drinking patterns that cause repeated problems for themselves and others.

- Acute alcohol intoxication—common in young adults.
- Alcohol as a component of deliberate self-harm—alcohol and paracetamol or antidepressants/benzodiazepines are commonly taken in combination. The risks are of respiratory depression and aspiration. The associated intoxication makes history-taking difficult and often results in a very uncooperative patient.
- Alcohol dependence as a cause of deliberate self-harm—either in the patient or in the patient's close family/partner.
- Acute alcohol withdrawal syndromes—delirium tremens, anxiety states, fits, acute thiamine deficiency.
- Alcohol-induced disease:
  - Alcoholic gastritis
  - Acute variceal bleeding

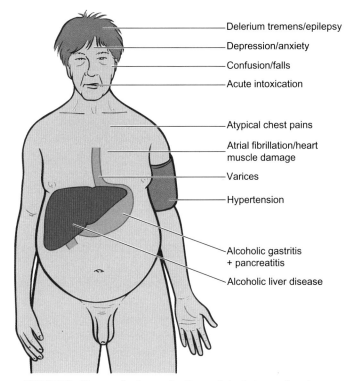

FIGURE 8.2 The medical complications of alcohol use disorder.

- Alcoholic liver disease
- Pancreatitis
- Other alcohol-associated medical conditions:
  - Unexplained vomiting
  - Atypical chest pain (often after binges)
  - Binge-associated acute atrial fibrillation
  - Hypertension
  - Unexplained falls and confusion in the elderly
  - Depression

How to Take a Drinking History

Although patients with alcohol-related problems do not usually welcome detailed enquiries into their drinking habits, an acute drink-related crisis in their health or personal life is often followed by a period of reflection and self-examination. During this time, the patient may accept for the first time that alcohol may be the root cause of their problem.

It is surprising how often the bland question *Do you think you may have been burning the candle at both ends?* leads to important disclosures and an initial acknowledgement of the critical issue.

It is important to establish the levels of consumption and dependence.

The Amount and Pattern of Drinking

1. How often do you drink (including 'stiffeners' added, particularly by the elderly, to tea and coffee)?
2. How much do you drink on a usual day (a unit is half a pint, a glass of wine or a single measure of spirits)? A regular consumption of more than 4 units a day puts the patient 'at risk'.
3. Have you had more than 5 units any day in the past month?
4. Have you had home, health or work problems in the last year due to drink?
5. Has anyone (including yourself) been harmed by your drinking?
6. Do you use alcohol to help solve your problems?
7. Has anyone suggested that you cut it down?

The Level of Dependence

1. Do you have difficulty controlling the amount that you drink once you start?
2. Do you have difficulty cutting down?
3. Do you have withdrawal symptoms (including early awakening and episodic anxiety)?
4. Are you drinking to avoid withdrawal symptoms?

These questions are distilled into a shortened form: the CAGE questionnaire. Two or more positive answers to the four questions suggest alcohol dependence.

- Have you felt you should Cut down?
- Have you been Annoyed by criticism of your drinking?
- Have you felt Guilty about your drinking?
- Do you ever have an Eye-opener in the morning to steady your nerves?

CAGE can be used on the patient to confirm any suspicions of alcohol dependence raised from an initial drinking history. The nature of the questions, however, means that it is not good for identifying problems in young adults or in the elderly.

Acute Alcohol Withdrawal Syndrome

Case Study 8.7 highlight some features of the acute alcohol withdrawal syndrome.

- It is important to recognise the clinical features of alcohol withdrawal in any patient admitted to hospital (Box 8.3). Timely sedation with benzodiazepines will prevent the onset of convulsions or progression to delirium tremens. The most effective regimen is to control the agitation, sweating and tremors with 'symptom-triggered dosing' using oral diazepam 10 mg every 2 h up to a maximum of 100 mg in 24 h. Antiemetics may also be required.
- Patients with alcohol withdrawal syndrome are often very apprehensive or frightened. They may be acutely disturbed and hallucinating. It is important to care for them in a well-lit room and provide a calm, reassuring environment.
- Severe acute alcoholic agitation can be managed with IV diazepam 5 to 10 mg or lorazepam 2 mg over 2 min. An infusion of clomethiazole (Heminevrin)

CASE STUDY 8.7 — Acute Alcohol Withdrawal Syndrome

CASE 1

A 35-year-old male was admitted, having had a grand mal fit. He had discharged himself from an AED a week before after a similar episode. He had been drinking cider heavily for 15 years, and since losing his father 6 months previously he had been drinking up to two bottles of vodka per day and had started antidepressants. He had recently had a normal endoscopy and colonoscopy for morning vomiting and episodic diarrhoea. On examination, he had severe shaking and sweating and was extremely agitated and anxious.

His liver enzymes were high and his alcohol levels were zero. His mean corpuscular volume was 103 mm^3. He was started on a regimen of chlordiazepoxide and high-dose parenteral vitamins. Within 36 h, he was much improved but insisted on discharging himself, with a promise that he would stop drinking 'through his own efforts'. He continued on a reducing regimen of chlordiazepoxide.

CASE 2

A 40-year-old male was admitted to hospital after a series of grand mal convulsions. He was a club steward on holiday in the area. While working, he would drink 'constantly' throughout the day and evening but would always stop completely on holiday. He was treated with thiamine and a benzodiazepine withdrawal regimen, and he made a full recovery.

BOX 8.3 ■ Symptoms of Alcohol Withdrawal

- Tremor
- Sweating
- Apprehension
- Nausea and vomiting
- Weakness and syncope
- Insomnia
- Auditory and visual hallucinations
- Fitting
- Severe confusion

is the traditional treatment for acute withdrawal states, but, while it can be effective, it carries a risk of respiratory depression. When taken long term, clomethiazole can itself lead to dependence and has in general been replaced by benzodiazepines.

- If the patient looks poorly nourished or is confused and unsteady on their feet, an acute Wernicke-Korsakoff syndrome (WKS) may be developing. WKS is a serious acute brain disturbance caused by thiamine deficiency and can be triggered in hospital by a carbohydrate load such as an infusion of dextrose. The clinical picture can be confused with that of acute intoxication, but the damage is permanent unless treated urgently with IV thiamine (in the form of high-dose vitamins B and C combination (Pabrinex): two pairs of ampoules three times a day for 5 days, each pair infused in 100 mL of normal saline over 30 min).

CASE STUDY 8.8 | **Acute Alcohol Intoxication**

A 16-year-old boy was admitted with a GCS of 3 and an unrecordable blood sugar, having been found lying in an outdoor play area. He had been drinking white cider and vodka outside with his friends. He recovered uneventfully over a period of 12 h, with attention to his airway and correction of his blood sugar.

Acute Alcohol Intoxication

- There is an increasing problem with young people binge-drinking out of doors, encouraged by the ready availability of 'designer drinks', including types of fortified wines and strong white ciders (Case Study 8.8).
- The main problems are hypoglycaemia, respiratory depression, airway protection and, in severe cases, fitting.
- The units of measurement are confusing and can lead to misinterpretation:
  - UK driving limit for blood alcohol levels is 16 mmol/L (80 mg/100 mL). It is 50 mg/100 mL in Scotland.
  - Severe intoxication 76 to 98 mmol/L (350–450 mg/100 mL).
  - Potentially fatal > 98 mmol/L (>450 mg/100 mL).

The management is that of any metabolic coma, with a number of important exceptions:

- Alcoholics are prone to head injuries while intoxicated:
  - Take a history from any witnesses.
  - Observe carefully for signs of trauma (bruising behind the ears, boggy swelling, etc.).
  - Low threshold for ordering a head CT.
  - Monitor the GCS—it is not appropriate to assume the patient will simply 'sleep it off'.
  - Failure to recover fully after a head injury may indicate impending WKS.
  - A cocktail of drugs and alcohol may have been taken—a situation that is particularly dangerous for patients with opioid use disorder.
  - In severe intoxication, start IV dextrose 10% 250 mL. If IV dextrose is being used in a patient with chronic alcohol use disorder, combine it with thiamine to avoid triggering the WKS. The management of severe intoxication in the familiar 'hardened' drinker who is unkempt and malnourished (and often disruptive) should include at least one pair of thiamine and vitamin C (Pabrinex) ampoules daily for the first 5 days.

Ethylene Glycol and Methanol: Antifreeze and Windscreen Washer Solution

Ethylene glycol and methanol can be ingested in error, as a deliberate act or, misguidedly, for recreational purposes. Both substances cause profound acidosis, acute multiorgan damage and, in the case of methanol, permanent blindness; they are extremely dangerous. The clinical picture can mimic diabetic ketoacidosis and the diagnosis may be overlooked. The intravenous drug Fomepizole inhibits the liver enzyme, which converts the two substances into highly toxic by-products (ethylene into oxalic acid and methanol into formic acid). Fomepizole is a highly effective antidote if given early.

Substance Use Disorder
COCAINE

Cocaine imparts its desired effects by stimulating the release of the stress hormones, noradrenaline (norepinephrine), adrenaline (epinephrine) and dopamine to inappropriately high levels. The effects are dramatic, as may be the side effects—notably, stroke, heart attack and aortic dissection. Cocaine is a major cause of drug-related death and any young fit adult admitted with unexplained cardiovascular or cerebrovascular emergencies should be asked about cocaine use (the maximum risk is within the first hour of a dose). The nature of the cardiac damage includes cocaine-related chest pain, acute coronary syndrome, acute myocardial infarction, acute arrhythmias and, with prolonged use, cocaine-induced heart muscle damage. The sudden changes in pulse rate and blood pressure can trigger cerebral infarction and cerebral haemorrhage and can tear major blood vessels (aortic and coronary artery dissection).

Treatment of all of these complications should follow conventional lines, except that β-blockers are contraindicated and that high-dose benzodiazepines may be needed to reduce cocaine-induced agitation.

Ecstasy

Ecstasy, or MDMA, has been a commonly used recreational drug for the past decade, particularly in the clubbing scene. Its amphetamine-like properties provide hyperstimulation, which, combined with the exertion of prolonged dancing, can result in:
- Dehydration and electrolyte disturbance
- Hyperarousal—agitation, tachycardia, hypertension
- Muscle breakdown (rhabdomyolysis) and kidney failure
- Hyperthermia up to 40°C
- Convulsions
- Acute liver failure
- Severe acidosis

MANAGEMENT

Reassurance and adequate IV fluids are the main measures. Hyperthermia is managed by active cooling and with IV dantrolene 1 mg/kg repeated as needed, to a maximum of

10 mg/kg. Acute agitation and convulsions respond to benzodiazepines. Acidosis may need correction with sodium bicarbonate.

Liquid Ecstasy

Liquid ecstasy is the drug GHB (gamma hydroxy-butyrate). Case Study 8.9 illustrates the use disorder of this substance.

Dystonic Reaction and Psychotropic Drugs

Case Study 8.10 describes psychotropic drug use disorder. The picture is typical of the abnormal posture and muscle spasms that occur in acute dystonic reactions to a variety of psychotropic drugs, including haloperidol, and various antiemetics, including metoclopramide. Problems with substance use disorder are widespread in the prison population.

CASE STUDY 8.9   **Liquid Ecstasy**

Two females aged 24 and 21 years who were at a nightclub each took four bottle-capfuls of a pink aniseed–flavoured liquid that they knew to be GHB. Within a few minutes, they developed euphoria that progressed over an hour to drowsiness and coma. They were carried out by bouncers, and the paramedics were called.
    On admission:

	Case One	Case Two
GCS	E1 V1 M1	E2 V2 M1
Pulse	30	42
Blood pressure	Unrecordable	70/40
Respiratory rate	6	8
Pupils	Normal and reactive	Pinpoint
Treatment	Atropine	Atropine
	Charcoal	Charcoal

The anaesthetists were called and oropharyngeal/nasopharyngeal airways were passed. Activated charcoal was administered down a nasogastric tube. Atropine 1 mg increased the pulse and blood pressures, and both patients regained consciousness within 3 to 4 h. According to the females, the desired effect is usually generalised tingling and a floating euphoria. This was the first time they had not spread the doses over 3 or 4 h.

CASE STUDY 8.10   **Dystonic Reaction**

A prisoner with a previous history of psychosis and IV amphetamine use disorder found a packet of tablets in a copy of a novel in the prison library. He took them for a buzz. A few minutes after taking them, he developed what he thought was a fit, with intense spasms of his jaw and neck and arching of his back.
    He was taken to casualty, and after an intramuscular injection of procyclidine 10 mg, his symptoms improved rapidly.

Synthetic Cannabinoid Receptor Agonists—'Legal' Highs

The use of synthetic cannabinoid receptor agonist (SCRAs), notably, spice, black mamba and similar branded products has reached epidemic proportions in certain groups—prisoners and the homeless. Apart from euphoria (their desired effect), they lead to agitation, convulsions, acute muscle damage, hallucinations and acute psychosis, hence the need to be familiar with them in the admission unit. They are now illegal so that generic mixes of herbal tobacco and SCRAs are marketed in anonymous small plastic bags—easily obtainable on the city streets and in prisons.

Heroin Use Disorder (Opioid Use Disorder)

Intravenous drug users (IVDUs) are often admitted acutely with multiple complex medical, social and behavioural problems. Previous experiences with the Health Service, characterised by stigmatisation and failed communication, commonly set the scene for a fraught clinical encounter—with patients often delaying seeking help. There is frequently a conflict between the perception of the patient that withdrawal symptoms and pain are not being addressed and that of the carers who view challenging behaviour as manipulative and 'drug seeking'. The key is an empathic approach that is non-judgemental and focuses on the key issues of communication, cooperation and confidentiality (sometimes with the need to set defined limits to behaviour). The patients should feel that they are in a secure environment and that their concerns will be heard. It is preferable to avoid the terms 'drug abuse' and 'drug addiction'—simply use 'drug use'.

Heroin use disorder is an increasing problem, particularly among the young, and is associated with several major health-related and psychosocial problems (Case Study 8.11):

- HIV
- Hepatitis C and B virus
- Superficial and deep soft tissue sepsis
- Venous thromboembolic disease
- Opiate overdose (often combined with temazepam, alcohol and diazepam)
- Social isolation
- Crime

METHODS OF HEROIN INGESTION

Chasing the dragon. An increasingly popular way of taking heroin, 'chasers' are younger, show less dependence and are less involved in the heroin culture than the more traditional IV user. Heroin is heated on tin foil and inhaled. Alternatively, it is smoked as a cigarette—'tooting'.

| CASE STUDY 8.11 | Heroin Use Disorder in a Young Girl |

A 17-year-old single girl was admitted with acute asthma because her inhalers had run out. She had been smoking heroin for 2 years, but in the last month her boyfriend, who was now in prison, had introduced her to intravenous heroin. She was using 1 g a day, which she funded by shoplifting. She had been thrown out by her mother and did not get on with her father. She wanted to sort out her life and her asthma.

Mainlining. In contrast to chasers, injectors are older and more likely to be male. They show high dependence and are likely to be using the drug in higher doses and on a daily basis. They are unlikely to have nonusers as friends and are steeped in heroin 'culture'. This group is increasingly turning to methadone treatment programmes. Many established users will have been injecting opiates for years: the average age at a methadone maintenance clinic will be around 35 years, with most starting to inject opiates at around the age of 20 years. More than 70% of these long-term addicts will test positive for the hepatitis C virus (HCV), around 50% will be positive for hepatitis B virus (HBV), and a significant proportion will be HIV positive. At least half will have shared injection apparatus.

Popping. Injecting directly into soft tissue rather than a vein. Popping is often complicated by localised cellulitis.

HEROIN OVERDOSE

Overdose may be due to simple error (especially if alcohol is also involved), inadvertent ingestion of a particularly pure batch of heroin, loss of tolerance following abstinence or a deliberate act of self-harm. Patients are usually deeply comatose, with pinpoint pupils. Treatment is with IV naloxone, the specific antidote, but reversal can be dramatic, leading to acute agitation, aggression and violence.

METHADONE THERAPY

Addicts who are admitted to medical wards often claim that they are 'registered' and, as such, they are 'entitled' to methadone or even to diamorphine.

- Only doctors who hold a special Home Office licence may prescribe diamorphine for the treatment of drug addiction.
- Since 1997, addicts are no longer registered with the Home Office (although there are voluntary anonymised regional and national Drug Misuse Databases for patients who first present with drug misuse).
- The addict may demand methadone in hospital because they realise that they are dealing with inexperienced staff who may comply with their wishes.
- Methadone can be abused and has a high value on the black market, particularly in tablet form (which can be crushed and injected) and in ampoules.

- The current recommendations for a methadone treatment programme include:
  - Only methadone syrup—oral solution 1 mg/mL, not tablets, should be prescribed.
  - Daily prescriptions should be given.
  - The effective maintenance dose should not exceed 60 to 120 mg of methadone daily.

Methadone programmes are carefully supervised and managed with a system of daily supply and directly observed ingestion. Apart from using methadone syrup (not tablets or injectable forms), effective treatment programmes monitor drug ingestion with blood and urine testing (the prevailing ethos for treating drug addiction is one of 'tough love').

Methadone treatment is not universally popular and some institutions, notably the prison service, use dihydrocodeine in long-acting preparations to aid withdrawal. Buprenorphine is a useful alternative heroin substitute, particularly as it has a low risk of causing respiratory depression if taken in excess. A typical regimen would be a rapidly tapering course of sublingual buprenorphine, starting at 4 to 16 mg per day, to be followed up longer term by the opiate blocker, naltrexone. In the future, a combination of sublingual buprenorphine with naloxone (the antidote to respiratory depression) will probably replace methadone treatment.

CLINICAL ASSESSMENT OF THE DRUG USER

- What drugs: how and in what quantity?
- Is the patient known to the Drugs Advisory Service?
- Is there a child at risk or is the patient pregnant?

Infections in Intravenous Drug Users

IVDUs are at risk from severe infections: they use contaminated equipment and drugs, clean injection techniques are the exception, and their levels of immunity are low, not necessarily due to HIV infection, often simply due to poor social circumstances and self-neglect. Typical clinical pictures include:

Skin and injection sites: Cellulitis, abscesses and necrotising fasciitis

Systemic infection: Sepsis and toxic shock syndrome

Respiratory tract: Pneumonia and empyema, infected pulmonary emboli

Vascular: Septic thrombophlebitis, deep vein thrombosis and 'pseudo' arterial aneurysms at the injection sites (often the groin)

Musculoskeletal: Joint infections (sternoclavicular, pelvis, spine and large joints)

Cardiac: Endocarditis of the tricuspid valve

Several unusual outbreaks have been caused by specific drug-related problems: botulism due to contaminated black tar heroin from Mexico, tetanus from heroin infected with *Clostridium tetani* and, most recently, anthrax from contaminated heroin in Scotland. It is therefore important to be vigilant for clusters of unusual infections among the IVDU population. Those with anthrax, for example, showed a specific severe soft tissue infection that progressed rapidly to necrotising fasciitis and overwhelming sepsis—others presented with an apparent subarachnoid bleed, which was actually the result of haemorrhagic meningitis, which is a feature of anthrax.

Infections in IVDUs often require prolonged antibiotic courses. A realistic expectation for severe infections would be a week of IV antibiotics followed by 4 weeks of oral treatment.

Special Risks to Members of Staff

The three most common work-related injuries in hospital staff are caused by falls, needle stick injuries and violent incidents.

Needle Stick Injuries

HIV, HBV (Hepatitis B) and HCV (Hepatitis C) are bloodborne infections that put at risk those lin the clinical team who are exposed to the blood and body fluids of infected patients.

THE NATURE OF THE RISK

A needle stick injury with HIV-infected blood carries a small but significant risk (1 in 300) of HIV infection in the recipient. Hepatitis is more easily transmitted than HIV: if the blood is from a patient with hepatitis, the risk can be as high as 1 in 10. The risks are lower after exposure of broken skin (e.g., severe eczema on a carer's hands) or mucous membranes (eyes or mouth) to infected blood or blood-stained body fluids.

Clinical Staff must be aware of the risks and systems of care should assume that bloodborne infection could be present in any or every patient. There must be a well-publicised local policy from Occupational Health, consistent with the most recent Department of Health Guidelines.

It is vital that staff know what to do in the event of a needle stick injury:

- Who do you contact during the day?
- Who do you contact at night and at weekends?
- Where are the starter packs for HIV prophylaxis?
- Could the system deliver HIV prophylaxis within 1 h of the incident?
- What blood specimens need to be taken from the patient and the staff member?
- Who can give expert advice?

OUTCOME

The outcome of the incident depends on four factors:

- Type of exposure
  - High risk—deep injury with a blood-stained sharp/used IV cannula
  - Low risk—injury with a subcutaneous injection needle

- Status of patient (HBV positive/HBC positive/HIV positive)
- Immunity of staff member (hepatitis B immunisation)
- Effectiveness and timeliness of the emergency measures

WHAT CONSTITUTES SIGNIFICANT EXPOSURE?

- Needle stick or blood-contaminated sharps
- Bite - causing skin puncture
- Mucocutaneous exposure to blood or blood-stained body fluids (high-risk fluids include cerebrospinal fluid, pleural and peritoneal fluids)

WHAT EMERGENCY ACTION SHOULD BE TAKEN?

1. Irrigate and wash (soap and water), encourage any puncture wound to bleed and irrigate an eye with saline or water before and after removing contact lenses.
2. Cover the wound with an impermeable dressing after washing.
3. Report the incident.
4. Attend the relevant department immediately (Occupational Health or the AED).

The important emergency interventions are the immediate (ideally within 1 h) institution of triple-drug antiretroviral therapy in a definite HIV exposure, and in the case of definite exposure to hepatitis B, instituting (depending on the carer's vaccination history) accelerated anti-hepatitis B vaccination or a booster dose of vaccine.

RISK ASSESSMENT TO IDENTIFY THE PATIENT'S INFECTIVITY

1. HBV (positive for hepatitis B surface antigen and E antigens—HBsAg, HBeAg)
2. HCV
3. HIV positive
4. Known to have HIV risk factors

Blood testing of the patient and storage of blood from the staff member. If there has been significant exposure, the patient should have the HBsAg checked urgently. If there are risk factors for HCV or HIV, consent should also be sought to check these. The possible outcomes are as follows:

1. Urgent testing of the patient (10 mL blood for HBsAg, HCV, HIV and storage).
2. Storage with delayed testing should it be necessary.
3. Baseline tests on the nurse and storage for later testing.

Documentation. Document the incident using an official incident form.

Hospital-Acquired Methicillin-Resistant *Staphylococcus aureus* Infections

Hospital-acquired methicillin-resistant *Staphylococcus aureus* (MRSA) is an increasing problem leading to unnecessary deaths and disability. Healthcare workers infect themselves by handling MRSA-positive patients and by touching adjacent contaminated surfaces. The staff then spread the organism from one patient to another. Spread is prevented by effective isolation, careful room cleaning and the use of universal precautions, of which by far the most important is thorough and frequent handwashing. The control of MRSA is based on universal screening of all admissions (nasal, throat, perineal and wound/ulcer swabs) followed by selective decontamination (5-day Hibiscrub body washes with 5-day nasal Bactroban tds).

Violent Incidents

The most common forms of violence in acute medical wards are those seen in severely agitated patients with acute confusional states who strike out, grab or scratch the medical or nursing staff, whom they misinterpret as posing a threat. Less common, but more dangerous, is the physical aggression that accompanies severe paranoid states due to an acute physical or psychiatric illness. The combination of drug or alcohol intoxication with a paranoid illness is particularly dangerous.

The principles of management include:

- Do not take risks.
- Any patient showing an obvious paranoid state should be asked if they are carrying any sort of weapon.
- Ensure your own safety and that of the patient.
- Seek immediate help from other staff members.
- Use the absolute minimum of force to control the situation.

PREVENTION

- Recognise the causes:
  - Acute anxiety and fear
  - Emotional distress and an unmet need
  - Alcohol and drug-withdrawal syndromes
  - Delirium
  - Dementia
  - Major psychosis, for example, paranoid schizophrenia
  - Uncontrolled pain
- Recognise the warning signs:
  - Agitation

- Shouting and pacing the room
- Misinterpreting any clinical interventions as personal threats
- Threats of violence and previous violent behaviour
- Paranoid ideas, fearing for their life
- Delirium/clouded consciousness

MANAGEMENT

The acutely disturbed and potentially violent patient should be cared for only by an appropriate number of trained, experienced and easily identified (uniformed) staff. It is critical that a medical assessment be made at an early stage to detect reversible causes of acute confusion, for example, hypoxia, infection and drug toxicity. The patient should be nursed in a quiet, well-lit room in which they cannot harm themselves. It can be calming to an acutely disturbed patient if you exhibit a relaxed but attentive manner and avoid anything that could be misinterpreted as being confrontational. As part of the de-escalation plan listen, explain and reassure. Remember that any physical contact may be misinterpreted as threatening behaviour, so explain very clearly what it is you are planning to do in terms of clinical observations and monitoring. If you are carrying out a procedure or observation—give a running commentary to the patient to avoid misunderstanding. If the situation deteriorates, you must obtain immediate help from the medical and security staff and, if serious violence is threatened, for example, with a weapon, the police.

There are situations in which common sense dictates that the patient should be restrained for their own safety: a clear example is someone with a severe toxic confusional state who has become acutely paranoid and is trying to escape through a window. Patients who are mentally disordered and putting themselves *or others* at risk can be treated in an emergency under Common Law without consent.

To calm an acutely disturbed or aggressive patient, intramuscular sedation can be used and repeated when necessary:

Lorazepam	2 mg IM repeat after 20 min
or	
Haloperidol	2.5 mg (0.5 mg in the elderly) IM combined with 50 mg of promethazine repeat after 20 min
or	
Midazolam	2 mg IV every 2 min up to 20 mg

If sedation is administered, the patient must be monitored carefully to prevent aspiration, respiratory depression and hypotension. Haloperidol is absolutely contra-indicated in Lewy Body Dementia

If, as a last resort, temporary restraining force is needed, there must be a sufficient number of experienced staff to apply it to an absolute minimum, ensuring the patient comes to no harm. Under these situations, it is essential to involve senior nursing and medical staff and subsequently to complete detailed clinical documentation. Urgent advice from Liaison Psychiatry may be needed for the complex issues of consent, capacity and the potential deprivation of liberty.

Further Reading

Humphreys, R.A., et al., 2014. When and how to treat patients who refuse treatment. British Medical Journal 348, 33–37.

National Poisons Information Centre: Toxbase. https://www.toxbase.org/.

NICE, 2011. Alcohol use disorders: diagnosis and management of physical complications. NICE Clinical guideline (CG100). Updated 2017. https://www.nice.org.uk/guidance/CG100.

NICE guideline (NG225) 2022. Self-harm: assessment, management and preventing recurrence. https://www.nice.org.uk/guidance/NG225.

Riddell, et al, 2015. Management of sharps injuries in the health care setting. British Medical Journal 350, h3733.

The 'Social Admission'

Introduction

Many acute medical assessment units have now abandoned the concept of age-related admission policies: on most units, 10% to 15% of patients will now be aged 80 years and above. This group of patients calls for particular skills in assessment and management, not least in the area of prioritising their care. Characteristically, the medical histories are complex, they involve several systems, and it is often difficult to establish which of their many conditions contribute most to the reason for admission. Many of these elderly patients are frail, presenting with non-specific ill health (off legs, falls, incontinence, unsteadiness and confusion) due to specific and treatable conditions (urinary tract infection, sepsis and pneumonia). To achieve an effective and lasting discharge, a comprehensive assessment must address medical, psychosocial and functional issues and must start from the point the patient is admitted.

The label of 'social admission', while acknowledging the issue of the home circumstances, is a disservice to this group of patients, as it inevitably means that less effort is paid to establishing exact diagnoses. In fact, a pure 'social' admission—one in which the patient is medically stable but in which the care input has failed—is a rare event and the term is generally *unhelpful*:

- It suggests a non-urgent or elective admission
- It denies a medical cause for admission
- It discourages a full medical assessment
- It implies a 'social' solution to the problems
- It suggests the patient can soon be shifted to hotel-type care
- The term falls into the same category as the unhelpful 'bed blocker' or even 'off legs and unable to cope', in which the emphasis suggests the unwelcome nature of the admission, rather than the challenge of returning an elderly person to their home with improved health

Common Errors and Omissions in the Admission of Elderly Patients

FAILURE TO OBTAIN AN ADEQUATE HISTORY

- Simple communication failure—patient too ill or too deaf to communicate
- Acute confusion/delirium
- Long-standing confusion
- Inadequate referral details, particularly from the deputising service or from a nursing home

FAILURE TO ESTABLISH A CORRECT DRUG HISTORY

It is important to establish:

- What the patient's doctors have prescribed
- What the patient has actually been taking
- When any changes in medication occurred

Common problems with the drug history include:

- New treatments that do not appear on a repeat prescription list
- Tablet bottles that contain a mixed assortment of drugs

- Medications that the patient does not consider to be a drug:
  - Eye drops and skin treatments
  - Etidronic acid (Didronel PMO; 'fizzy drink')
  - Monthly (e.g., B_{12}) or weekly (e.g., methotrexate) treatments
  - Insulin
- Non-compliance with multidrug regimens (more than three different medications)
- Failing to mention PRN drugs, especially analgesics
- Confusion concerning the doses of diuretics and the correct use of inhaled medication
- Not realising the DOAC (direct acting anti-coagulant) is an anticoagulant

FAILURE TO MAKE AN ADEQUATE REVIEW OF THE PATIENT'S PREVIOUS HOSPITAL RECORDS

Readmissions in this age group are common. Hospital notes are helpful, but they can be difficult to track down. Some of the patient's problems may have been identified already: examples include septicaemia due to known kidney stones or gallstones, recurrent angina or dizzy episodes due to arrhythmias and falls due to alcohol.

Inadequate Clinical Assessment

- Failure to assess the musculoskeletal system
- Missed crush fracture of the spine
- Missed fracture of the long bones
- Missed joint infection
- Missed shoulder injury following a fall
- Missed broken skin over pressure areas
- Failure to diagnose 'silent' myocardial infarction
- Silent pneumonia
- Silent septicaemia
- Faecal impaction as a cause of worsening confusion in a patient with dementia
- Failure to take an alcohol history (alcohol problems in the elderly present with depression, confusion and falls)
- Missed retention with or without overflow incontinence

Taking the History
TAKING A HISTORY FROM THE PATIENT

Elderly unwell patients often have considerable difficulty in recalling the time course of the symptoms that brought them into hospital. For many, the point at which new symptoms took over from the chronic symptoms of generalised ill health and multiple pathologies will be far from clear. For many elderly patients the process of giving a

| CASE STUDY 9.1 | Failure to Give Adequate Time to a Patient |

An 84-year-old male was admitted under the chest physician with immobility due to painful feet. He was frustratingly slow to give a rambling history, but after having successful dermatological treatment to his cracked and fissured soles he slowly mobilised. He was referred for rehabilitation and seen briefly at the end of very rushed ward rounds as ' ... and just the sore-foot man waiting to go to elderly care'. On a less hectic round, he mentioned that he, too, had worked in a hospital and proceeded with a detailed account to a chastened chest consultant about the 20 years he had spent nursing in one of the country's earliest cardiothoracic surgical units, how fierce the matron was and, in his day, how precise the bed alignment had to be prior to consultant ward rounds.

history, often more than once when they are already feeling unwell, can be a considerable ordeal. The tendency is for staff to rush them rather than sit and listen (Case Study 9.1).

- Every patient has their own life story and, with patience, you will learn more from them than they will from you.
- Piece together the history and try and find something of the person rather than simply the 'admission problem'.
- In the elderly, you are more likely to encounter atypical symptoms in commonplace conditions: dizziness as a presentation of myocardial infarction, 'off legs' as a result of a urinary tract infection and acute confusion as a side effect of a change in drug treatment.
- It is important that efforts are not duplicated and that the patients are not subjected to unnecessary repetition.
- It is critical to obtain a history from a third party: a close relative, a professional carer or the patient's general practitioner.

Pain

It can be difficult to separate symptoms from different systems. The problem of referred pain and the inability of some elderly patients to describe and localise their pain clearly can make it challenging for the listener. Examples include bandlike abdominal pain attributable to collapsed thoracic vertebrae, upper abdominal pain due to acute myocardial ischaemia with cardiac failure and diffuse abdominal pain due to a strangulated femoral hernia. To complicate the issue, many patients have pre-existing chronic pain from joint degeneration, from poorly controlled angina and from chronic arthritis of the spine. Pain in patients with dementia can be difficult to recognise, presenting as increased confusion, changes in pulse and blood pressure, emotional distress, withdrawal or simply a refusal to eat and drink.

TAKING A HISTORY FROM A THIRD PARTY

The patient's description of the home circumstances and their level of dependence must be supported by evidence from other sources. Without a detailed background, the assessment is seriously flawed:

- The patients may be unforthcoming because of confusion, anxiety or depression.
- The patients may minimise their disability.
- Carers may have a different perspective on the situation.
- Late information cannot contribute to the critical initial diagnostic process and will probably delay the eventual discharge.

Where to Go for Information

1. Relatives
2. Paramedic records (especially the initial National Early Warning Score 2 [NEWS2])
3. The previous hospital, medical and nursing notes
4. GP—early liaison with primary care will save a lot of time
5. Community nurse
6. Nursing home staff
7. Health visitors
8. Neighbours
9. Home care services
10. Social services

Dealing With Relatives

- Many relatives fear that an elderly person may be written off at an early stage and may therefore be defensive about their normal level of dependence. Just because someone is 85 years old, it is wrong to assume that either the relatives or the patient will take a philosophical view about having had a 'good innings'. Some of the most serious allegations of substandard care concern this area. Relatives often assume that, in the chaos of an acute unit, the elderly are given lower priority.
- Be sure who you are dealing with and what input they have in the care of the patient. It is not helpful to have an early detailed discussion with a niece who happens to be on the ward, before speaking to the daughter who has been sacrificing her sanity and her marriage to look after her confused elderly father for the past 5 years.
- Be sensitive to family dynamics, particularly in the issues of chronic dependence and dementia. The admission may have been the culmination of months of severe family stress in trying to cope with an increasingly difficult situation. The elderly spouses of patients with dementia often show evidence of significant stress-induced ill health. A straightforward and tactful information-gathering exercise is all that is needed in the early stages.

A Team-based Approach

Communication among the admitting clinicians is of paramount importance in the management of the elderly. Apart from minimising the ordeal for the patient of repeating the same information to different staff members, there is critical information that *must* be shared at the outset:

- The patient's baseline level of dependency
- The presence and time course of any confusion
- The list of current medication
- Any suspicion of a head injury or a fracture
- The relatives' main immediate concerns
- Any particular risk of falling

Excellence in Communicating With the Relatives

1. Establish the depth of personal knowledge. Is the history from a third party due to personal familiarity with the patient, or is it hearsay?
2. When was the patient last well, and from that point, how did the symptoms first develop? (Giving an approximate order)
3. What is the level of dependence and when did this change?
4. Establish the usual mental state, and if there is a component of confusion/loss of short-term memory, when did it first develop and how has it progressed or changed over time?
5. When you are doing your assessment, try to picture the patient in their own environment.
6. In particular—'Who are they?' and 'What matters to them?'

Frailty and Frailty Syndromes

Frailty describes a patient's situation in which their body has been failing in a variety of ways, making them vulnerable to the added burden of even a relatively minor acute illness. Given its many facets, frailty requires a coordinated multidisciplined approach, which depends on immediate recognition and rapid interventions. All acute admissions over the age of 65 should therefore be screened with the Clinical Frailty Scale (CFS). This is an overall judgement based on information collected on admission from the patient, from family and carers and from medical records. CFS has nine grades, from Very Fit (1) to Terminally Ill (9). The threshold for immediate intervention (ideally within 30 min of admission) is usually Grade 6—'Living with moderate frailty'. Such a patient needs help with all outside activities, housework and some aspects of personal care (notably bathing). Intervention takes the form of a Comprehensive Geriatric Assessment (CGA)—a team-based approach to optimise the medical, psychological and functional aspects of the patient's condition.

There are five frailty syndromes which need to be identified and managed:

- Falls
- Immobility
- Delirium
- Incontinence
- Medication interactions and adverse effects

Falls

Falls are a common and important cause for acute medical admission. Almost 10% of patients aged 70 years and above will attend the Accident and Emergency Department (AED) at least once per year with injuries caused by a fall, and a third of these will be admitted to hospital. Apart from a 10% risk of a fracture, falls have long-term consequences, particularly if they are recurrent:

- They lead to a loss of confidence.
- They are a threat to independence, particularly when they are recurrent.
- Hospital admission after a fall often triggers a slow general decline.

Despite their importance, patients are often not adequately assessed to establish the causes or the effects of their fall. Many will have attended on several previous occasions: a first-time faller has a greater than 50% chance of falling again within 12 months. In a significant proportion, the cause is reversible or the risk factors can be reduced.

The Cause of Falls

Fig. 9.1 and the following case studies illustrate the many factors that increase the risk of falls.

Most falls are caused by a combination of *internal* problems with balance, vision and posture, and *external* factors such as loose rugs, poor lighting and cluttered living space. The fall may be triggered by new medication leading to dizziness or confusion, or the effects of an intercurrent acute illness such as anaemia, heart failure or infection. Case Study 9.2 illustrates such falls.

Patients will be admitted after a fall if:

- They fail to make a full recovery.
- They have injured themselves.
- They are in need of care that is not available at home.
- A serious medical cause for the fall is suspected.
- The patient has been lying for a long time.

Assessment After a Fall
CRITICAL CLINICAL TASKS IN ASSESSMENT AFTER A FALL

Ensure the safety of the patient: ABCDE. Assess the vital signs and, if the patient is acutely ill, correct oxygen saturation, exclude hypoglycaemia, examine the pulse for bradycardia or tachycardia and measure the core temperature (hypothermia or fever). Always search for postural hypotension: *a fall in the systolic blood pressure of 20 mm Hg or more on standing upright* (postural changes can be identified in the immobile from recordings taken when the patient sits up with the feet dependent over the side of the bed).

Fear of falling

Poor vision + hearing

Postural hypotension

Bradycardia/
tachycardia

Arthritic joints

Muscle weakness

Painful neglected feet

Cerebral
ischaemia

Vertigo

Cognitive
dysfunction

Urinary
incontinence
(stress or urgency)

Environmental
hazards?

Parkinson's
disease

Drug history

FIGURE 9.1   The patient with recurrent falls.

 CRITICAL CLINICAL TASKS IN ASSESSMENT AFTER A FALL

- Ensure the safety of the patient: ABCDE
- Look for injury
- Has this been a stroke?
- Arrange for an urgent electrocardiogram (ECG) and cardiac monitor

Look for injury. Pain is the main clue to injury, although acute confusion can mask pain completely. Note the sites of pain—they will need to be x-rayed if there is tenderness, deformity or swelling. Inspect the scalp for bruising and look behind the ears (Battle sign; p. 111). Is there bruising around the hips? Look for pain on moving the wrists, shoulders, hips and elbows. Pleuritic pain may be due to fractured ribs. Deep pain in the lower back or groin is seen after pelvic fractures. If the patient has been lying in one position, there may be soft tissue pressure damage (bruising, discolouration and swelling) or burns.

CASE STUDY 9.2	Causes of Falls

CASE 1

A 90-year-old female was started on the antidepressant, dothiepin: one tablet in the morning and two at night. She was also already taking atenolol 100 mg a day, β-blocker eye drops and bendroflumethiazide. She had fallen and lain against the radiator, suffering a full-thickness burn to the right shoulder. On admission, her systolic blood pressure fell by 30 mm Hg when she stood up from lying, associated with unsteadiness. She was otherwise well.

- Drug treatment is a common and treatable factor in falls.
- Half of all elderly fallers cannot get back on their feet unaided.

CASE 2

An 86-year-old female was visiting her daughter at Christmas. She tripped in her bedroom and was in the line of a fan-heater. She was unable to move and suffered extensive burns to both lower legs.

- Falls are more common in unfamiliar surroundings, particularly those encountered when staying in cluttered or poorly lit spare rooms. People become used to their own frayed carpets and unsafe stairs, but these pose a threat to an elderly guest.

CASE 3

An 83-year-old male was admitted having been found on the floor with extensive occipital bruising. He had signs of a chest infection, but with treatment made a good recovery. Mobilisation, however, was very slow. He had generalised stiffness, had a tremor and was very reluctant to move his feet due to fear of falling. A diagnosis of Parkinson's disease was made and he was started on treatment.

Falls are common in Parkinson's disease:

- Patients tend to topple backwards.
- They are slow to correct any imbalance.
- There is often an associated postural hypotension.

If there is any pain around the neck or radiating around to the jaw, consider high cervical spine injuries (fractures can occur here in the elderly even with minor, low-impact falls). CT of the cervical spine may be necessary.

Has this been a stroke? Examine for one-sided weakness, facial droop or an obvious speech disorder. Confusion must not be confused with dysphasia. If a stroke is suspected, check the safety of the airway and of the swallow. A head CT or MRI will be needed if the patient is on anticoagulants.

Arrange for an urgent ECG and cardiac monitor. This is to exclude a myocardial infarction or arrhythmia as the cause of the fall.

HOW TO IDENTIFY POSTURAL HYPOTENSION

The supine blood pressure is the value obtained after the patient has been lying quietly for 5 min. The standing blood pressure is the value obtained after the patient has been standing for up to 5 min. The blood pressure should therefore be checked every minute of standing for 5 min. A drop in the systolic pressure of 20 or more or if the systolic pressure falls below 90—particularly if accompanied by symptoms—indicates postural hypotension. The change in posture can also be accompanied by a marked increase in heart rate (by 30 or more beats/min or to a rate >120 beats/min) which may also be associated with symptoms of dizziness and can be the culprit in some cases of syncope.

IMPORTANT CLINICAL TASKS IN ASSESSMENT AFTER A FALL

Obtain an Adequate History

- What were the circumstances? A fall, often forwards and causing facial injury, in which there is no warning and no loss of consciousness, suggests a *drop attack*. A 'draining away', particularly on standing with greying vision and fading voices, suggests *syncope*. It should be remembered that the elderly may not realise that they have lost consciousness and can have significant postural hypotension in the absence of symptoms. Dizziness with the room spinning, especially if triggered by sudden turning or neck extension, suggests *vertigo*. If the patient has acute vertigo and cannot stand without support, and particularly if there is also slurring of the speech and focal weakness, a posterior circulation stroke is the likely cause. Head injuries, particularly in males, are frequently associated with excessive alcohol intake.
- What is the drug history? The main culprits are nitrates, diuretics and antihypertensives—all causing postural hypotension—and psychotropics, notably, long-acting benzodiazepines (e.g., nitrazepam), anticonvulsants and antidepressants, affecting balance and causing drowsiness.

Assess Mobility

- Gait and balance disturbance predict the likelihood of further falls. Establish the patient's existing mobility and cross-check their account with that of a relative: patients often overestimate their usual level of function.
- For a more objective assessment, there are three simple tests that can be tried once the patient has recovered from the immediate effects of the fall:
  - 'Get up and go'—the patient who can rise from a chair, stand steadily, walk across the ward, then turn and return to the chair without help does not have an immediate problem with mobility or balance. This can be combined with a measurement of gait speed.
  - Can the patient stand on one leg for 10 s? This will give a rapid global assessment of balance, power in the lower limbs and difficulty with weight bearing due to, say, problems with arthritic knees.
  - Does the patient stop walking when talking? Patients who are beginning to find mobility an increasing problem, for whatever reason, have to marshal their resources when dealing with the challenge of walking. This is apparent if a conversation is started while the patient is on the move—they will stop walking to talk.

IMPORTANT CLINICAL TASKS IN ASSESSMENT AFTER A FALL
- Obtain an adequate history
- Assess mobility
- Assess cognitive function
- Speak to the carers and close family

Assess cognitive function. This is an important part of any assessment of the elderly patient, but in the particular case of recurrent or unexplained falls, cognitive impairment will have a profound effect on the plans for discharge.

The Abbreviated Mental Test Score (AMTS) (Box 9.1) is simple to administer: a score of less than 7 out of 10, assuming this is not due to a simple communication problem, suggests cognitive impairment. The AMT4 is even shorter, only asking for the DOB, age, year and place. Any wrong answer indicates probable cognitive impairment.

The next step is to establish from the relatives' history whether this is a recent or long-standing problem.

SPEAK TO THE CARERS AND CLOSE FAMILY

- Obtain an overall picture of the patient in their home, with an emphasis on mobility, vision and the immediate domestic environment. Confirm the drug (and alcohol) history. Check the input from family and professional carers.
- Has there been evidence of cognitive impairment: memory loss and difficulty with complex tasks?

ADDITIONAL ASSESSMENT ON EXAMINATION

- Look at the feet and lower limbs. Examine for generalised arthritis, particularly of the knees. Knees that are swollen, arthritic and stiff are often associated with thigh muscles that are weak and wasted through disuse. Is there generalised weakness of

BOX 9.1 ■ The Abbreviated Mental Test Score

1. How old are you now?
2. What time is it now (to the nearest hour)?
3. I will give you an address and ask you to repeat it later on: 42 West Street.
4. What year is it now?
5. Can you tell me where you are now?
6. Can you tell me who (two persons) these people are?
7. Can you tell me the date of your birthday (day and month)?
8. What were the dates of World War II?
9. Who is on the throne at present?
10. Can you count from 20 to 1 backwards?

the legs? Are the feet well cared for or are they misshapen, with overlapping toes, bunions, painful fissures and huge uncut nails?

- Assess the hearing and vision. Sensory deprivation leads to a loss of balance, a loss of the compensatory mechanisms needed to maintain equilibrium and a reduction in the level of self-confidence. Ensure hearing aids and glasses are brought in soon after admission.
- Evaluate and localise any pain and ensure appropriate analgesics are prescribed and given.

Answering Relatives' Questions in Patients Who Fall

Will everything be all right? You should be guarded about the prognosis until more information is available. The outlook after a fall can be poor, for example, a fall followed by a lie on the floor for an hour or more carries a 6-month mortality rate of 50%.

Why do the falls keep occurring? The majority of elderly patients who fall will fall again. However, while some risk factors cannot be corrected some, such as drug side effects and environmental factors, can be addressed.

What can we do to prevent it? Our assessment will identify any reversible medical cause for the falls, and part of the rehabilitation will involve an evaluation of the situation at home.

Shouldn't the patient now be in a nursing home? We cannot possibly take the patient into our house. One of the outcomes of this admission will be an assessment of the domestic situation, to assess the patient's personal needs and to look at what support is available. Any eventual discharge will take all these factors into account as well as your views and those of the patient.

Does the patient need all those tablets? We will take this opportunity to re-evaluate all the medication—what is prescribed, what is actually taken and what is really needed.

Why did the patient fall in the ward? Patients who are unsteady on their feet are more likely to fall in unfamiliar surroundings, particularly if an acute illness has led to confusion. We will try to prevent further falls by treating the underlying problems, and in the meantime, it may be helpful to bring in glasses/supportive footwear/usual walking aids.

Can't you use sedation or cot sides? Sedation or physical restraints are the absolute last resort—and only then if the patients are a danger to themselves. Their use causes increasing confusion, and there is no evidence that they are effective in preventing falls: indeed, they may slow down mobilisation.

What are the chances of this happening again in hospital? Recurrent falls are quite common at this age, even if all possible precautions are taken. There is always a balance to be struck between safety and encouraging the patient to maintain independence. There are effective ways of reducing the chances of falling again: a detailed risk assessment of all the factors that may be contributing to the falls, leading to a management plan to reduce these and special targeted exercise programmes to improve balance, gait, posture and muscle strength.

Excellent Care for Patients Who Fall

- Are the staffing levels appropriate for the dependence levels in your patients?
- Are your elderly patients assessed according to a protocol?
- How much unnecessary duplication is there?
- Are the relatives and carers interviewed on admission?
- Do you use an AMTS/AMT4 as routine in assessing the elderly?
- Can you identify the 'high-risk faller'?
- Is there a protocol for the prevention of falls/use of cot sides?
- Have you audited falls in the acute ward?
- How safe is your ward for the unsteady elderly?
  - Bed to chair or commode
  - Chair to bathroom
  - How cluttered is the space around the beds?
  - How well do their pyjama bottoms fit?
- How soon after admission do you start planning for discharge?

Immobility

Increasing immobility can have many important causes, as illustrated by these case studies (Case Studies 9.3–9.6).

'*Off legs and unable to cope*' is the commonplace label for immobility and should be ignored. Immobility is either part of a slow global deterioration in function or, more commonly on the admitting ward, it occurs suddenly over days or weeks and signifies an acute illness of some form.

The common causes of recent onset immobility are as follows:

- Stroke
- Parkinson's disease
- Heart failure
- Acute exacerbation of chronic obstructive pulmonary disease (COPD)
- Musculoskeletal disease (arthritis and osteoporosis)

CASE STUDY 9.3 — Advanced Malignant Disease Presenting as Increasing Immobility

An 86-year-old female presented with an 8-week history of increasing immobility, anorexia and reduced fluid intake. She had previous admissions to elderly care for respite care. She denied any particular complaints and said she was able to walk with a stick.

On initial assessment, she appeared frail and cachectic. Her AMTS was 4/10. She had a productive-sounding cough and evidence of left lower lobe pneumonia.

The initial diagnosis was 'poor mobility and a chest infection'.

Immediate blood tests showed that she was anaemic and also had abnormal liver function tests. An ultrasound showed a large right-sided renal cancer, with secondary spread to the liver.

- When elderly patients become ill, their history cannot be relied on.
- Malignant disease rather than 'frailty of old age' is often the cause of progressive deterioration.
- Early investigations mean that an appropriate management plan can be instituted soon after admission.

CASE STUDY 9.4   **Infection as a Cause of Acute Immobility**

A 78-year-old widower took to his bed because he was too weak to walk. His only complaint was of burning on passing urine. He was unable to recall any of his medication, but his daughter later provided a list, which included prednisolone, oral nitrates and atenolol.

Coliform bacteria were cultured from his urine and blood. Within 4 days of starting antibiotics, he was feeling well and was fully mobile.

Infection, particularly urinary infection, can lead to generalised ill health. It is important to identify those regular medications that must not be stopped suddenly. These may include:
- Steroids (acute steroid insufficiency)
- β-Blockers (rebound angina)
- Anticonvulsants (recurrence of fits)
- Benzodiazepines (withdrawal syndromes)

CASE STUDY 9.5   **Immobility Due to Drugs**

CASE 1

An 85-year-old female with Alzheimer's disease came to the AED and had her dislocated shoulder reduced under sedation with IV diazepam. Two days later, she was admitted with an impaired conscious level, having taken to her bed with aspiration pneumonia. She had a productive cough and a Glasgow Coma Score (GCS) of 5. She responded to physiotherapy and IV antibiotics.
- Patients' psychosocial circumstances must be assessed fully before discharge.
- There is a major risk in sending an elderly infirm female with dementia home from the hospital immediately after sedation.

CASE 2

A 73-year-old female with diabetes and a previous history of strokes was admitted with a gradual deterioration, lethargy and increasing immobility. She was a 'dead weight' and her husband was unable to cope. Nothing specific was found. She was transferred to elderly care where she was noted to be on two sedatives, antidepressants and nitrazepam. These were gradually withdrawn. She made a spontaneous recovery and was rapidly (over 3–4 days) able to mobilise with a Zimmer frame and support.
- In any immobile patient, the drug history is critical.
- A third of admissions in the elderly is related to drug toxicity.
- Polypharmacy increases the chances of interactions, drug duplications and non-compliance.

These may be accompanied or triggered by:
- Depression or grief
- Anxiety, especially associated with a fear of falling
- Pain
- Underlying cognitive impairment

CRITICAL CLINICAL TASKS IN ASSESSING IMMOBILITY

Immediate safety of the patient: ABCDE
- Exclude hypothermia: a core or tympanic membrane temperature <35°C
  - Hypothermia causes confusion and incoordination.

CASE STUDY 9.6	**Difficulties in Predicting the Outcome in the Elderly Immobile**

An 80-year-old male with a known history of chronic heart failure and atrial fibrillation was admitted with sudden generalised deterioration and confusion.

On assessment, his AMTS was unrecordable, he was unable to stand unsupported and was incontinent of urine. His speech was slurred and he was slumped in bed with a respiratory rate of 30 breaths/min. His blood pressure was 235/122 mm Hg and his oxygen saturation was 85%. His initial blood tests showed dehydration. The diagnosis was 'acute confusion'.

Two hours after admission, he was found on the floor, having fallen from his bed and bruised his shoulder. The next morning on reassessment he appeared dysphasic rather than confused and was slumped to one side with definite evidence of unilateral weakness. Further blood tests showed high digoxin levels but nothing else of note.

By 24 h, his GCS had fallen from 15 on admission to 6, and his respiration had become laboured and irregular (Cheyne-Stokes respiration). An urgent CT scan showed a large cerebral bleed related to his severe hypertension. A diagnosis of stroke complicated by aspiration pneumonia was made. He was started on IV ampicillin and metronidazole. The neurosurgeons advised that there was no indication for surgery.

By the eighth day of admission, he was sitting up cheerfully in bed with mild functional impairment and was starting to mobilise. His blood pressure was controlled with cautious use of antihypertensives.

- Stroke presents as confusion.
- Dysphasia may be mislabelled as confusion.
- Always look for evidence of weakness down one side (the family will often notice this first).
- Outcomes are difficult to predict in the elderly, who can have excellent powers of recovery (patients who reach the age of 80 years have a proven track record of survival!).

- Triggers include alcohol and psychotropic drugs.
- It can result in dehydration and pneumonia.
- Active rewarming is indicated.

Assessing the cause: establish the full history

- From the patient *and* a third party
- Establish the sequence of events: acute/chronic/acute on chronic
- A comprehensive list of medications
- What is the patient's normal level of mobility?
  - How did the immobility develop: progressive/sudden onset/stuttering?
  - Is there musculoskeletal disability?
  - How are hearing, sight and balance?
  - Are there recurrent falls?
  - Have you accessed previous nursing or medical notes?

 CRITICAL CLINICAL TASKS IN ASSESSING IMMOBILITY

- Ensure the safety of the patient: ABCDE
- Assessing the cause: establish the full history

IMPORTANT CLINICAL TASKS IN ASSESSING IMMOBILITY

Assess the overall condition

- Does the patient look well for their age? (grooming/foot care/state and cleanliness of the skin)
- Is there evidence of neglect? (underweight/poor hygiene/chronic changes to the skin and feet)

Is the patient in pain? Pain, particularly on movement, leads to immobility and commonly arises from the musculoskeletal system—either chronic arthritis or vertebral collapse. Severe osteoporosis is a major cause of increasing immobility, with loss of height, spinal deformity and severe pain from fractures of the thoracic and lumbar vertebrae. When bones are osteoporotic, even minor falls can lead to fractures of the hip, wrist, pelvis and ribs.

IMPORTANT CLINICAL TASKS IN ASSESSING IMMOBILITY

- Assess the overall condition
- Is the patient in pain?
- Look at the areas of risk
- Look for evidence of malnutrition and dehydration
- Examine the patient's mobility
- Is there any evidence of urinary incontinence?
- Should the patient be catheterised?
- Are time-critical drugs (in particular anti-Parkinson medication) easily available?

Look at the areas at risk

- Examine skin creases and groin
- Record any changes over the pressure areas
- Remove any dressings and note the findings
- Examine and record any areas of bruising, redness or tenderness

Look for evidence of malnutrition and dehydration. The risk factors for malnutrition are as follows:

- Poverty
- Depression
- Social isolation
- Dementia
- Recent bereavement
- Anorexia
- Ill-fitting dentures and sore mouth

There may be signs of vitamin and protein deficiency—but the main clue remains the patient's weight: *a body mass index (BMI) (weight in kg/height in metres squared) of less than 19 indicates likely malnutrition* (to estimate height in the bed-bound or those who have lost height, double the distance from fingertip to mid sternum). These patients should be referred immediately for nutritional assessment and dietetic support.

Examine the patient's mobility.

Note: Remember the risk of postural hypotension.

- What do you anticipate from the history you have already?
- Is the patient well enough to try to stand?
- Can the patient sit up unsupported with good balance?
- Is there any obvious one-sided weakness in the face, arms or legs?
- Can the patient lift each foot, in turn, 3 in (8 cm) or more off the bed?
- Can the patient sit on the edge of the bed unsupported?
- Can the patient transfer to a chair?
- Can the patient 'get up and go'?

If there is evidence of urinary incontinence, what is the time course?

Long-standing incontinence. Chronic incontinence is common in the elderly, particularly those with cognitive impairment: one in five nursing home residents is incontinent during the day. However, even in established incontinence, there may be reversible causative factors such as immobility or overuse of diuretics. The acute admission provides an opportunity to review possible underlying causes.

Recent onset urinary incontinence. There are five mechanisms that can interact to result in acute urinary incontinence:

- **Impaired cognition.** This is seen in delirium, stroke and oversedation, all of which are potentially reversible.
- **Reduced mobility.** An elderly patient with bladder irritability may have to urinate every hour or so. Any cause of sudden immobility can therefore result in incontinence.
- **Excessive fluid challenge.** Overuse of diuretics or excessive osmotic diuresis from uncontrolled diabetes can both overwhelm an ageing bladder and lead to temporary incontinence.
- **Bladder instability.** A common problem in the elderly is the additional effect of urinary infection or faecal impaction on the bladder which will produce urgency and incontinence.
- **Retention** with overflow. Especially in elderly males.

Should the patient be catheterised? Catheterisation is associated with short-term complications, impairment of early mobilisation and reduced chances of regaining continence. Situations in which it may be justified include:

- With terminal illnesses when there is distress from bladder distension or incontinence.
- To allow healing when incontinence has produced skin excoriation or ulceration.
- In critical illness in which measurements of the hourly urine output are required.
- Patients in coma.

Delirium

Cognitive impairment is a common and challenging problem in the acute medical unit (AMU), with current estimates that, among those over 65 years admitted as an emergency, it will be a significant issue in 20%. In half of these, the picture is of chronic confusion (dementia) and in the other half there will either be an acute confusional state (delirium) occurring de novo or a combination of long-standing confusion with a sudden worsening, coinciding with the hospital admission.

Delirium is an acute confusional state with these features:

- A fluctuating conscious level—the patient is unable to stay awake or is difficult to arouse, this may alternate with periods of agitation and anxiety
- A reduced level of attention—questions have to be repeated
- Disorganised thinking—rambling, incoherent and slurred speech
- Visual or auditory hallucinations

Delirium is classified as hyperactive (restless and agitated) or hypoactive (withdrawn and drowsy) although frequently there is a mixed picture.

Delirium occurs in around one in five elderly patients after hospital admission:

- It carries a significant mortality risk.
- It can mask pain and acute illness.
- It delays rehabilitation and discharge.
- It can take weeks to resolve.

There are six important risk factors:

1. Existing cognitive impairment
2. Sight and hearing impairment
3. Immobility
4. Acute physical illness
5. Dehydration
6. Sleep deprivation

There are five major causes in the AMU:

1. Infection
2. Hypoxia
3. Metabolic upset (particularly dehydration)
4. Major organ failure
5. Drug therapy

PRINCIPLES OF MANAGEMENT

- Make an immediate comprehensive assessment (Fig. 9.2)
- Establish exact baseline health and functional status
- Treat any acute medical condition
- Prevent deterioration in existing function through enforced immobility, lack of communication and unfamiliar surroundings

- Prevent infliction of harm through unnecessary drug therapy, neglect, falls or premature discharge from hospital

Case Study 9.7 presents some of the problems encountered with confused patients.

Critical Clinical Tasks in Assessing the Confused Elderly

The critical clinical tasks in the acutely confused elderly patient are similar to those in a seriously ill younger patient. Although there are differences in the way in which problems present, the essential priorities are the same: addressing basic resuscitation using the ABCDE system and maintaining the immediate safety of the patient.

Fig. 9.2 summarises the assessment of acute confusion.

HYPOXIA

- The most common cause of hypoxic confusion in the elderly is pneumonia with sputum retention. The chest sounds wet on coughing, but the patient is often too weak to expectorate. Chest pain after a fall may be due to fractured ribs and can severely inhibit deep inspiration and coughing. The pain must be addressed before the patient can have effective chest physiotherapy. It is important to recognise that pneumonia may be complicating another event: a fall with an unrecognised fracture or a stroke with aspiration. The only signs of pneumonia may be an increased respiratory rate and confusion; the temperature may be normal or only increase after admission.
- The other main cause of hypoxic confusion is acute left ventricular function (LVF), which can be very difficult to distinguish from pneumonia or even COPD. Examination can be unhelpful in this age group, and chest films are difficult to interpret. Initial emergency management will often be a compromise by targeting both the heart and the lungs: combining nebulised bronchodilators and antibiotics with diuretics and nitrates.

Management of Hypoxia

- Sit the patient up.
- Encourage the patient to cough. If it sounds productive, arrange urgent physiotherapy. Ensure there is effective analgesia, without the risk of further sedation or confusion.
- Administer oxygen to increase saturations to between 94% and 98% (using nasal cannulae or a simple face mask).
- Organise an ECG to exclude an acute myocardial infarction or arrhythmia (acute atrial fibrillation is very common in this age group).
- Patients should be catheterised if intensive diuretic therapy is planned, particularly as the confused patient is likely to be incontinent: it is kinder for the patient and the output can be accurately assessed during the critical first 24 to 48 h.

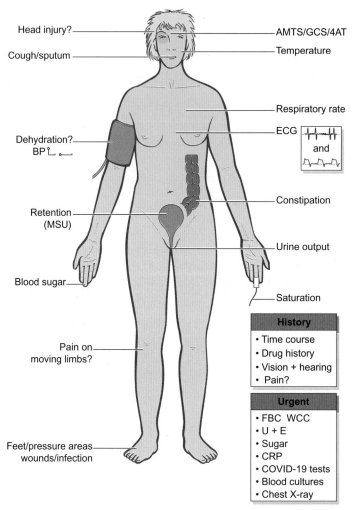

FIGURE 9.2 Assessing the patient with acute confusion. *4AT*, 4A Test; *AMTS*, Abbreviated Mental Test Score; *BP*, blood pressure; *CRP*, C-reactive protein; *ECG*, electrocardiogram; *FBC*, full blood count; *GCS*, Glasgow Coma Score; *MSU*, midstream specimen of urine test; *U + E*, urea and electrolytes; *WCC*, white cell count.

 CRITICAL CLINICAL TASKS IN ASSESSING THE CONFUSED ELDERLY

- Address basic resuscitation: ABCDE
- Maintain the immediate safety of the patient
- Identify and correct hypoxia
- Exclude hypoglycaemia
- Consider head injury
- Consider hyponatraemia

CASE STUDY 9.7 | Confusion

CASE 1

An 83-year-old female was admitted from a nursing home. The background was a diagnosis of Alzheimer's disease with 2 years of progressive memory loss. Before her recent deterioration, she was fully mobile and able to dress, but she needed some help with personal needs and was failing to recognise close family members. For 48 h, she had taken to her bed with increasing restlessness and confusion.

The patient was admitted to the AMU at midnight. She was not initially assessed, and at 1:00 a.m., she fell from the bed onto the floor, sustaining extensive superficial grazes above her eyes and an abrasion to her face. Subsequent examination showed an AMTS of 3/10 and evidence of recent urinary incontinence. She was restless and unable to give an account of herself but was apyrexial. By the next day her respiratory rate had increased to 25 breaths/min, she had a wet, productive-sounding cough and remained incontinent of urine. She was sitting anxiously picking at the bedclothes and was clearly distressed but unable to say why.

With physiotherapy, she produced green sputum. The head wounds healed uneventfully and she slowly returned over the subsequent few days to her previous state.

The diagnosis was of an initial urinary infection complicated by a fall.

Should Cot Sides Have Been Used?

Probably not: There is little evidence that cot sides are helpful in acute confusion, indeed, they increase the potential height of any fall. The main value of cot sides is in combination with pillows to maintain a safe position, in patients with a depressed conscious level.

History

It is important to obtain a history from a nursing home and relatives, although it is common for elderly females to have no close relatives available at the time of admission.

Should Antibiotics Be Used Blindly?

Antibiotics should not be given blindly in acute confusion and incontinence on the assumption that there may be a urinary tract infection. Treatment should be reserved for proven infection associated with any of these:

- Fever
- Dysuria
- Lower abdominal pain
- New incontinence
- Frequency/urgency

Pneumonia can be difficult to recognise in the elderly, but an increased respiratory rate and a productive cough are sufficient evidence of infection to start antibiotics.

Alzheimer's Disease

Patients with Alzheimer's disease have a low threshold for developing a superadded confusional state in response to even minor acute illnesses. Patients should not be sedated but they must be maintained in a safe environment to reduce the risk of self-injury through falling.

CASE 2

An 82-year-old female with dementia was admitted to hospital 'off legs and vomiting'. No history was available from the patient as her AMTS was 1/10. She was weak, incoherent and febrile. The day after admission, she became poorly responsive and more febrile. The patient then rallied and became brighter, but her speech was noted to be incomprehensible. She was, however, said to be 'back to her normal self'. The patient was transferred to elderly care for rehabilitation. There she required full nursing care. On medical review, she was found to be dysphasic, with some receptive problems. The new diagnosis of a stroke was discussed with her son, who with great frustration said the family had been saying that all along but no one was listening.

(Continued)

CASE STUDY 9.7   Confusion—cont'd

Care must be taken with the label of dementia and particular attention must be paid to the preadmission functional level and to the family's account of their relative's normal state of health and of how the illness developed.

CASE 3

A 72-year-old female was admitted with coffee-ground vomiting and hallucinations. She was also mildly dysphasic. The history was limited, but her hallucinations were addressed at the expense of her vomiting, and a referral was made to the psychogeriatricians, who felt her social circumstances needed sorting out. She was transferred to elderly care, where a subsequent endoscopy showed pyloric stenosis and significant ulceration.

The hallucinations had coincided with initiating opiate analgesia. This was stopped and at a later date, fentanyl patches were effectively introduced for what turned out to be severe postherpetic neuralgia. She mobilised well and after a successful home visit was discharged from hospital.

This patient did not undergo a comprehensive initial assessment. In her case there was a combination of physical conditions and cognitive impairment—these are impossible to sort out without full background information from a third party. In particular, there must always be a full drug history, which should include any sedation, anticonvulsants and analgesics, as these may accumulate, causing toxicity and contributing to confusion.

CASE 4

A 94-year-old female who lives alone was found on the floor unable to get up. Apparently, she had fallen before. On admission, she was confused, with a productive cough, a temperature of 38.5°C and an AMTS of 2/10. The oxygen saturation was low, at 88%, and she had signs of a chest infection. She was treated with IV fluids and antibiotics but remained confused.

Six days after admission, her neighbour brought in her hearing aid. Her AMTS improved immediately to 8/10 and she complained of persistent severe back pain. The fall had resulted in a crush fracture of a thoracic vertebra. With analgesia, she was able to cooperate with physiotherapy and started to make a good recovery. On further assessment, she had a long-standing tendency to fall backwards, which was probably related to the development of mild Parkinson's disease.

- Always look for hearing problems when assessing confusion
- Have hearing aids brought in urgently
- Recurrent falls usually have a clear cause
- Falls followed by enforced immobility on the floor can lead to serious complications (and carry a significant mortality rate):
  - Hypothermia
  - Unrecognised fractures
  - Pressure damage to soft tissue and muscle
  - Pneumonia
  - Deep vein thrombosis

Hypoglycaemia. In this age group, hypoglycaemia is seen only in patients with diabetes who are on insulin or (and) oral hypoglycaemics and occasionally after a heavy drinking binge. Longer-acting oral hypoglycaemics such as glibenclamide and chlorpropamide are particularly dangerous in the elderly. If drug interaction with oral hypoglycaemics is suspected (and it should be whenever a patient is taking four or more drugs), contact the ward pharmacist for advice. Be aware of the possibility of a self-administered insulin overdose in an elderly patient with masked depression.

Head injury. Head injuries are a very important cause of reversible confusion—a trivial injury can result in a subdural haemorrhage and the history will not be forthcoming in a delirious patient. If there is a fluctuating conscious level or a progressive fall in the GCS, it is vital to consider a CT scan (particularly if the patient is on anticoagulants) before the situation becomes irretrievable. Even the very elderly can benefit from neurosurgical intervention in the appropriate circumstances. Important clues, apart from the all-important history, are facial bruising, scalp wounds, bruising behind the ears and 'raccoon eyes'.

Hyponatraemia. Hyponatraemia (low serum sodium) is a less pressing but nonetheless important and common cause of confusion in the elderly. It is often due to excessive urinary salt loss from diuretic therapy, particularly if the patient also loses excessive fluid, say from acute diarrhoea. The signs in these patients are hypovolaemia (high pulse rate and postural hypotension) and treatment is with saline. This is not the only cause of hyponatraemia: in some patients, it can be due to inappropriately high levels of antidiuretic hormone (ADH)—a hormone that stimulates the kidneys to retain salt-free water and hence dilute the blood. ADH secretion is vital as the normal response to dehydration, but in this group of patients, the trigger for ADH secretion is either an adverse drug reaction (especially psychotropics) or, occasionally, cancer of the lung. Treatment of inappropriate ADH secretion is with fluid restriction.

IMPORTANT CLINICAL TASKS IN ASSESSING THE CONFUSED ELDERLY

- Assess the degree of cognitive impairment
- Exclude infection and dehydration
- Administer subcutaneous fluids
- Assess constipation
- Assess the social circumstances and dependence
- Have hearing aids and glasses brought in

Important Clinical Tasks in Assessing the Confused Elderly

Assess the degree of delirium/cognitive impairment. Provided the patient can hear and is not dysphasic, the 4 A Test (4AT) is a quick and easy tool for the initial identification of delirium and cognitive impairment. It combines a simple four-point cognitive assessment (AMT4) with a measure of alertness, attention and, critically for the diagnosis of delirium, identification of an acute or fluctuating change in these components over the previous week. The 4AT complements NEWS2 which provides regular surveillance for the development of new confusion.

Exclude infection and dehydration. The main sources of infection are the chest, urine and soft tissues. Generalised infection, and even septicaemia, may have very nonspecific findings in the elderly:

- Increased respiratory rate of >15 breaths/min
- Tachycardia

- Hypotension
- Mild confusion

Patients with infected wounds may be confused because of the development of septicaemia or spreading soft tissue infection. Any wound should be fully exposed in a good light to determine and document its depth and extent and to look for elements such as critical limb ischaemia or gas gangrene. In difficult cases, it is preferable that the wounds are exposed to the combined team of nursing staff and doctors. A management plan can then be produced on admission, rather than taking dressings down three or four times during the first 24 h for a selection of doctors and nurses of varying expertise and experience.

- If there are skin breaks, wounds or ulcers that concern you, ensure that these are all accessible and highlighted on the consultant's ward round. Consider referral to the Tissue Viability Team.

Dehydration can be difficult to identify without blood tests showing increases in the urea and creatinine. The most reliable signs are as follows:

- Postural hypotension
- Tachycardia
- Decreased level of consciousness
- Urine output of less than 50 mL/h

Subcutaneous fluids. It can be difficult to give sufficient fluids to an acutely confused patient. Drinks will be refused and infusions will be pulled out. Subcutaneous fluids are often the key, particularly in the first 48 h until the patient improves. Up to 1.5 L of isotonic saline or 5% dextrose can be given every 24 h. In the very agitated patient, siting the 'butterfly' posteriorly below the shoulder blade can reduce the risk of it being pulled out.

Assess constipation. In the elderly, faecal impaction causes acute confusion, worsens existing cognitive dysfunction and is a reversible factor in urinary incontinence. It can be suspected from a full history and stool chart but can only be diagnosed by a combination of a rectal examination and an abdominal x-ray.

Assess the social circumstances and dependence. Gain information from both patient *and* carers—do not let the carers leave the ward until they have been seen or telephone them at the end of the initial clerking for further information.

1. Does the patient live alone?
2. Does the patient care for someone else?
3. What is the degree of family and/or neighbour support?
4. Is the property secure?
5. Are there pets at home?
6. What are the levels of input?
   a. District nurse
   b. Warden
   c. Social services and meals on wheels
   d. Home help
   e. Voluntary help
   f. Social worker

Dementia

Dementia commonly complicates acute medical conditions in the elderly: it obscures the immediate diagnosis, impairs recovery and has an obvious impact on planning for the patient's discharge.

Sixteen per cent of all females and 6% of all males who reach an average life expectancy will develop dementia—a rate equivalent to around one in five people over the age of 80 years. Of these, 80% will have Alzheimer's disease, in which there is a progressive continuous deterioration; 10% will have multi-infarct dementia, in which the deterioration is stepwise punctuated by a series of mini strokes; and 5% will have dementia against a background of Parkinson's disease, in which the picture is complicated by immobility and drug-induced side effects and, particularly in Lewy body dementia, visual and auditory hallucinations.

In some cases, there will be another psychiatric disorder present: depression, acute anxiety or an alcohol-related problem. This will need to be recognised and addressed.

THE DIAGNOSIS OF ALZHEIMER'S DISEASE

As Alzheimer's disease progresses, the history becomes less reliable due to memory loss. It is unusual for patients to complain directly of memory disturbance—the first indications are usually the onset of problems with complex tasks and difficulties with the challenge of new or unexpected events. Specific common examples include:

- Managing medication
- Using the telephone
- Using transport
- Coping with a household budget

Complications of Dementia That Can Occur in the AMU

Psychoses. These usually take the form of acute paranoia and can be triggered by any acute medical illness. Classically, they are seen after acute myocardial infarction. Patients become intensely suspicious of the staff and often accuse them of being plotters or poisoners. Mobile patients may actively try to flee from the ward to escape this 'persecution'. Acute paranoid states need urgent psychiatric assessment and the warning signs require urgent action.

Aggression. This is also seen in dementia as a complication in acute illness and may be a result of drug toxicity or dehydration. Treatment with sedation is usually unhelpful in the acute situation. Traditional management with haloperidol 2 mg every 8 h leads to drug accumulation and can lead to parkinsonian side effects and oversedation. If there is no alternative for a severely disturbed patient, a short-acting benzodiazepine such as lorazepam is the drug of choice. Any prescription for sedation must be reviewed at least every 12 h to ensure the patient is not over-sedated.

CLINICAL OBSERVATIONS FOR A PATIENT WHO HAS REQUIRED SEDATION

- Hourly checks of conscious level: GCS
- Is the airway safe? (Use the recovery position.)
- Respiratory rate (<8 breaths/min: oversedation? > 20 breaths/min: developing pneumonia?)
- Pulse and blood pressure
- Oxygen saturations: maintain at 94% to 98%

Any sudden change in behaviour is likely to have a cause—metabolic disturbance, pain, drug toxicity or acute events such as pneumonia or myocardial ischaemia.

Haloperidol and lorazepam. Haloperidol is a strong antipsychotic drug traditionally used in acutely disturbed medical patients but it can be hazardous to use. In the elderly, it can trigger an acute parkinsonian reaction with sudden rigidity and swallowing difficulties leading to aspiration and death. This is a major risk in Lewy body dementia in which it should *never* be used. The safe dose of Haloperidol in the frail elderly is 0.5 mg orally or IM with a maximum of 2 mg in 24 h.

Lorazepam is a short-acting benzodiazepine which is easily reversed with flumazenil. The dose is 0.5 mg orally or 1 mg IM with a 2 mg maximum in 24 h.

Nursing Home Admissions

Dependence levels in patients who are admitted from a nursing home vary tremendously. One patient may have been bed-bound and totally dependent for all their needs for a number of years, whereas another from the same home may be mobile and dependent on nursing care only for specific areas of needs. The majority will be dependent for several basic functions, at least half will have cognitive impairment and as many will have chronic urinary incontinence. *The exact level of baseline dependence must be established from the home in every case.* Particular care is needed in patients who have come to the nursing home within recent weeks—there may not have been time to identify any reversible causes of confusion or ill health. Their admission to the nursing home may have been triggered by an unrecognised but reversible physical illness.

Common problems in this group of patients are as follows:

- Falls
- Dehydration during acute illness
- Sepsis
- Pressure sores and contractures
- Delirium
- Incontinence
- Hearing problems
- Sight problems

- Depression
- Dementia

During influenza outbreaks and the recent COVID-19 pandemic, many nursing home residents were admitted with cardiac failure, increasing breathlessness, wheezing and toxic confusion caused by pneumonia.

It cannot be assumed that every admission from a nursing home is for terminal care (Case Study 9.8). However, one of the current features of nursing home care is that frail patients are seen out of hours by on-call deputising medical services and admitted to hospital. There may be pressure from relatives that 'something must be done', equally there may be dismay that a seemingly natural progression towards death is punctuated by an unnecessary trip to an unfamiliar noisy ward in the middle of the night. It is critical to speak to the relatives immediately when the patient is admitted.

- What is the level of dependence?
- What is the time course of the deterioration?
- What are their expectations of the outcome?
- Have they got any particular concerns or worries (this often involves uncontrolled pain/seeing their relative suffer)?
- Have they got an opinion on what the patient may want?
- Has the patient been discharged from hospital recently?

CASE STUDY 9.8 **Admissions From Nursing Homes**

CASE 1

An 85-year-old female was admitted from a nursing home. She had been mobile with a walking frame, but had a 3-day history of increasing breathlessness. She remained very distressed and it was impossible to differentiate between bronchopneumonia and LVF. She was treated with oxygen, a combination of antibiotics, furosemide and low-dose opiates, on which she settled. She recovered fully.

CASE 2

An 81-year-old female was admitted from a nursing home. She had been to the pain clinic within the previous 3 months because of unremitting backache and had been started on fentanyl patches. She had become progressively dependent, and 1 month before admission had been transferred from a rest home into a nursing home, where she had continued to deteriorate and had taken to her bed.

On examination, she had a GCS of 15 and was lying rigidly in bed continually moaning, yet denying on direct questioning any discomfort or pain. Assessment was very difficult: there was no evidence of drug side effects despite the fentanyl, and she appeared to have adequate levels of pain relief. She was screened for sepsis; the nursing home was contacted to make absolutely sure there were no other drugs that may have given a Parkinson's disease-type of side effect; and her fentanyl was reduced slightly in case this was an opiate-induced state.

None of this made any difference, but a rectal examination 24 h after admission revealed severe faecal impaction. She was treated with Microlax enemas and stool softeners with a good result and appeared less distressed. Nonetheless, she remained very dependent and was eventually transferred back to the nursing home.

It is far better to treat a patient aggressively in the early stages, particularly while the normal level of functioning or degree of reversibility is unclear. There is increasing use of the NEWS2 in nursing home residents—to establish the baseline clinical condition, to trigger an early escalation plan involving general practice or urgent hospital transfer, and, most importantly, to establish a 'common clinical language' between the nursing home, general practice, the ambulance service and the hospital.

Ethical Issues and the Elderly Sick

This is a very difficult area, in which even the most experienced medical and nursing staff can be left feeling very uncertain as to whether the correct decisions have been made. The fundamental issue for the individual patient is how far to pursue medical and supportive treatment or, having started them, whether they can be withdrawn:

- Cardiopulmonary resuscitation?
- Ventilatory or renal support?
- Surgery?
- Antibiotics?
- Artificial nutrition?
- Fluids?

WHO SHOULD DECIDE?

- **The patient?** The patient has the basic right to give consent for (and refuse) treatment, but in the very situations in which the decisions are most hard to make—the elderly with delirium, dementia or severe illness—the patient is least able to contribute. Advance directives, living wills and the ReSPECT documentation are increasingly used in the United Kingdom, and it is becoming more common for a patient to have had prior discussions concerning their resuscitation status particularly if they have undergone repeated hospital admissions.
- **The doctor?** Although the medical staff have traditionally adopted this role, this may not be ideal. Their paternalistic role has become less acceptable to the public. Studies also show that doctors may systematically underestimate the pre-existing quality of life in their patients, as well as being poor at predicting the patient's own wishes concerning treatment.
- **The patient's advocate?** This is an onerous task—weighing up the burdens and benefits of any proposed intervention and trying to predict what the patient would have wanted can prove too much for many close relatives: indeed, it may be unfair to burden some with such a difficult decision. Often, they may simply want reassurance that 'everything possible is being done'.

Most of these very difficult issues can be resolved with effective sharing of information between the health professionals and the family (Box 9.2). This can be particularly

> **BOX 9.2** ■ **Providing Clear Information to the Family**
>
> - What is the diagnosis and what is the prognosis?
> - What are the goals of management?
>   - Simple prolongation of life (e.g., nutritional support in irreversible coma)
>   - Maintaining or improving function (e.g., successful defibrillation)
>   - Providing comfort (e.g., subcutaneous morphine in advanced cancer pain)
> - What are the prospects for reaching these goals with and without treatment?
> - What is the burden associated with treatment?
>   - Discomfort and side effects (e.g., trauma of intubation and ventilation)
>   - Survival with severe disability (e.g., postarrest anoxic brain damage)
>   - What are the alternative treatments? (e.g., oxygen and physiotherapy but not ventilation)

important within the first 48 h of admission, when the medical condition can change rapidly. It can be very helpful to contact the family or to have them on the ward, at the times that key assessments are completed:

- Soon after admission
- During the registrar's ward round
- During the consultant's round

WITHHOLDING VERSUS WITHDRAWING TREATMENT?

The decision to withhold treatment may be appropriate if the treatment would do more harm than good—prolong suffering, increase discomfort or shorten life. Withdrawing treatment can be more difficult unless it is clear that the original treatment goals—say to improve ventilation and relieve respiratory distress—cannot be reached. It is therefore important for everyone—carers, family and patient—to be clear about what can and cannot be achieved by the intervention in question before it is started.

Like many difficult issues on the ward, the key is to keep open the best possible lines of communication between the medical and nursing staff, the relatives and, most importantly, the patient.

COVID-19 IN THE OLDER PATIENTS

Older patients have fared badly in the COVID-19 pandemic—75% of the deaths have occurred in the over 75s. The diagnosis in the elderly can be difficult as it is clouded by atypical features (such as extreme lethargy, gastrointestinal symptoms and acute renal failure) or it may simply present as acute delirium (often appearing as decreased responsiveness rather than restlessness). Frailty, as a major risk factor, must be quantified at an early stage (Clinical Frailty Scale) as it impacts the chances of recovery and must be taken into account in decisions concerning escalation plans and ceilings of care. Comorbidities, in particular dementia, add to the difficulties in making informed management plans. Ideally, an early CGA, which will include discussions with the patient and the family, will identify whether or not there is a realistic chance of recovery. Interestingly, a previous COVID-19 infection and/or four or more COVID-19 vaccinations have a major benefit in reducing the risk of a COVID-related death.

Unsurprisingly, the combination of acute illness, isolation in unfamiliar surroundings and visiting restrictions contributes to high rates of delirium in older patients with COVID-19. This is distressing for the patient, their family and the staff and, if the patient is wandering and uncooperative, puts others at risk. Current guidelines have therefore recommended that sedation is considered at a much earlier stage than is usual in non-COVID-19 delirium (assuming that reversible causes such as retention, constipation, drug reaction and coexistent infection have been addressed). Importantly, delirium in COVID-19 is associated with mortality rates approaching 50% so its early recognition and treatment is critical.

The Emergency Admission of Patients With a Terminal Disease

Ninety per cent of patients with advanced malignancy spend most of their last year at home and the majority would like to die there. In fact, only 25% will die at home—many are admitted as emergencies prior to death because there is a change in their condition (often uncontrolled pain, increased confusion or a diminished level of consciousness) or because exhausted carers can no longer cope. The situation requires the utmost sensitivity and clinical skills:

- No one is likely to know the patient's case: the carers will be keenly aware of this.
- The patient will be on a complex regimen, probably including a carefully tailored analgesic regimen.
- The usual EAU approach: urgent tests, empirical antibiotics and IV fluids, may be entirely inappropriate in the setting of a patient at the (predicted) end of their life.
- The relatives and the patient may have unrealistic expectations of a same or next-day discharge back home. Given the usual circumstances of such admissions, a finite time is usually required to maximise the drug regimen, fine-tune the care packages and marshal the appropriate resources in the community.
- Communication is based on the principle that patients have the right to be involved in decisions regarding their care and to understand as much as they want to concerning their prognosis.

It is critically important to bring in the 'home team' who know the patient and their family and also to urgently involve the hospital palliative care service.

Maintaining hydration: Except in exceptional circumstances (e.g., patient choice) end-of-life care includes the avoidance of dehydration with oral or parenteral fluids—the aim is not to prolong life but to avoid the possibility of thirst. Particular attention must be given to mouth care.

End-of-life nausea and vomiting: Levomepromazine (Nozinan) is invaluable for symptom control in the terminally ill. It is a potent anti-emetic, one subcutaneous dose (6.25 mg) can be effective for hours and it can be given as a subcutaneous infusion (12.5–25 mg per 24 h). Its sedative effect calms terminal agitation and restlessness.

End-of-life pain: Most patients will already be taking oral morphine and may need conversion to a subcutaneous diamorphine infusion. Charts are used to calculate appropriate dose conversions: the dose of diamorphine in a 24-h syringe driver is one-third of the patient's usual 24 h morphine dose—and is prescribed with one-sixth of this diamorphine dose, up to one hourly, as a breakthrough treatment. Opiate naive patients should start on diamorphine 10 mg per 24 h with 2.5 mg as needed for breakthrough therapy. Fentanyl patches should be continued and combined with breakthrough subcutaneous diamorphine at one-fifth of the 'patch dose' (e.g., 50 mcg/h patch = 10 mg diamorphine breakthrough dose).

Terminal breathlessness, restlessness and excessive airway secretions: Excessive airway secretions can be controlled with hyoscine hydrobromide, 400 mcg subcutaneously followed by a subcutaneous infusion of 1.2 mg per 24 h. Breathlessness responds to subcutaneous midazolam 2.5 to 5 mg followed by 10 to 20 mg per 24 h as a subcutaneous infusion. Alternatives, with a less sedating effect, are hyoscine butylbromide (20 mg subcutaneously stat and 60 mg per 24-h infusion) and haloperidol (2.5 mg subcutaneous stat and 5 mg per 24 h).

End-of-life delirium: Fear, anxiety and agitation associated with repetitive behaviour such as plucking at bed coverings suggest end-of-life delirium. While this may be reversible by, for example, switching opioids or pushing fluids, in most cases, it is a symptom of dying. For severe agitation in a frightened patient, palliative sedation to control the distress of dying may be required. Carefully titrated midazolam, haloperidol and levomepromazine, alone or in combination, can provide effective relief.

These regimens need review adjustment to ensure patients remain symptom-free yet at an appropriate level of sedation—relatives will often express concerns if the level of symptom control becomes inadequate (commonly this occurs during the night). This can become the major issue in the last hours of a patient's life.

Further Reading

NICE, 2010. Delirium: prevention, diagnosis and management. NICE Clinical Guideline. https://www.nice.org.uk/guidance/cg103.

NICE, 2013. Falls in older people: assessing risk and prevention. Clinical Guideline. https://www.nice.org.uk/guidance/cg161.

NICE, 2015. Care of dying adults in the last days of life. NICE Guideline. https://www.nice.org.uk/guidance/ng31.

NICE, 2016. Multimorbidity: clinical assessment, management. NICE Guideline. https://www.nice.org.uk/guidance/ng56.

Transition between inpatient hospital settings and community or care home settings for adults with social care needs. https://www.nice.org.uk/guidance/ng27.

Multisystem Failure

Shock: The Basic Mechanisms

Shock is the clinical condition in which a generalised reduction in tissue perfusion reduces the blood supply to vital organs, notably the kidneys and brain. Untreated, shock leads to cell death and multiple organ failure. It is therefore important to recognise the early warning signs and start immediate corrective action. Restoring the blood pressure and improving oxygenation are the priorities in shock; establishing its exact cause may have to wait.

In the *early stages*, the extremities are cool as blood is diverted to more important areas, the pulse increases and the blood pressure starts to fall.

Once *established*, shock causes cold clammy skin, tachycardia and increased respiratory rate. Oxygen saturations decrease. The urine output is reduced due to impaired blood flow to the kidneys. The release of lactic acid (measured by the serum lactate) from ischaemic, poorly perfused tissues leads to acidosis. Acidosis in turn impairs cardiac function and leads to further falls in blood pressure. Serial measurements of the lactate levels are used to assess whether treatment is successful.

In *severe shock*, reduced perfusion to the brain leads to agitation, restlessness and eventual coma. By this stage, the reduced blood supply to the kidneys means there may be little or no urine output.

The classical features of shock are listed in Box 10.1 and illustrated in Fig. 10.1.

There are three forms of shock: cardiogenic shock, hypovolaemic shock and redistributive (low-resistance) shock.

> ## BOX 10.1 ■ The Classical Features of Shock
>
> - A systolic blood pressure of less than 90 mm Hg
> - Tachycardia
> - An increased respiratory rate (above 20 breaths/min) and reduced oxygen saturations
> - Mottled, cool and clammy skin
> - Evidence of hypovolaemia: dry mouth, dry axillary skin, postural hypotension, thirst
> - Low urine output (less than 0.5 mL/kg/h)
> - National Early Warning Score 2 score of 5 or more
> - Confusion or agitation progressing to coma

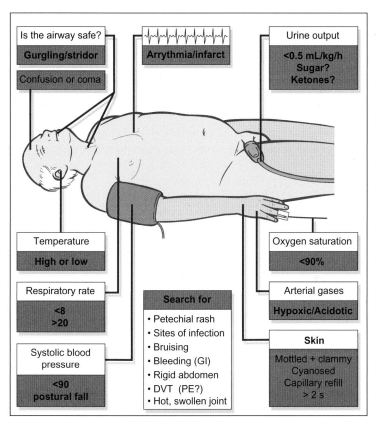

FIGURE 10.1   Features of shock. *DVT,* Deep vein thrombosis; *GI,* gastrointestinal; *PE,* pulmonary embolism.

CARDIOGENIC SHOCK

In cardiogenic shock, the heart as a pump fails to propel blood around the circulation. The common causes of cardiogenic shock include the following:

1. **Heart muscle damage**—A myocardial infarction severe enough to damage a large part of the left ventricle will reduce the cardiac output sufficiently to produce shock.

2. **Severe arrhythmia**—An acute rapid arrhythmia, most commonly atrial fibrillation, can reduce the blood pressure enough to cause shock. This commonly occurs in the setting of a pre-existing acute illness such as diabetic ketoacidosis (DKA) or pneumonia.

3. **Valve disease**—Acute valve failure is an important reversible cause of cardiogenic shock. Sudden mitral regurgitation can complicate myocardial infarction, and acute aortic incompetence can complicate bacterial endocarditis.

4. **Output obstruction**—This is seen in massive pulmonary embolus: the output from the right side of the heart is suddenly cut off by a clot lodging in the main pulmonary arteries, leading to sudden profound shock. A similar clinical picture is seen in a tension pneumothorax in which a sudden increase in pressure inside the chest prevents blood from returning to the heart.

Cardiogenic shock is treated with inotropic and vasopressor support possibly supplemented by intensive therapy unit (ITU) ventilation and ventricular assist devices if there is a potentially reversible cause or urgent transplant is an option. After a cardiac arrest, patients who are in cardiogenic shock *even if they have not regained consciousness* should be considered for urgent percutaneous intervention (PCI) if there is evidence of a recent myocardial infarct as their heart muscle function may still be salvageable.

HYPOVOLAEMIC SHOCK

Hypovolaemic shock is probably the most important type to recognise; it is relatively easy to treat and is rapidly fatal if allowed to progress. In hypovolaemic shock, there is a reduction in the circulating blood volume due to either external fluid loss or 'internal loss' by fluid being sequestrated within the body's internal compartments.

Common medical causes of acute external fluid loss include the following:

- Upper gastrointestinal bleeding (Table 10.1)
- Severe diarrhoea and vomiting
- Diabetic ketoacidosis

TABLE 10.1 ■ Hypovolaemic Shock: The Effects of Blood Loss on the Patient

Blood loss	Percentage of Total Blood Volume	Clinical Observations				
		BP	Pulse	Respiratory Rate	Mental State	IV Therapy
750 mL	15%	Normal	90	Normal	Thirsty	Saline
1500 mL	30%	Low	120	>20 breaths/min	Anxious confused	Blood

Internal fluid loss is seen in:

- Acute pancreatitis
- Severe paralytic ileus

REDISTRIBUTIVE (LOW-RESISTANCE) SHOCK

Redistributive shock is due to the effect of circulating toxins disturbing the normal distribution of blood flow within the body. Some vessels, notably, those in the skin, open up and provide little or no resistance to blood flow. Other vessels shut down in a pattern in which organs such as the kidneys are starved of blood. In contrast to the other forms of shock, in redistributive shock the overall resistance to blood flow is reduced: the cardiac output is therefore high, the pulse is bounding and the peripheries are warm. The patient appears flushed and warm rather than grey and clammy. Without treatment, however, the progression is the same as that in other forms of shock—to kidney failure and to increasingly severe acidosis.

The main causes of redistributive shock are as follows:

- Sepsis, especially from gut and renal tract infections
- Anaphylaxis

Acute Severe Hypotensive Collapse

Clinically, patients with shock present to the acute medical unit (AMU) as a problem of acute severe hypotensive collapse. Given this clinical situation, there are five groups of conditions to consider:

1. Cardiorespiratory collapse (Case 1 in Case Study 10.1)
2. Massive pulmonary embolus
3. Septicaemia (Case 2 in Case Study 10.1)
4. Hypovolaemia (Case 3 in Case Study 10.1)
5. Anaphylaxis

Importance of Immediate Resuscitation

Resuscitation from hypotensive collapse is frequently inadequate on the AMU and instituted too late. Several problems can arise:

- There are delays before the patients are first seen.
- Priority may not be given to the sickest patients.
- Abnormalities in the basic vital signs—*oxygen saturation and blood pressure*—are not corrected.
- The results of urgent investigations are either not seen or ignored.

These deficiencies in the first critical hours of admission have an impact on the patient's chance of recovery, especially, as in Case Study 10.2, where there is sepsis. Once

CASE STUDY 10.1	Three Examples of Shock

CASE 1

A 70-year-old female is admitted with collapse.

Initial observations

She is coughing frothy sputum and cannot lie flat. She has a pulse of 160 beats/min, blood pressure of 90/60 mm Hg, saturations of 80%, respiratory rate of 35 breaths/min and temperature of 37.4°C.

- This is pulmonary oedema due to acute heart failure—cardiorespiratory collapse.
- She needs to be sat up and given immediate oxygen.
- Her low blood pressure and high pulse are due to the heart problem.

CASE 2

An 80-year-old male with a urinary catheter is admitted with new confusion and rigours.

Initial observations

He is hot and delirious, with rigours. He has a pulse of 115 beats/min, blood pressure of 70/40 mm Hg, saturations of 82%, respiratory rate of 30 breaths/min and temperature of 38.5°C.

- This is septicaemic shock.
- He needs urgent oxygen, IV fluids and immediate antibiotics.
- Progress can be judged from the blood pressure and urine output.

CASE 3

A 50-year-old male has collapsed after vomiting a large amount of fresh blood.

Initial observations

He is cold, clammy and very restless. He has a pulse of 130 beats/min, blood pressure of 100/50 mm Hg lying and unrecordable on sitting, saturations of 88%, respiratory rate of 40 breaths/min and temperature of 36.5°C.

- This is hypovolaemic shock.
- He needs urgent oxygen, a large cannula, rapid IV fluids and then blood.
- Progress can be judged from the falling pulse rate and increasing blood pressure.

CASE STUDY 10.2	Delayed Resuscitation

A patient came in at 1:30 p.m. and was clerked in at 4:30 p.m. Although the NEWS2 documentaion records record a blood pressure of 90/40 mm Hg, this is not recorded in the doctor's clerking. Blood gases were taken on admission, but the results were not recorded in the notes. The chest x-ray showed a right upper lobe pneumonia.

At 7:30 p.m. the registrar was asked to see the patient because of persistent hypotension. A blood pressure of 60/40 mm Hg was noted, as were the abnormal blood gases and a high creatinine (indicating a renal problem). Intensive IV fluids were started.

The patient had a central line put in at 1.30 a.m., 12 h after admission and was transferred to the ITU. Noradrenaline (norepinephrine) was needed to restore the blood pressure. By the second day, the whole of the right upper lobe had consolidated due to the rapid progression of pneumococcal pneumonia. The pneumococcus bacterium was grown in two sets of blood cultures taken on admission.

the condition deteriorates to septic shock, the mortality rate approaches 50%. In this case, the priority should have been to correct the oxygen saturation and try and restore blood pressure within the first half hour of admission. The admitting clinical team must share their information from the initial assessments to draw up an effective management plan. Communication must employ the SBAR approach as outlined in Chapter 1 and use the National Early Warning Score 2 (NEWS2) as the universal clinical currency.

There are critical time intervals between admission and the

- First dose of antibiotics—within 1 h
- Treatment with oxygen—immediate
- Initiation of IV fluids—immediate
- Correction of the blood pressure—within the first hour

RESUSCITATION OF THE PATIENT WITH HYPOTENSIVE COLLAPSE

It is important to identify the patient who needs a high priority for resuscitation. This is carried out by the triage system, ABCDE. In these critically ill patients, resuscitation will commence before the full diagnosis is apparent.

Rapid Assessment in the Critically Ill: the Importance of ABCDE

AB: The airway and breathing. If the patient can respond appropriately to 'Are you okay?', then it can be assumed that the blood is reaching the brain and that the upper airway is clear.

Look. A respiratory rate of <8 breaths/min (depressed respiration) or >20 breaths/min suggests a serious problem.

- Remember that an increased respiratory rate is seen in any cause of shock, even if the lungs are normal.
- Measure the oxygen saturation: a level below 90% indicates severe hypoxia (even, as may frequently occur in COVID-19 pneumonia, the patient is not distressed).
- Does breathing look like hard work or is the patient tired and losing interest?
- Does this look like acute asthma?

In left ventricular failure (LVF), the patient will be sitting upright and coughing frothy sputum.

Fit the patient with an oxygen reservoir mask at 15 L/min pending further assessment.

Remember that an unresponsive patient is critically ill and if a patient is not breathing or having occasional gasps, start cardiopulmonary resuscitation (CPR).

Listen. Gurgling indicates aspiration and needs urgent aspiration of the mouth and oropharynx (attempting to aspirate the larynx or trachea may trigger laryngospasm) with a rigid Yankauer suction catheter.

- A crowing sound or harsh inspiratory stridor suggests acute upper airway obstruction, which is seen in acute epiglottitis or severe tonsillitis.
- Snoring suggests an unsafe airway and is seen in coma or stroke.
- Wheezing occurs in chronic obstructive pulmonary disease (COPD), asthma, LVF, acute anaphylaxis and massive pulmonary embolus.

Feel. A finger sweep may be needed to clear an airway or obstruction. Well-fitting dentures can be left, as they will make it easier to apply a mask and maintain an airway.

C: The circulation. An impalpable pulse suggests a systolic blood pressure of less than 80 mm Hg. Hypotension is the major finding in shock and, if severe, will be associated with an increased respiratory rate, anxiety and confusion due to reduced blood flow to the brain. Other features of low blood pressure will be cool and clammy skin, reduced capillary refill and a low hourly urine output (<0.5 mL/kg/h). Capillary refill time provides an important assessment of the state of the circulation: after digital pressure has been applied to a fingertip for 5 s, the capillaries should refill in less than 2 s—a delay indicates an impaired circulation and is a useful sign, especially in hypovolaemic shock.

Important: An increased pulse rate may only appear as a late sign of shock, especially in otherwise fit young patients, and occasionally the response to a major internal bleed may be a slowing of the pulse. An increase in respiratory rate is frequently the first sign of shock.

D: Disability. Check the conscious level quickly using the ACVPU score (**a**lert, **n**ew confusion, responding to **v**oice/**p**ain, **u**nresponsive; Chapter 4: Acute Neurological Problems). Use the Glasgow Coma Score (GCS) for a later more detailed assessment if the conscious level is impaired. Check the blood sugar.

Shocked patients are restless and often uncooperative due to impaired circulation to the brain.

E: Exposure. Examine for sites of infection, sites of skin/soft tissue damage and for the characteristic rash of meningococcal septicaemia. Shock complicated by extensive bruising suggests widespread intravascular clotting (termed DIC or disseminated intravascular coagulation)—an uncontrolled clotting response to tissue injury and is a very serious complication. A leg swollen from the ankle to the groin would suggest an extensive iliofemoral DVT and a possible pulmonary embolus. Anaphylaxis is associated with an urticarial rash and swelling of the face, lips and tongue.

Common Examples of the Critically Ill

Cardiac arrhythmia. A male comes in with very rapid atrial fibrillation and hypotension after suffering a painless myocardial infarction at home.

Massive pulmonary embolus. An obese female in her 20s collapses with breathlessness, syncope and hypotension a week after a caesarean section.

Anaphylaxis. A young male with nut allergy collapses with wheeze and hypotension after inadvertently consuming peanuts during a Chinese meal.

Gastrointestinal bleed. A male in his 40s vomits a pint of fresh blood and passes a large melaena stool. He comes in with hypotensive collapse.

Acute abdomen. A female aged 35 years, known to have gallstones, comes in with a 12-h history of increasing abdominal pain, hypotension and signs of acute pancreatitis.

Septicaemia. An elderly lady has a week's history of vomiting and diarrhoea and is admitted to hospital with hypotension and renal failure. Her blood cultures yield Salmonella.

Pneumonia. A 35-year-old male becomes increasingly breathless and confused during an influenza epidemic. He is hypotensive and hypoxic. The chest film shows pneumonia.

Soft tissue infection. A 60-year-old female with multiple sclerosis is admitted with hypotension and drowsiness. She has necrotic infected sacral pressure sores and positive blood cultures.

Recognition of a deteriorating patient. Chapter 1 outlined the basis of using simple clinical observations in the NEWS2 scoring system which is used to recognise the patient who is deteriorating and is at risk. The score is used to document clinical progress and to trigger corrective measures, particularly through the involvement of critical care outreach teams.

The assessment aims to recognise what is initially reversible that, unless corrected, will progress to:

1. Persistent hypotension
2. Increasing acidosis (and a rise in lactate levels)
3. Kidney failure
4. Cardiorespiratory failure
5. Cardiorespiratory arrest

Box 10.2 summarises the clinical findings that need urgent attention on the AMU.

CRITICAL CLINICAL TASKS IN ASSESSING HYPOTENSIVE COLLAPSE

Maintain the safety of the patient. Secure the airway and maintain oxygenation.

BOX 10.2 ■ What Needs Immediate Action in the Acute Medical Unit

NB: Patients who have a cardiac arrest often go through a warning period of unrecognised deterioration in their vital signs.

Threats to the airway

- Impending obstruction: anaphylaxis with swollen tongue, epiglottitis
- Unsafe airway: impaired conscious level or stroke

Respiratory failure

- Respiratory arrest
- Respiratory rate low (<8 breaths/min) or very high (>30 breaths/min)
- Poor arterial gases: pO_2 less than 8.0 kPa on at least 60% oxygen; pCO_2 more than 6.5 kPa; pH less than 7.2

Circulatory failure

- Pulse less than 40 or greater than 140 beats/min
- Systolic blood pressure less than 90 mm Hg
- Urine output (i.e., circulation to the kidneys) of less than 0.5 mL/kg/h

Falling level of consciousness

- GCS of less than 12 or a fall of 2 or more

Measure the respiratory rate and the oxygen saturations. Choose the most appropriate oxygen delivery system to bring the saturations above 90%. When there is doubt, administer continuous high-flow oxygen at 15 L/min through a tight-fitting mask with a reservoir bag. The patient requires urgent blood gas measurements to:

- Assess the adequacy of the oxygen therapy
- Look at the degree of acidosis (low pH and low bicarbonate)
- Use the CO_2 levels as a measure of adequate ventilation
- Measure the blood lactate levels (high) as evidence of poor overall tissue perfusion

These critical results must be shared within the clinical team.

Measure the radial and apical pulse rates. If the pulse is weak, use the monitor or an electrocardiogram (ECG) trace. Rapid atrial fibrillation will give a deficit between the apical and radial pulses.

Measure the lying blood pressure and look for any postural decrease. Hypotension will, in general, require IV fluid replacement or drugs to support the heart. A patient with a systolic blood pressure of less than 90 mm Hg will show signs of reduced blood flow to the brain—restlessness, confusion and a reduced conscious level. Reduced blood flow to the kidneys results in reduced hourly urine output.

Ensure large-bore venous access. Venous access must be obtained immediately, as the priority in shock is often the need for urgent fluid replacement.

Obtain an immediate 12-lead ECG. This will exclude myocardial infarction and acute arrhythmias as the cause of the hypotension.

CRITICAL CLINICAL TASKS IN ASSESSING HYPOTENSIVE COLLAPSE

- Maintain the safety of the patient
- Measure the respiratory rate and oxygen saturations
- Measure the radial and apical pulse rates
- Measure the lying blood pressure and look for any postural decrease
- Ensure large-bore venous access
- Obtain an immediate 12-lead ECG
- Keep the relatives on the ward

Keep the relatives on the ward. You may require urgent information concerning:

- The recent history (in the elderly, any sudden deterioration can be due to sepsis)
- Previous health and levels of dependence, history of substance or alcohol use disorder
- Details of medications and allergies
- Information to inform future discussions regarding resuscitation status

IMPORTANT CLINICAL TASKS IN ASSESSING HYPOTENSIVE COLLAPSE

Monitor the heart. For the best trace, use adhesive electrodes placed over bony prominences. The skin should be shaved and cleaned with alcohol. The red electrode should be placed below the right clavicle, the yellow one in the same position on the left and the green electrode below the left rib margin.

Assess the site and severity of any pain. Examples of pain in sudden hypotensive collapse include the following:

- Severe chest pain: myocardial infarction or pulmonary embolus
- Severe abdominal pain: perforation/acute pancreatitis/leaking abdominal aneurysm, ruptured ectopic pregnancy
- Effective pain relief is critically important

Reassure the Patient About the Management Plan and Initiate Symptom Relief

- Make sure that you supply adequate analgesia. There is no place for withholding analgesia on the basis that it may mask the development of complications—pain needs pain relief.
- Relieve breathlessness: give oxygen and sit the patient up if the patient wishes to (unless hypovolaemic).
- Ensure the mask is comfortable and tight fitting and that the patient understands that it must be kept on.
- Prepare the patient for possible further procedures:
  - Blood gas sampling (wrist arterial puncture)
  - Central venous line placement (via internal jugular or subclavian veins)
  - Urinary catheterisation
  - Further tests (endoscopy, CT, ultrasound). It is critical that resuscitative measures are not compromised while the patient is off the ward.

IMPORTANT CLINICAL TASKS IN ASSESSING HYPOTENSIVE COLLAPSE
- Monitor the heart
- Assess the site and severity of any pain
- Reassure the patient about the management plan and initiate symptom relief
- Explain
- Speak to the relatives
- Access further information

Explain. Explain what has gone wrong and what will be the signs of improvement, for example:

- Acute LVF: less dyspnoeic, falling pulse, good diuresis
- Upper gastrointestinal bleeding: less thirsty, less light-headed, no further vomiting, clearing of melaena

Speak to the Relatives

- Explain what they will see: drips, monitors, urinary catheters, masks
- Explain the management plan

- Explain the signs of improvement or deterioration
- Forewarn the relatives that the patient may need to be transferred to a high-dependency unit

Access further information. Obtain the previous hospital records and any previous laboratory results urgently.

An example of the immediate management of hypotensive collapse in a male with abdominal pain is given in Case Study 10.3.

CASE STUDY 10.3   Hypotensive Collapse

A 30-year-old male was admitted with a 3-day history of upper abdominal pain. He was reluctant to give many details and denied any significant past history, but he was clearly in considerable discomfort and was very agitated. His wife was with him and added that he had been drinking a litre of strong cider a day for several years and that, 6 months previously, he had been investigated for alcohol-related liver damage and told that he should stop drinking for good.

The initial assessment was of a wasted male lying restlessly in bed with severe upper abdominal pain. His GCS was 15, but he scored only 7/10 on an abbreviated mental test score. His respiratory rate was 30 breaths/min and oxygen saturation was 88%. His pulse rate was regular at 120, and his blood pressure was 90/70 mm Hg lying and 70/50 mm Hg sitting up. On general exposure there was scattered bruising, and he appeared moderately jaundiced. His abdomen was distended, tense and silent but only moderately tender. The BM stix was satisfactory at 7.0 mmol/L.

1. He was given high-flow oxygen at 60% with immediate improvements in his saturation to 98%.
2. Venous access was obtained with difficulty and blood was taken for:
   a. Full blood count (FBC)—to look for bleeding (low Hb) and infection (high white cell count)
   b. Platelets—he is bruised, and alcoholics have low platelet counts
   c. Culture—to identify sepsis
   d. Biochemistry:
      i. To check for dehydration (urea and electrolytes)
      ii. To exclude acute pancreatitis
      iii. To check the liver function tests
      iv. Lactate to identify sepsis
   e. Clotting—bruising can indicate a serious coagulation disturbance.
3. Arterial blood gases were taken to look at the oxygen and carbon dioxide levels and to identify acidosis (a common problem resulting from hypotension in the setting of an acute serious illness).
4. Initial resuscitation was started with a rapid infusion of a litre of 0.9% saline.
5. While awaiting initial results, a small dose of IV opiates was administered to provide immediate pain relief, and he was reassured that further analgesia would be available once the test results had been seen.

The investigations showed a very high amylase (1500 IU), abnormal liver function and early kidney failure. Combined with the clinical assessment, the overall picture was of acute pancreatitis complicated by *redistributive shock*:

- Hypotension
- Confusion
- Hypoxia
- Poor kidney function due to hypotension

| CASE STUDY 10.3 | Hypotensive Collapse—cont'd |

BASIC MANAGEMENT PLAN

- Administer continuous oxygen immediately
- Provide effective analgesia
- Bring up the blood pressure urgently
  - Assess the IV fluid requirements with a CVP line
  - Administer sufficient IV fluid to bring the CVP up to 15 cmH$_2$O of water
  - If this does not bring up the blood pressure consider *inotropic support*
- Use the urine output to assess the response to the improved blood pressure (catheter)
- Rest the gastrointestinal tract with nasogastric intubation on free drainage

CLINICAL OBSERVATIONS TO MONITOR THE RESPONSE

- Hourly urine output to aim at >50 mL/h
- Hourly pulse
- Hourly blood pressure
- Hourly pain score
- 2-Hourly oxygen saturations
- 2-Hourly temperature (shock, central lines and the underlying disease can all lead to sepsis)
- Careful charting of input and output
- Continuous cardiac monitoring

In this man's case, the initial urine output was 10 mL in the first 3 h despite vigorous fluid replacement and his blood pressure remained low. He was therefore started on IV dopamine at 5 μg/kg/min. His blood pressure responded, followed after 2 h by an increase in his urine output.

WHEN DO WE USE DOPAMINE, DOBUTAMINE AND NORADRENALINE (NOREPINEPHRINE) IN PATIENTS WITH SHOCK?

The priority in shock is to maintain the circulation by normalising the blood pressure. The key to this is to give adequate IV fluids. This may require several litres in the first 24 h but if, after 2 or 3 L, the blood pressure remains low, the next stage is to use IV inotropes: drugs that directly increase the blood pressure and improve the blood flow to the kidneys.

Which One to Use?

Dopamine. Dopamine is used in the range of 2–20 mcg/kg/min. At the lower dose it acts to improve kidney perfusion (although the clinical value of this is questionable), in the midrange it also begins to stimulate the heart, and at the higher doses, it begins to constrict peripheral arteries to produce additional beneficial effects on the blood pressure. It is the most widely used 'general purpose' inotrope. It is usual to start with the lower dose and increase accordingly.

Dobutamine. Dobutamine only stimulates the heart and tends to be reserved for cardiogenic shock.

Noradrenaline (Norepinephrine). In the range of 0.5–5 mcg/kg/min, noradrenaline (norepinephrine) has a marked effect on the peripheral vessels and will bring up the blood pressure, but it does not stimulate the heart. It is the drug of choice in septic shock.

How to Monitor Their Effectiveness

- The blood pressure
- The mental state (brain blood flow)
- The hourly urine output (kidney blood flow), which should be kept above 0.5 mL/kg/h
- The blood lactate levels (lactate levels fall as tissue perfusion improves)

There are two adverse effects that must be identified:

1. If the vasoconstrictor effect on the peripheral vessels is too strong, the patient can develop ischaemic tips to their fingers and toes, that is, fixed blue/black discolouration.
2. The cardiac stimulation can lead to marked tachycardia and then arrhythmias: these patients need close cardiac monitoring.

Ensuring Adequate Oxygen Delivery to Vital Organs: Maintaining the Oxygen Saturation and the Blood Pressure

OXYGEN THERAPY

The main indications for emergency oxygen therapy include the following:

- Oxygen saturations of less than 90%
- Systolic blood pressure of less than 100 mm Hg
- Respiratory distress (respiratory rate of more than 20 breaths/min)
- Cardiac or respiratory arrest
- Acidosis on blood gas results

There is understandable anxiety about the correct dose of oxygen in patients with COPD, but in general, the problem in acutely ill medical patients is not giving too much oxygen, but giving too little. *The aim, whatever the circumstances, should be to give sufficient oxygen to raise the oxygen saturation above 90%.* Oxygen is a drug and, unless in an emergency, it should be prescribed—the prescription should specify the mask, the flow rate, and, in the case of the Venturi mask, the oxygen concentration. A target oxygen saturation should also be specified. The aim should be for a normal saturation (94%–98%) in most acutely ill medical patients and for saturations of 88%–92% in those (usually patients with severe COPD) who are at risk from Type II (hypercapnic) respiratory failure. The different techniques of oxygen administration are illustrated in Fig. 10.2.

Oxygen Masks

- **High-flow (Venturi) masks**—these give fixed percentages of oxygen from 24% to 60%, depending on the property of the individual mask. Masks are colour-coded and the appropriate flow rate is clearly marked on each mask. A green Venturi valve delivers 60% oxygen (flow rate set to 15 L/min) and a blue valve delivers 24%

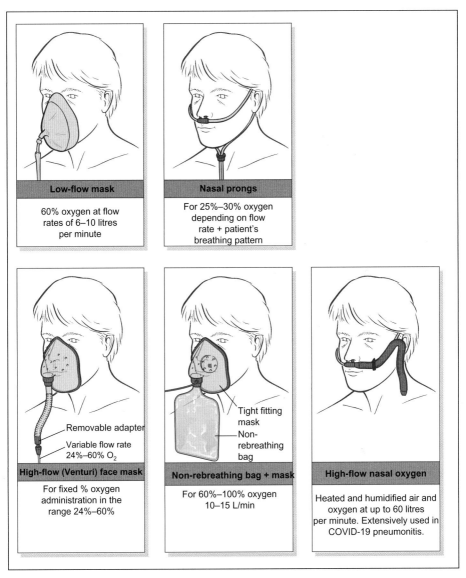

FIGURE 10.2   Techniques of oxygen administration. (For continuous positive airway pressure and high-flow nasal oxygen, see Chapter 3.)

oxygen (flow rate set to 2 L/min). The flow rates are chosen to ensure there is sufficient gas flow into the patient's lungs during each breath. Changing the flow rate does not alter the % oxygen. In patients with COPD who are breathing quickly (>30 breaths/min), the stated flow rates are too low and should be increased from

2 up to 3 or 4 L/min (24% mask) and from 4 up to 6 L/min (28% mask). Venturi masks are used when the oxygen concentration has to be precise, such as in the patient with unstable COPD (24% or 28%) or one with severe asthma (60%).

- **Simple face masks (Hudson masks, MC masks)**—these provide up to 60% oxygen at flow rates of 6–10 L/min, but underperform at rates of less than 5 L/min. These masks are suitable for most situations in which emergency oxygen is needed.
- **Nasal prongs**—the percentage of oxygen delivered by nasal prongs at 2 L/min is between 24% and 28%. At 4 L/min around 30% will be delivered and around 50% at 5 L / min. Nasal prongs are less intrusive than masks and tend to be better tolerated in uncooperative patients. Although oxygen delivery with nasal prongs may be inadequate for a critically ill patient, they are suitable for most situations in which emergency oxygen is needed.
- **Reservoir mask (Non-rebreathing mask with reservoir bag)**—depending on their fit, these masks can administer from 60% to 100% oxygen with flow rates set at 15 L/min. Proper use requires some expertise because the mask must fit tightly, the reservoir bag must be filled before the patient starts to breathe, and the flow rate requires adjustment to ensure the bag remains at least half full throughout the respiratory cycle. Reservoir masks are used in the critically ill to correct severe hypoxia.
- **Escalating the oxygen delivery in COVID-19**—Collective expertise from the first 2020 COVID-19 wave has generated explicit protocols for correcting the oxygen saturations in severe acute COVD lung involvement. Thus if saturations of 94% or greater (or 88% in COPD) cannot be achieved with a 40% Venturi mask, patients escalate to CPAP or High Flow Nasal Oxygen (HFNO) with or without proning (Chapter 3 and Fig. 10.3).
- **Oxygen therapy during nebuliser treatment**—in patients with acute asthma, the nebuliser can be driven by oxygen at 6 L/min or by compressed air combined with nasal prongs to maintain target saturations. In COPD, oxygen should not be used to drive the nebuliser but nasal prongs at 2 L min during air-driven nebulisation should keep the saturations between 88% and 92%.

THE BLOOD PRESSURE

There are two main reasons why the blood pressure can suddenly fall in the critically ill. Firstly, the heart may start to fail as a pump—examples would be an acute myocardial infarction or the toxic effects of septicaemia. Secondly, there may not be enough fluid returning to the heart to fill it sufficiently; examples would be rapid blood or fluid loss or the sudden loss of vascular tone seen in overwhelming sepsis. Improving the circulation of the blood by restoring the blood pressure is as important as correcting the amount of oxygen contained in it. It is critical to ensure there is sufficient circulating volume to carry any additional oxygen to the tissues. If there is hypotension and evidence of inadequate tissue perfusion—notably, oliguria, poor capillary refill and impaired conscious level—*an urgent challenge with 500–1000 mL of IV saline should be considered.*

WHEN IS A CENTRAL LINE USED?

- To assess the state of the circulation from the central venous pressure (CVP)
- To gain access to major veins:
  - When there is no peripheral access
  - For administration of irritant infusions or drugs, for example, dopamine and amiodarone
- To insert a temporary pacemaker

Inserting a central venous line: subclavian and internal jugular venous cannulation. These are the two preferred sites for inserting central venous lines. Placement involves the Seldinger technique, in which the vein is first cannulated with a needle, through which is pushed a guide wire. The needle is removed, leaving the wire in place and then the cannula is fed into the vein over the guide wire, which itself is then withdrawn. Success rates have improved and complications are less common with the use of portable ultrasound machines to locate the central veins before cannulation.

The Procedure

1. Are the results of clotting studies available to the operator?
2. This is a sterile procedure: masks, gowns, drapes, gloves and full skin preparation are required.
3. Two percent aqueous chlorhexidine is more effective as a skin disinfectant than povidone-iodine.
4. The patient must be 20 degrees head-down to prevent air from entering the cannula (air embolus) during insertion.
5. The operator must check the trolley and packs before starting the procedure.
6. The infusion should be run through and ready.
7. If a multilumen catheter is inserted, the staff must be prebriefed about its correct use.
8. Decide beforehand what dressings are to be used to secure the site.
9. Explain and reassure the patient (and the relatives) about the procedure:
   a. The rationale for needing a central line
   b. The fact that it is a routine method of monitoring/administering certain treatments
   c. Local anaesthetics will be used.
   d. The clinicians will provide an appropriate level of information on the benefits and risks.
   e. It would be normal practice to obtain written consent if the patient is well enough.

Complications. The two main complications are puncturing the lung and puncturing an artery. Pneumothorax is much more common with cannulation of the subclavian vein. The approach is from below the clavicle and the route into the vein skirts the apex of the lung. There must always be a postprocedure chest film, which must be seen and interpreted by the person who put the line in or a designated deputy (lines tend to be put in at the end of work shifts). If a patient deteriorates acutely with breathlessness or hypotension immediately after the procedure, it is important to consider a pneumo-thorax. Arterial bleeding is more likely during internal jugular vein cannulation, as the carotid artery is adjacent to the point of entry. Such bleeding is not dangerous, but it will need 10 minutes of firm digital pressure before it will stop.

The central venous pressure. The CVP is a simple measurement that gives important information about the overall state of the circulation, and specifically about the degree of hydration. The measurement is taken from the height of a vertical column of fluid that is in free communication with a central venous catheter (Figs. 10.3 and 10.4). If the patient is lying flat, the reference point from which the measurement is made is in the mid-axillary line at a point vertically below the sternal angle. This coincides with the position of the right atrium.

The normal CVP is from 0 to +8 cmH_2O.

The CVP is abnormally high in congestive cardiac failure and in overtransfusion; it is too low in hypovolaemic and septic shock, in which values of -3 cmH_2O or less will be found.

FIGURE 10.3 Measuring the central venous pressure (CVP).

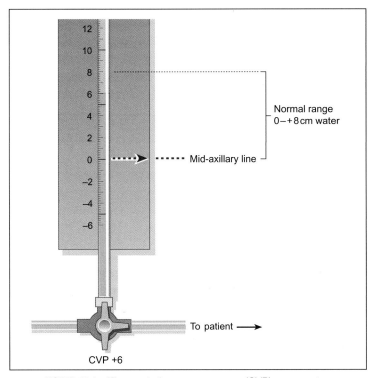

FIGURE 10.4   The central venous pressure (CVP) manometer.

In a sick patient with low blood pressure, the CVP provides invaluable information on the fluid requirements, which may not be obvious from simple observation. In particular, patients who are septic tend to be dehydrated:

- They have a poor intake.
- They have been sweating.
- The respiratory rate is increased, so there is increased respiratory fluid loss.
- Patients with sepsis often have diarrhoea.

In these patients, a fluid challenge can be given with confidence if there is a combination of hypotension and a low CVP. Conversely, if the blood pressure is low but the CVP is high, the cause may be cardiac and a fluid challenge would be inappropriate.

INTRAVENOUS FLUID RESUSCITATION AND FLUID CHALLENGE

Hypovolaemia is the most likely cause of a low blood pressure in the critically ill patient. The signs of significant fluid depletion include the following:

- Systolic blood pressure of less than 100 (and a postural drop)
- Capillary refill of >2 s
- NEWS2 score of 5 or more
- A respiratory rate of 20 or more

- Cold peripheries
- Low CVP
- Improved blood pressure with 45 degrees passive leg raising

In these circumstances, once the airway is secured and oxygen saturations are corrected, the circulating volume is expanded using relatively large amounts of fluid over a short period of time. The term 'fluid challenge' applies to the combination of aggressive volume expansion and a careful assessment of its effect on the patient. A crystalloid, 500 mL of isotonic saline (or Hartmann's), is given over 15 min and if necessary repeated. A reasonable challenge would be a total 20 mL/kg in the first hour. The response is evaluated using the mental state, NEWS2, capillary refill, serial lactate measurements and urine output. The patient is observed for signs of fluid overload: overfilling of the neck veins (increased jugular venous pressure [JVP]) and new-onset breathlessness with wheezing and crackles (pulmonary oedema) at the lung bases.

Which Critically Ill Patients May Need Transfer to Intensive Care Unit/High-Dependency Unit?

- **Patients with a threat to the safety of the airway**—this may be due to a poor conscious level or due to a local inability to protect the airway, such as respiratory muscle weakness with a feeble cough.
- **Patients who have had a respiratory arrest**—these patients remain at marked risk until the underlying problem (pneumonia, asthma, etc.) has been treated.
- **Patients with a respiratory rate of less than 8 or more than 40 breaths/min**—extremes of respiratory rate indicate severe illness with impending cardiorespiratory arrest.
- **Patients with oxygen saturations that remain less than 90% despite at least 50% oxygen by mask**—these patients will need extra respiratory support, possibly even intubation and ventilation of the lungs.
- **Patients after a cardiac arrest**—particularly if the arrest was in the setting of a critically ill patient rather than as a 'simple' early complication of an acute myocardial infarction.
- **Patients with a pulse rate of less than 40 or greater than 140 beats/min despite treatment**—this can be evidence of circulatory failure, although clearly straightforward uncontrolled atrial fibrillation would not come into this category.
- **Patients with a systolic blood pressure that stays below 90 mm Hg despite fluid replacement**—this suggests established shock and may need support with inotropic drugs.
- **Patients with an unexpected and sudden fall in the conscious level**—(a fall in GCS of more than two points.) This may be a manifestation of falling cerebral blood flow due to persistent shock.
- **Patients with increasing arterial carbon dioxide tension with acidosis**—deteriorating blood gases despite treatment is a warning of impending respiratory arrest.
- Any patient giving cause for concern (to the clinical team or the close relatives) in whom there is a reasonable expectation of recovery.

Surviving Sepsis

'Sepsis' describes the clinical situation in which the major organs start to fail due to the body's overwhelming immune response to infection. Sepsis can deteriorate to septic shock if the blood pressure does not respond to IV fluids and requires inotropic support—septic shock carries a mortality rate of 40%. There is increasing concern about the rising incidence of sepsis as a cause of critical illness and death—a trend which can be reversed with earlier recognition and timely protocol-based intervention.

There are clear guidelines on screening for diagnosing and treating sepsis based on the initial NEWS2 score and the level of suspicion that infection is present:

Sepsis can be strongly suspected:

- If there are clinical concerns (particularly if there are also concerns from relatives/carers)
- When the NEWS2 score is 5 or more
- When there are risk factors
  - IV lines in place
  - Intravenous drug users (IVDUs)
  - Broken or damaged skin
  - Diabetes
  - Immunosuppressed (recent chemotherapy, steroid use, etc.)
  - Aged over 75 years

The following 'Red Flags' each warn of impending deterioration and indicate the need for immediate action:

- New confusion
- Systolic blood pressure 90 or less
- Pulse over 130
- Respiratory rate over 25/min
- Oxygen required to maintain saturations at or above 92%
- Lactate 2 mmol/L or above
- Urine output—nil passed for 18 h or less than 0.5/mL/h
- Ashen, mottled or blue extremities

SEPSIS SIX

Taking the above into consideration there are six interventions which must be carried out immediately:

- Oxygen to keep the saturations at 94%–98% (high flow reservoir mask)
- IV access and blood cultures (plus lactate etc), wound swabs, MSU, etc.
- IV fluid challenge if systolic blood pressure is 90 or less
- IV antibiotics within an hour of the suspected diagnosis
- Accurate urinary output (catheterisation)
- Hourly NEWS2 and serial lactate measurements to confirm a response

Failure of the blood pressure to recover within 6 h of adequate fluid replacement (e.g., 20 mL/kg in the first hour with a 6 h total of 30 mL/kg) indicates septic shock and the need to escalate management.

2024 NICE SEPSIS GUIDELINES

The updated guidelines stress the use of NEWS2 scores in stratifying patients at presentation in to their risk of severe deterioration or death. The guidelines aim to standardise the early recognition of deterioration and address the timing of the first antibiotic dose in terms of the patient's level of risk (giving time in all but the sickest patients to elicit further diagnostic information)

- A NEWS2 score of 7 and above represents a high risk of severe illness or death
  - Antibiotics within an hour.
  - Re-score and review every 30 min
- A NEWS2 score of 5 or 6 represents a moderate risk
  - Antibiotics within 3 h
  - Re-score and review every hour
- A NEWS2 score of 1 to 4 represents a low risk
  - Antibiotics within 6 h
  - Re-score and review every hour
- A NEWS2 score of 0 represents a very low risk
- A score of 3 in any measurement (regardless of the total score) indicates the need for an urgent clinical review and a decision on antibiotic treatment.

Anaphylactic Reaction

Anaphylaxis is the term used for a severe generalised allergic reaction in which there are critical threats to the airway and circulation. Allergic diseases in general are on the increase, and a growing number of acute anaphylactic reactions are now being seen—often in patients with a history of asthma.

The most common causes are as follows:
- Foods, especially nuts
- Insect stings
- Drugs, especially antibiotics, aspirin and ACE inhibitors
- Latex allergy, especially in healthcare workers

From 5 min to 1 h after exposure, the patient suddenly develops a generalised reaction with swelling, redness and itch (urticuria). In cases of oral ingestion in food allergy, the swelling usually starts in the mouth and tongue and progresses to upper airway obstruction. Often accompanied by an itchy, blotchy rash (urticaria) and swelling of the lips and face, these features alone, without airway or circulatory problems, do not constitute an anaphylactic reaction.

The time course depends on the route of exposure: it may take 30 min for latex to be absorbed sufficiently by the skin to trigger a reaction. Occasionally, the delay from

CASE STUDY 10.4 — Acute Anaphylaxis Due to Nut Allergy

Ten minutes after finishing a bowl of cereal, a 30-year-old female developed sudden itching and discomfort in her throat. Within a further few minutes, there was a generalised itchy red blotchy rash and she started to wheeze. She felt faint and collapsed on the kitchen floor. Her husband dialled 999.

In casualty, she was still wheezy and distressed, with a widespread urticarial rash. She was given IV piriton, hydrocortisone and nebulised salbutamol and then she was admitted to hospital.

On admission to the AMU, this initial assessment was made:

ABCDE: THE SAFETY OF THE PATIENT
- The patient was drowsy but responding to the spoken voice.
- The face, lips and tongue were swollen and the voice was hoarse.
- The patient was having difficulty swallowing her saliva.
- There was a loud harsh wheeze.
- The oxygen saturation was 85% on air and the respiratory rate was 35 breaths/min.
- Pulse was 105 beats/min, with a lying blood pressure of 75/40 mm Hg.
- There was a widespread raised urticarial rash.

The assessment was of acute anaphylaxis with impending upper airway obstruction (unable to swallow, swollen tongue, voice change). There was bronchospasm, hypoxaemia and circulatory collapse.

Management

The patient already had venous access. High-flow 60% oxygen was given. Intramuscular adrenaline (epinephrine), 0.5 mL of 1:1000 (0.5 mg), was administered immediately. This was followed by IV chlorpheniramine and hydrocortisone. A litre of 0.9% saline was given over 30 min, followed by 1 L over 1 h.

The recovery was uneventful, but the patient was referred to the allergy service as a case of probable nut allergy and was fully assessed and advised appropriately before discharge. She now wears a Medicalert bracelet and carries two EpiPens to self-administer adrenaline (epinephrine) should it be necessary.

It should be noted that steroids and antihistamines are no longer recommended as part of the first-line treatment of anaphylaxis.

---

exposure to reaction is as long as 6 h, or there may be an early reaction that clears, to be followed by a delayed reaction 1–2 days later.

This is accompanied by two potentially fatal complications:

- Airway obstruction (laryngeal obstruction and an asthmatic reaction; Case Study 10.4)
- Circulatory collapse (severe hypotension with syncope)

In atypical cases, the skin and mucus membrane changes may not be prominent and patients can also have abdominal symptoms—vomiting, pain and explosive diarrhoea. The picture may be dominated by circulatory collapse, syncope and wheeze (not dissimilar to a large pulmonary embolus).

MANAGEMENT OF ANAPHYLACTIC SHOCK

The basic approach of ABCDE is used as in any other acutely ill patient—correcting the most critical problems first (usually the airway) (Fig. 10.5). Lay the patient flat and elevate the legs. If the picture is dominated by breathlessness the patient may be more comfortable sitting up. Do not make any sudden changes in the patient's position.

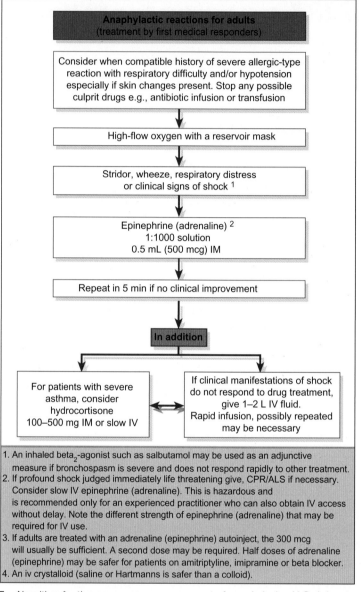

FIGURE 10.5   Algorithm for the emergency management of anaphylaxis. *ALS*, Advanced life support; *CPR*, cardiopulmonary resuscitation.

Intramuscular adrenaline (epinephrine) (Box 10.3). Adrenaline (epinephrine) is the most important part of the management and must be given early. It is important to be familiar with the different preparations of adrenaline (epinephrine) and to understand that in anaphylaxis the preferred route is intramuscularly (with a green or blue needle) and *not* subcutaneous or intravenous—and that the dose is *not* 'one ampoule' but 0.5 mL (0.5 mg) of 1:1000 strength adrenaline (epinephrine). The injection can be repeated every 5–10 min.

> ### BOX 10.3 ■ Emergency Treatment of Anaphylaxis
>
> - Intramuscular adrenaline (epinephrine) 0.5 mL of 1:1000 (0.5 mg or 500 µg)
> - Repeat the adrenaline at 5-min intervals until improvement (or IV adrenaline is started)
> - Intravenous fluids
> - Oxygen
> - Immediately administer intramuscular adrenaline into the anterolateral midthigh.

Intravenous adrenaline (epinephrine)? Severe bronchospasm, increasing upper airway obstruction or continuing hypotension are indications for the careful use of IV adrenaline (epinephrine). This requires specialist input and very careful monitoring. One millilitre (1 mg) of 1:1000 adrenaline is added to 100 mL of 0.9% saline and infused at an initial rate of 0.1 mL (1 mcg)/min building up to 10 mcg/min.

Oxygen. The patients are hypoxic and shocked so a reservoir mask at 15 L/min is required.

Fluids. Intravenous fluids and adrenaline (epinephrine) should restore the blood pressure. Give 500–1000 mL of 0.9% saline as a rapid fluid challenge if there is hypotension (systolic pressure less than 100). In resistant cases, very large volumes of IV fluid are needed to restore the blood pressure (when Hartmann's solution is the preferred fluid).

Bronchodilators. Patients can die from the asthmatic component of the anaphylactic reaction: treatment follows the acute asthma guidelines with nebulised salbutamol or, in the critically ill, IV aminophylline. If the obstruction is mainly in the upper airways, nebulised adrenaline 5 mg (5 mL of 1:1000 strength) is recommended.

Antihistamines. This will clear the rash and the itch but is not an immediate priority.

Steroids. Steroids will not have an immediate effect but will help any asthmatic component and prevent a prolonged or delayed response. However, it should be noted that in the most recent guidelines steroids and antihistamines are no longer recommended as part of the emergency treatment of anaphylaxis.

Prevention. There must be effective education in allergen avoidance and good control of any underlying asthma by optimising the use of prophylactic antiinflammatory treatment with inhaled steroids. Many patients with food allergies are supplied with adrenaline (epinephrine) auto-injectors (EpiPen) and trained in their use. After any severe anaphylactic reaction, referral to the specialist allergy service is mandatory.

Answering Relatives' Questions in Shock

What do you mean by shock? This is not the same as emotional shock. By shock, we mean a drastic change in the overall function of the body due to a fall in the patient's blood pressure. The kidneys are not producing enough urine to flush out waste products, and the brain is at risk of being starved of oxygen.

What is the cause? The most common cause is dehydration due to blood loss or loss of other body fluids. Two other common causes are shock complicating a heart attack and shock complicating an overwhelming infection.

What else can go wrong? The damage to some of the organs could become more serious. The kidneys and lungs are at particular risk and we are paying particular attention to these.

How are you treating the main causes? We are using drugs and intravenous fluids to try and keep the blood pressure up. The extra oxygen is to make up for the problems with the circulation. We are giving antibiotics to combat infection, and we are replacing any lost blood or body fluids.

How will we know that the patient is going to recover? Within 24–48 h of starting treatment, we should see a general improvement: less drowsiness, a better urine output and an increase in the blood pressure. Any fever should start to fall and you may see that we are easing off on the drugs and the intensity of the clinical observations.

What can we do to help? It is reassuring to have somebody familiar at hand, particularly if, as commonly happens in shock, there is an element of confusion. Try and keep the patient calm. Keep the oxygen mask in place and explain what it is for. Keep visitors down to a few very close relatives because for the first 48 h there will be a lot of clinical activity going on in the form of observations, changing drip bags, administering drugs and so forth.

Emergency Blood Transfusion in Shock

There are two main indications for transfusion on the AMU: to treat acute blood loss and to improve oxygen transport in patients with anaemia.

- **Acute blood loss**—this is the most common indication and may require massive transfusion, with its associated risks. Recently, the concept of 'restricted transfusion' has been adopted, particularly in upper gastrointestinal and variceal bleeding. Unless there is life-threatening blood loss, transfusion is limited to maintaining a Hb of 70 to 90 g/L.
- **Improving oxygen transport in patients with anaemia**—this is of uncertain benefit in the acute situation unless the haemoglobin levels are particularly low—probably down to less than 70 g/L with post transfusion targets of 70–90 g/L (or 80–100 g/L in patients with acute coronary syndromes).

Transfusion is often regarded with suspicion by patients and their relatives. This has been exacerbated by the recent discovery that two patients have developed a new variant of Creutzfeldt–Jakob disease (CJD), transmitted in blood from infected donors. Fortunately, the risks associated with transfusion are surprisingly low. The chance of catching AIDS through transfusion is less than one in a million. In fact, patients are 100 times more likely to be given the wrong blood (as a result of human error), but even this risk is extremely low. The most common reactions are minor febrile reactions and rashes that require symptomatic treatment and reassurance. The risks involved in blood transfusion are listed in Table 10.2.

It is important to reassure the patient and provide adequate information (if the patient is well enough to discuss it):

- Indications for and purpose of the transfusion
- Risks to the patient

TABLE 10.2 ■ **Risks Involved in Blood Transfusion**

Risk/Reaction	Risks per Unit
Urticarial rash	1 in 50
Febrile reaction	1 in 100
Pulmonary oedema	1 in 5000
Wrong blood	1 in 30,000
Bacterial contamination	1 in 50,000
Hepatitis B	1 in 100,000
Hepatitis C	1 in 200,000
Major reaction	1 in 600,000
HIV	1 in 3,000,000

- Benefits to the patient
- The patient's right to refuse
- Alternative treatments to transfusion
- A National Transfusion Service information leaflet should be given to the patient or relatives

Transfusion Reactions

CLINICAL FEATURES AND BASIC MANAGEMENT

It is important to monitor transfusion using a standard protocol. The patients must be told to report:
- Shivering
- Rashes
- Flushing
- Breathlessness
- Loin and limb pains

The temperature, pulse and blood pressure are recorded before the start of the transfusion, after 15–20 min and at the end of delivery of each unit of blood. This information is recorded and dated separately from the routine observations. Most transfusion reactions start within 15 min of starting the blood, so early observations are critical.

Urticarial rashes. Urticarial rashes may occur during transfusion. If the patient develops an acute allergic response to any protein in the donated blood product, urticaria, an intense itchy red eruption, will develop. It is more common with platelet transfusions or fresh frozen plasma (FFP) than with whole blood. Urticaria is frightening for the patient but not serious. The best treatment is IV chlorpheniramine 10 mg, an antihistamine. Provided that the reaction is not associated with major symptoms or changes in the pulse or blood pressure, the transfusion does not have to be stopped. The observations should be increased to hourly.

Febrile reactions. These may occur towards the end of a transfusion or within hours of its completion. The patient reacts against the white cells in the donated blood. It can be simply treated with paracetamol to bring the temperature down. If patients have had reactions before, they can be premedicated with antihistamines. Rarely, a patient can develop signs of septic shock during transfusion—hypotension, increased respiratory rate and fever—which is due to bacterial contamination of the blood; platelet transfusions are the most likely to be contaminated.

Pulmonary oedema. This is not always due to overtransfusion—there is a form of acute transfusion-related lung injury that is a direct toxic effect of stored blood. The symptoms are the same as cardiac pulmonary oedema: increasing breathlessness, increased respiratory rate, tachycardia and hypoxia. Platelets and FFP are the most dangerous in this regard.

Wrong blood. Within the first few millilitres of the transfusion, a reaction may occur that is due to the patient rejecting the blood. Usually, this is a case of AB blood being incorrectly given to an O-group patient. It is vital to recognise this type of transfusion reaction.

CLINICAL ASSESSMENT TO IDENTIFY A SEVERE TRANSFUSION REACTION

When to Suspect a Reaction

- The patient complains of symptoms.
- The basic observations change (pulse, temperature and blood pressure).

What action to take. Any of these may lead you to suspect a severe reaction:

- A reaction starts within minutes of the start of blood.
- An error is discovered.
- The patient develops acute loin or limb pain.
- There is fever, hypotension and tachycardia.

In this situation, it is imperative that you act.

1. Stop the blood and call a senior team member.
2. Change the giving set and put up slow saline to keep the vein open.
3. Tell the blood bank and return the blood.
4. Start 15-min observations of pulse, blood pressure and temperature.
5. Observe the volume and colour of any urine passed.

Avoiding human error. The most important risk in blood transfusion is that of simple human error leading to the administration of the wrong blood. The mistakes are predictable:

- When blood samples are taken for cross-matching they are mislabelled at the bedside.
- The wrong blood is collected from the blood bank.
- The blood is given to the wrong patient (identification bracelets must be fitted on admission).

It is important to work to the defined protocols for taking blood for cross-matching, collecting the correct blood from the bank, receiving the correct blood on the ward and administering it to the correct patient.

An example of good practice. Take the transfusion request form to the patient.

1. Ask the patient to give their name and date of birth.
2. Confirm this with the identification bracelet.
3. Check these details and the hospital number with the form.
4. Take blood and then label the tube at the bedside, but not with an addressograph label.
5. Use electronic patient identification systems to eliminate human error.

Transfusion should start as soon as the blood is delivered to the ward. If blood has been out of the refrigerator for more than 30 min and is not about to be used, the hospital blood bank should be consulted and the blood returned.

The *bedside* check before the start of the transfusion is vital. There must be exact matches:

Patient → blood transfusion compatibility report form → compatibility label on blood pack → prescription or fluid balance chart → medical notes.

Keep the blood transfusion compatibility report form readily available during the transfusion, in case there is a reaction.

Massive Blood Transfusion

Acute massive blood loss on the AMU is usually due to upper gastrointestinal bleeding. The term is usually used when a patient loses around half his blood volume (1500 to 2000 mL) over 2–3 h. Surprisingly, there is a tendency to underestimate the total volume loss. Massive blood loss requires large-volume transfusions with cross-matched blood. In extreme life-or-death situations, blood from 'universal donors'—group O rhesus negative, delivered through a warming device—can be used while awaiting the emergency cross-match (saline or polygeline (Haemaccel) may be used while awaiting blood).

The aim of emergency transfusion is as follows:

- To normalise the blood pressure and
- To maintain a urine output of at least 30 mL/h

Stored blood carries very little clotting factor, and so massive transfusion can lead to a clotting deficiency. This is compounded by the exhaustion of the patient's own clotting factors in trying to stem the blood loss.

- Full clotting studies (platelet count, prothrombin time, Kaolin cephalin clotting time (KCCT) and fibrinogen levels) must be checked before the start of the transfusion.
- These are repeated every 30 min until the bleeding stops.
- The prothrombin time and KCCT must be kept at no more than 1.5 times the normal value using FFP—a concentrated source of clotting factors—giving a unit of FFP for every 2 units of blood. (*Note:* FFP takes 30 min to thaw out).

- Platelets will need to be replaced to keep levels above 100,000 per 10^9.
- Low fibrinogen levels will need correction with cryoprecipitate.
- Calcium is mopped up by the stored blood and may need replacing.

Occasionally, rather than a clotting deficiency, massive transfusion triggers off spontaneous clotting within the small arteries and veins—this is disseminated intravascular coagulation (DIC). There are five reversible factors that increase the risk of DIC and that are, to some extent, amenable to standard resuscitation measures:

- Massive blood loss
- Hypoxia
- Hypovolaemia
- Administration of excessively cold fluids
- Failure to correct the clotting factors and platelets

Acute Kidney Injury

The term acute kidney injury applies to situations where there is a risk of acute renal failure and also to situations where renal failure is fully established. The term AKI has replaced acute renal failure to emphasise the progressive loss of renal function that occurs if urgent preventative action is not taken. There are three stages in the deterioration from 'at risk of' to 'established' renal failure. They are defined by the urinary output (Table 10.3) or by the increases in the serum creatinine—a rise in the patient's creatinine of 26 μmol/L or more above the baseline level within a 48-h period, or a 50% increase within the previous 7 days, indicates that there is at least the first stage of AKI.

Critically, preventative action at the 'risk' stage will avoid the progression to acute renal failure—this action may include appropriate volume replacement, withdrawal or avoidance of nephrotoxic drugs, treatment of sepsis and the relief of any obstruction to urinary flow.

To function, the kidneys require:

1. An adequate blood pressure
2. Sufficient functioning glomeruli to filter the blood
3. Intact renal tubules to reabsorb water and exchange electrolytes
4. An unobstructed urinary tract leading from the kidneys to the outside of the body

Fig. 10.6 summarises the basic mechanisms of AKI.

TABLE 10.3 ■ The Three Stages of Acute Kidney Injury

Stages of Acute Kidney Injury	Urine Output
1. Risk	<0.5 mL/kg/h for > 6 h
2. Injury	<0.5 mL/kg/h for > 12 h
3. Failure	<0.3 mL/kg/h for > 24 h or anuric for 12 h

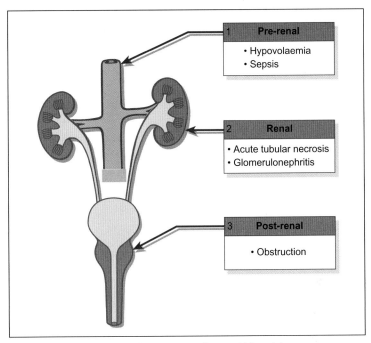

FIGURE 10.6   The causes of acute kidney injury.

In the AMU, problems with kidney function are commonly the result of inadequate blood pressure—*pre-renal failure*—which occurs in the setting of acute fluid depletion. A useful concept is 'volume-responsive' AKI as it will usually respond to fluid replacement.

Uncorrected pre-renal failure may progress to *acute tubular necrosis*. Acute tubular necrosis can also be the result of direct renal toxicity from drugs such as non-steroidal anti-inflammatory drugs (NSAIDs), from the products of acute muscle damage (rhabdomyolysis) and from sepsis.

Urinary tract *obstruction* is clearly important because it is easy to treat and is a fully reversible cause of kidney failure.

Diseases of the glomeruli—acute *glomerulonephritis*—are rare causes of acute renal failure on the AMU, although they are important to recognise because the patients usually need specialist assessment and care.

While AKI is an important clinical area, it is often handled with limited confidence in the AMU. Once a set of very abnormal kidney function tests comes back from the biochemistry laboratory, the tendency is to phone the renal unit and hope that they will take the problem over. This is unfortunate because many of the cases are straightforward and will recover—with fluid replacement, with catheterisation or simply with time—provided that immediate problems of electrolyte disturbance and fluid balance are addressed.

WHICH PATIENTS ARE AT PARTICULAR RISK FROM ACUTE KIDNEY INJURY?

- Patients with fluid depletion—with severe diarrhoea, major upper gastrointestinal bleed or poor access to fluids, for example, cognitive impairment, stroke
- Patients with septic shock
- Patients with a vulnerable blood supply to the kidneys—acute and chronic heart failure, vascular disease, hypertension, diabetes
- Patients taking diuretics, NSAIDs, ACE inhibitors and those undergoing chemotherapy
- Patients who already have chronic renal failure
- The elderly frail and those who have several medical conditions, particularly if those include diabetes and hypertension
- Patients with falling NEWS2 scores
- Patients with a urine output of less than 0.5 mL/kg/h

ILLUSTRATIVE CASE STUDIES

The following case studies (Case Studies 10.5–10.7) illustrate the typical presentation and immediate management of acute renal failure. The main features of emergency management of acute renal failure are summarised in Fig. 10.7.

Management of Acute Kidney Injury

Management follows the same principles that govern other medical emergencies:
1. ABCDE: ensure the immediate safety of the patient.
2. Complete a full clinical assessment.
3. Identify priorities and institute a management plan.
4. Provide the patient and the relatives with reassurance and an explanation.

ENSURING THE SAFETY OF THE PATIENT

The safety of the patient is established with attention to the airway, oxygenation and circulation. There are two life-threatening complications that require urgent action: hyperkalaemia and pulmonary oedema.

CASE STUDY 10.5   Rapid Deterioration in Severe Pneumonia

A 34-year-old female was admitted with bilateral pneumonia. On admission, the temperature was 35.5°C, blood pressure was 90/60 mm Hg, pulse was 100 beats/min and respiratory rate was 15 breaths/min; the saturations were 90% on high-flow oxygen. On admission, the WCC was 1.2×10^9/L, urea 10.7 mmol/L and creatinine 102 µmol/L. She was treated with fluids and antibiotics but was markedly oliguric, passing less than 10 mL/h. Within 24 h, her WCC had increased to 28.2×10^9/L, her urea had increased to 24.3 mmol/L and her creatinine was 259 µmol/L. Her respiratory rate increased to 25 breaths/min and she was transferred to the ITU with a view to ventilation.

CASE STUDY 10.6 | **Renal Tract Obstruction**

A 70-year-old female was awoken in the early hours of the morning with severe constant pain in the right loin. This was described as being as severe as labour pain. Her pain persisted for 72h, during which time she developed rigours and passed absolutely no urine. In the past, she was known to have a chronically damaged left kidney from childhood infections.

She was admitted to hospital where she was found to be pyrexial and dehydrated, with a pulse rate of 110 beats/min and a blood pressure of 70/60mm Hg when lying. On palpating her abdomen, there was an enlarged tender right kidney. Investigations showed a high WCC (15×10^9/L) and a low platelet count. There was mild renal insufficiency. An urgent ultrasound confirmed hydronephrosis (an obstructed kidney) due to a large stone blocking off the ureter.

She was treated with fluid replacement and IV antibiotics. Her subsequent management included an emergency nephrostomy to allow drainage of urine from the obstructed right kidney, followed some time later by surgical removal of the stone.

CASE STUDY 10.7 | **Acute Poststreptococcal Glomerulonephritis Presenting as Oedema and Cardiac Failure**

A 50-year-old male with a 2-week history of malaise was admitted because of swelling of his eyes and ankles. Three weeks previously he had an acute sore throat.

On admission, there was generalised oedema. His blood pressure was 202/114mm Hg. His ward urine testing was strongly positive for blood and protein. A subsequent MSU showed red cell casts.

His chest film showed mild pulmonary oedema. His creatinine was 128 μmol/L, urea 11.6mmol/L. The total 24-h urinary protein excretion of 1.14g. His ASO titre was greater than 800 units/mL (indicative of a recent streptococcal infection).

He was treated with furosemide and fluid restriction. At follow-up 3 months later, his creatinine had fallen to 105 μmol/L, his urea to 6.9mmol/L and his blood pressure was normal. His urine testing showed microscopic haematuria.

Hyperkalaemia. Hyperkalaemia, or an increase in the serum potassium level, is the most serious complication of acute renal failure because it has a dramatic effect on the heart. Levels above 6.0mmol/L lead to cardiac arrest. It is critical to measure and document serial changes in the potassium in any patient with established or threatened kidney failure. Hyperkalaemia produces characteristic changes on the ECG (peaking of the T waves and slurring of the QRS complexes), if these are present with a potassium level of 6.0mmol/L (or above 6.5mmol/L even if there are no ECG changes), urgent action must be taken to protect the heart and to bring the potassium concentration down.

Emergency Management of Hyperkalaemia

1. Give 10mL of 10% calcium gluconate over 5 min and repeat until the ECG starts to improve. Calcium gluconate protects the heart but does not reduce

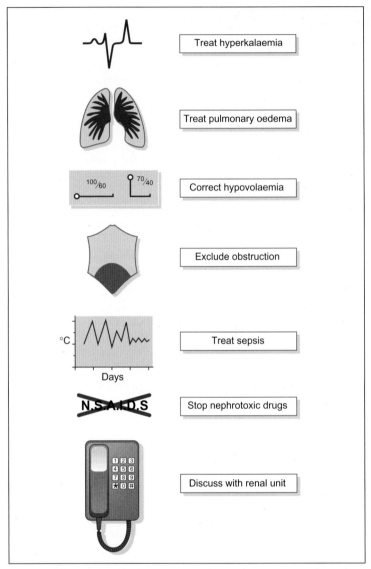

FIGURE 10.7 The emergency management of acute kidney injury. *N.S.A.I.D.S.*, Non-steroidal anti-inflammatory drugs.

the potassium. It can be repeated at 5-min intervals for a maximum of four doses.

2. Give 10 units of neutral insulin solution (Actrapid) in 50 mL of 50% glucose over 15 min. This will reduce the potassium level by 2.0 mmol/L over 1 h. The capillary blood sugars must be monitored.

3. Give 15 g of calcium resonium orally every 6 h. This takes 4 h or more to work.

Pulmonary oedema. This occurs because of the inability of the failing kidney to get rid of fluid. Pulmonary oedema is often triggered by over-enthusiastic IV fluid replacement in the critically ill, particularly if saline has been used and the CVP has not been monitored. The evidence for pulmonary oedema will be obtained from the initial assessment of a patient whose blood tests have shown kidney failure:

- Low oxygen saturation
- Increased respiratory rate
- Unable to lie flat because of breathlessness
- In advanced pulmonary oedema, the patient is restless and confused

The management is the same as for other types of pulmonary oedema:

- Sit the patient up
- Administer high-flow 60% oxygen
- Diuretics (often in high doses) and consider low-dose IV opiates
- Consider a GTN infusion (1–10 mg/h)

COMPLETING THE CLINICAL ASSESSMENT

Assessing fluid balance:

- What fluid has been lost?
    - Is there a history of vomiting, diarrhoea, gastrointestinal bleeding?
    - Is there internal fluid loss, as in acute pancreatitis?
- Is there any postural hypotension on sitting the patient up?
- What is the CVP?
- What is the urine output?

Is there evidence of obstruction?

- There may be a history of prostatism:
    - hesitancy in starting
    - poor stream
    - terminal dribbling
    - frequent small amounts
- A distended bladder may be palpable.
- Sudden complete cessation of urine output or overflow with constant dribbling.
- Pain over the kidneys due to distension and back pressure.
- If the patient has a catheter—is it blocked? (gentle flush and aspiration with sterile water.)

What was the previous kidney function?

- Examine old notes and laboratory reports.
- The GP's surgery may have results of prior renal function.
- A flowchart of results and their dates is invaluable.

Is there a comprehensive drug list? In particular:

- Diuretics
- NSAIDs
- ACE inhibitors

What does ward urine testing show? Urine testing is usually negative in pre-renal failure. In acute tubular necrosis, there is usually a combination of light to moderate proteinuria and microscopic haematuria. In acute glomerulonephritis, the characteristic findings are haematuria and heavy proteinuria. Should a fresh MSU also show copious red cells that have been moulded into the shape of the renal tubules (red cell 'casts'), the diagnosis is acute glomerulonephritis and a specialist opinion will be required. Send a spot urine sample for osmolality ('concentration') and urinary sodium. In hypovolaemia, the kidneys are trying to retain fluid and sodium to keep up the blood pressure—osmolality will be high (over 450 mosmol/L) and sodium low (less than 10 mmol/L). The reverse occurs once acute tubular necrosis becomes established (osmolality less than 300 mosmol/L and sodium more than 20 mmol/L). The finding of leucocytes and nitrites suggests a urinary infection.

ESTABLISHING A MANAGEMENT PLAN

Assuming there has been emergency treatment of acute hyperkalaemia and pulmonary oedema, the priorities include the following:

- **To correct hypovolaemia**—If hypovolaemia is present, prompt fluid replacement should immediately increase the blood pressure and increase the urine output to more than 0.5 mL/kg/h. Depending on the patients' frailty and cardiac status, fluid replacement may require between 250 and 1000 mL of isotonic saline, aiming for a systolic blood pressure of 100 mm Hg. If the urine output remains poor despite adequate hydration, a fluid challenge may be indicated.
- **To remove any obstructive component**—This will range from bladder catheterisation to percutaneous drainage of an obstructed kidney. There should be 24 h access to renal ultrasound as obstruction must be recognised and treated immediately especially if an infected kidney is suspected.
- **To stop any nephrotoxic drugs**—This relies on a full drug history, with details from both hospital and GP sources. The ward pharmacist will advise on nephrotoxicity and the need for dose modifications in the presence of renal failure.
- **To identify and treat sepsis**—Sepsis is an important cause of renal failure and is easy to miss, especially in the elderly. Symptoms may simply consist of an abrupt change in health. Sites for 'hidden' sepsis include the perineum, the joints, the spine and the soft tissues, including infected bedsores. It is important to take at least two sets of blood cultures if sepsis is suspected: each set consists of 5 mL into each of the two culture bottles—one aerobic and one anaerobic.

CRITICAL CLINICAL TASKS IN ACUTE RENAL FAILURE

 CRITICAL CLINICAL TASKS IN ACUTE KIDNEY INJURY

- Prepare to start treatment for hyperkalaemia
- Carry out basic management of pulmonary oedema
- Identify sepsis: strong clues are fever, malaise, rigors and perhaps dysuria
- Identify hypovolaemia:
  - Symptoms of thirst and dizziness
  - Signs of postural fall in blood pressure
  - Low CVP

IMPORTANT CLINICAL TASKS IN ACUTE KIDNEY INJURY

Confirm that the problem is not a simple outflow obstruction

- Enlarged tender bladder
- Blocked catheter

Take a full history

- Is there any history to indicate hypovolaemia?
  - Severe diarrhoea
  - Vomiting
  - Bleeding
- Is there any history to suggest sepsis?
  - Dysuria
  - Rigors
  - Fever
- Is there any history to suggest obstruction?
  - Absolute anuria
- Past history
  - Chronic kidney disease
  - Diabetes
  - Hypertension
- Drug history
  - NSAIDs
  - ACE inhibitors
  - Diuretics

Exclude rhabdomyolysis in prolonged immobility/coma

- Be aware of this possibility in coma, alcoholics and overdoses.
- Look for tense swollen legs and areas of bruising, suggesting soft tissue damage. In rhabdomyolysis, the blood creatinine kinase level will be very high.

IMPORTANT CLINICAL TASKS IN ACUTE KIDNEY INJURY

- Confirm that the problem is not a simple outflow obstruction
- Take a full history
- Exclude rhabdomyolysis in prolonged immobility/coma
- Check the urine
- Ensure that there is a system for reviewing the abnormal urea and electrolyte results on the ward

Check the urine

- Appearance (e.g., a muddy appearance is typical of myoglobinuria—rhabdomyolysis)
- Dip for blood and protein (In rhabdomyolysis, the urine is positive for blood on the dipstick but no red blood cells are seen on microscopy.)
- Send for microscopy to look for casts (Hyaline casts are from normal urinary constituents and occur in pre-renal failure because the urine is concentrated. Red cell casts indicate glomerulonephritis; granular casts indicate acute tubular necrosis.)

Ensure that there is a system for reviewing the abnormal urea and electrolyte results on the ward. There should be flowcharts that follow sequential tests in a critically ill patient. The most common cause for a delayed diagnosis of renal failure in the AMU is a failure to see and act on the abnormal results when they come back to the ward.

Answering Relatives' Questions in Acute Kidney Injury

What does acute kidney failure mean? The kidneys filter impurities from the blood, so they need a constant bloodstream and an effective filtering mechanism. If anything too drastic happens to either mechanism, the kidneys become inefficient and eventually, as a result, impurities build up and poison the body—this is known as kidney failure.

Will the kidneys recover? The kidneys have good powers of recovery, particularly if they were working normally before this happened. We are checking previous hospital records and blood tests to see if the kidneys were completely normal up until the present illness. In many cases of acute kidney failure, the kidneys start to show signs of recovery within a few days of starting treatment.

Why are you not sending the patient to a kidney unit? The doctors use the unit for advice during the initial period of stabilisation. If the kidneys do not show the expected rate of recovery or if complications occur that could be more effectively dealt with in a kidney unit, we can transfer the patient at that stage.

Have the patient's drugs damaged the kidneys? Couldn't the patient's own doctor have seen this coming? Some drugs—especially diuretics and antiinflammatories—can damage the kidneys or make them more vulnerable, particularly in older patients. It is not always easy to anticipate problems with the kidneys, and most people who take these drugs have no particular problem. You may want to discuss this with the doctors when the present episode is over and we can give you more information as to the exact cause of the kidney failure.

Sudden Collapse and Cardiac Arrest

It is important to understand the events that can precede and progress to a cardiac arrest.

- A respiratory arrest may lead to a cardiac arrest and vice versa. In most arrest situations, the term cardiorespiratory arrest is appropriate.
- Most cardiac arrests occur as an early complication of myocardial infarction. These have the most successful outcomes.
- However, cardiorespiratory arrest should also be viewed as an endpoint in acute illnesses other than myocardial infarction. Examples include acute severe asthma, septicaemic shock and uncorrected acidosis. By recognising and treating them at an early stage, the risk of progressing to cardiorespiratory arrest can be reduced. Several studies have now shown that 'sudden death' on AMUs is often preceded by a period of potentially reversible deterioration—most notably, unrecognised hypoxaemia and hypotension. Competent assessment and early intervention in the critically ill (Chapter 1) should prevent this sequence.

COMMON CAUSES OF THE SUDDEN COLLAPSE

Cardiac. In 80% of cases, sudden pulseless collapse is due to ventricular fibrillation (VF) or ventricular tachycardia (VT). In the remainder, the problem is a severe bradycardia or asystole. Pulmonary embolism is a classical cause of sudden severe collapse.

Respiratory

- Tension pneumothorax
- Aspiration/upper airway obstruction; this can cause a major deterioration, especially in a coma
- Massive haemoptysis, usually as a terminal event in lung cancer

Gastrointestinal. A catastrophic bleed, usually from oesophageal varices. A ruptured abdominal aortic aneurysm.

Anaphylaxis. A characteristic setting with a recognised trigger, wheeze, oropharyngeal swelling and severe hypotension.

ASSESSMENT OF COLLAPSE

What is the setting in which it occurred (Fig. 10.8)?

1. A new patient just arrived on the ward: this could be anything.
2. A patient admitted earlier in the day with unexplained breathlessness: pulmonary embolus.
3. A patient with known heart disease/chest pain: a major arrhythmia.
4. A patient admitted with deliberate self-harm: an arrhythmia or a respiratory arrest.

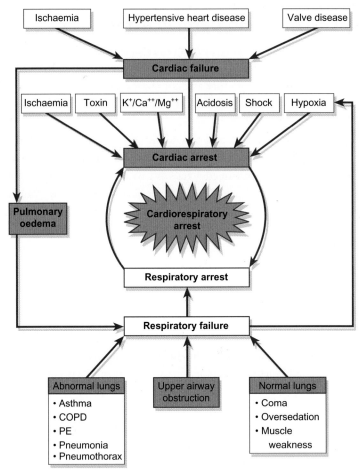

FIGURE 10.8 Cardiorespiratory arrest: an overview of causes and interactions. *Ca*, Calcium; *COPD*, chronic obstructive pulmonary disease; *K*, potassium; *Mg*, magnesium; *PE*, pulmonary embolism.

DIAGNOSING CARDIAC ARREST

Look at the patient and the monitor if it is available, but *treat the patient, not the monitor*. A patient who has collapsed with no apparent signs of life has had a cardiac arrest. Occasionally the sudden cessation of a blood supply to the brain following a cardiac arrest can lead to a convulsion—and obscure the true clinical picture.

There are four common scenarios in cardiac arrest:

1. Pulseless and collapsed with VF or VT—cardiac arrest
2. Pulseless and collapsed with a flat trace—cardiac arrest
3. Pulseless and collapsed but with an electrical rhythm (pulseless electrical activity [PEA])—cardiac arrest
4. Flat trace but the patient looks well—has an electrode come off?

If this is a pulseless cardiac arrest, the cause is almost certainly VF or VT. With immediate defibrillation, these patients have a 23% chance of survival. If VF deteriorates into asystole or the initial rhythm is asystole (a flat trace) or PEA, the chances of survival decrease to 2%.

The Chain of Survival

This is the term used to describe the sequence of events from prevention, in the form of the recognition and treatment of the critically ill patient, through early resuscitation integrating CPR and urgent defibrillation to the final link of effective post resuscitation care. The key to survival is the immediate recognition of a cardiac arrest and the institution of basic life support (BLS). The aim is to keep the patient alive and neurologically undamaged (to 'buy time') until defibrillation can be carried out to restart the heart.

BASIC LIFE SUPPORT

BLS describes the process of:
- The initial assessment of the collapsed patient
- The techniques to keep the airway open
- The use of expired air ventilation and chest compression—CPR

The equipment used in BLS comprises a simple airway and a face mask to facilitate mouth-to-mouth breathing.

If the cause of the collapse is a respiratory arrest, then BLS alone may succeed. In most cases, however, the patient has had a cardiac arrest, the rhythm is VF (VF arrest) or pulseless VT, and *BLS is a holding operation until the defibrillator arrives and the process moves into that of advanced life support (ALS)*. ALS involves following established management algorithms for treating resistant arrhythmias and for maintaining ventilation with endotracheal intubation or other airway adjuncts.

Providing immediate and effective BLS markedly increases the chances of success in a cardiac arrest:
- *A 2 or 3 min' delay will halve the chances of survival.*
- *A 3 or 4 min' delay will result in brain damage.*
- *Interruptions to chest compression must be kept to an absolute minimum. For example, using a manual defibrillator, the pause between stopping and restarting chest compression while the shock is being administered should be no more than 5 s.*

BLS must be started at the time of the arrest and, except during defibrillation, it must be continued throughout the resuscitation procedure until the return of a spontaneous circulation.
- Start BLS
- The primary helpers continue active resuscitation
- Secondary helpers may need to:

- Fetch the crash trolley
- Make the referral letter and the medical and nursing notes readily available
- Ensure laboratory results are fed back to the arrest team
- Make recent radiology imaging available (is this a pneumothorax?)
- See to other patients in the ward and move any patient if appropriate
- Make the paramedics' assessment documents available
- Send for any old hospital notes
- Handle the relatives: phone calls and direct contact

SEQUENCE OF ACTIONS IN BASIC LIFE SUPPORT

1. Ensure the safety of the rescuer and patient (Fig. 10.9).
2. Shout for help. Check the patient and see if there is a response: gently shake the patient's shoulders and ask loudly, 'Are you all right?'
3. If the patient responds by answering or moving:
   a. Place the patient in the recovery position

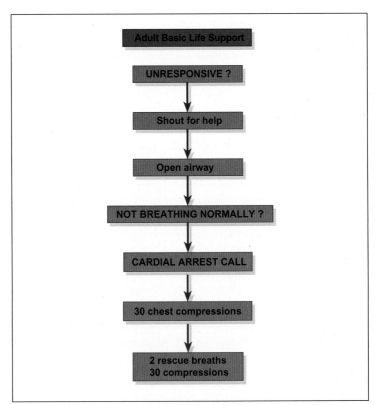

FIGURE 10.9 The basic life support algorithm. (*Reproduced with the kind permission of Resuscitation Council UK.*)

   b. Check the patient's condition (ABCDE), give oxygen, secure IV access and attach monitors

   c. Reassess the patient regularly, recording vital signs

   d. Hand over to the emergency medical team using a standardised communication framework (e.g., RSVP: **R**eason, **S**tory, **V**ital signs, **P**lan of management)

4. If the patient does *not* respond:
   a. Turn the patient onto their back
   b. Open the patient's airway by tilting their head and lifting their chin:
      i. Place your hand on their forehead and gently tilt their head back, keeping your thumb and index finger free to close their nose if rescue breathing is required
      ii. At the same time, with your fingertip(s) under the point of the patient's chin, lift the chin to open the airway
      iii. Remove any visible obstruction from the patient's mouth, including dislodged dentures, but leave well-fitting dentures in place

5. Keeping the airway open, look, listen and feel for normal breathing (occasional gasps, slow and laboured or noisy breathing are abnormal):
   a. Look for chest movements
   b. Listen to the patient's mouth for breath sounds
   c. Feel for air on your cheek
   d. Look, listen and feel for no more than 10 s before deciding that breathing is absent

6. If the patient is breathing normally or if you are in any doubt (occasional, irregular ('agonal') gasps commonly occur after a cardiac arrest and must not be confused with normal breathing):
   a. Turn the patient into the recovery position
   b. Check for continued breathing

7. If the patient is *not* breathing normally:

8. Assess the patient for signs of circulation and for signs of life:
   a. Look for any movement, including swallowing and coughing
   b. Check the carotid pulse
   c. Take no more than 10 s to do this

9. If you are *confident* that you can detect signs of circulation within 10 s (i.e., this is a respiratory arrest):
   a. Start rescue breathing (Box 10.4) if necessary until the patient starts breathing on their own
   b. Every 10 breaths, check for circulation, take no more than 10 s each time
   c. If the patient starts to breathe on their own but remains unconscious, turn the patient into the recovery position. Check their condition and be ready to turn them onto their back and restart rescue breathing if the patient stops breathing.

BOX 10.4 ■ Techniques of Mouth-to-Mouth Ventilation

The Laerdal Pocket Mask (Fig. 10.10A)

Rescue breathing is usually started with a Laerdal Pocket mask, which is an acceptable and safe way to administer mouth-to-mouth ventilation until the self-inflating bag mask and reservoir are available.

- The patient is approached from behind the head.
- The thumbs and index fingers press and seal the mask onto the face.
- The remaining fingers perform the jaw thrust to keep the airway open.
- Blow through the inspiratory valve for 1 s and watch the chest rise.
- Apply oxygen to the input valve at 10 L/min.

Guedel or Oropharyngeal Airway

The Guedel airway is used with head tilt and jaw thrust to ensure the airway remains patent. It will not be tolerated by a conscious patient. In the correct position, it stops the tongue from falling back and blocking the upper airway.

1. Select the size (from small 2, medium 3 or large 4) by matching an airway to the vertical distance between the incisors and the angle of the jaw.
2. Remove any loose material from the patient's mouth.
3. Insert the airway upside down and, when it is in position with the flat part between the patient's teeth, turn it the right way up.

The Self-Inflating Bag Mask and Reservoir (see Fig. 10.10B)

During resuscitation, expired air alone supplies the patient with only 16% oxygen. This can be significantly enriched using a Laerdal mask, but only with a bag mask and reservoir can the levels approach 100%. The technique, however, requires two people: one to secure a tight seal and maintain a clear airway using the Laerdal mask technique, and the other person, utilising both hands, to squeeze the bag. Ventilation at 10 breaths/min can be continued without interrupting chest compression.

---

10. If there are *no* signs of circulation or signs of life, or you are at all unsure:
   a. Start chest compression rather than initial ventilation (Fig. 10.11):
      i. Place the heel of one hand in the centre of the victim's chest (in the middle of the lower half of the sternum)
      ii. Place the heel of the other hand on top of the first hand
      iii. Interlock the fingers of both hands. Ensure that pressure is not applied over the patient's ribs. Do not apply any pressure over the upper abdomen or bottom tip of the sternum
      iv. Position yourself vertically above the patient's chest and, with your arms straight, press down on the sternum to depress it 5–6 cm
      v. Release the pressure without breaking contact between the hands and the sternum, then repeat at a rate of about 100–120 times a minute (a little less than two compressions a second). Compression and release should take an equal amount of time
   b. Combine rescue breathing and compression:
      i. After 30 compressions, tilt the head, lift the chin and give two effective breaths—these should be normal-sized breaths (600–700 mL) each given

FIGURE 10.10 Techniques for (A) mouth-to-mask and (B) two-person and mask ventilation.

without force over 1 s with an equal time allowed for expiration (this recommendation applies to any form of CPR ventilation including bag valve and mask). The two breaths should take no more than 5 s. Add supplemental oxygen as soon as possible.

ii. Return your hands immediately to the correct position on the sternum and give 30 further compressions, continuing compressions and breaths in a ratio of 30:2.

c. When using two-person BLS, these points should be noted:

i. When changing from single-person to two-person BLS, the second rescuer should take over chest compressions after the first rescuer has given two

FIGURE 10.11 The correct hand position for cardiac massage.

rescue breaths. During these rescue breaths, the incoming rescuer should determine the correct position on the sternum and should be ready to start compressions immediately after the second rescue breath has been given. It is preferable that the rescuers work from opposite sides of the patient.

ii. A ratio of 30 compressions to two rescue breaths should be used. By the end of each series of 30 compressions, the rescuer responsible for rescue breathing should be positioned ready to give a breath with the least possible delay. It is helpful if the rescuer giving compressions counts out aloud '1-2-3-4-5 …'.

iii. Chin lift and head tilt should be maintained at all times. Each rescue breath should take the usual 1 s, during which chest compressions should cease; they should be resumed immediately after inflation of the chest, waiting only for the rescuer to remove their lips from the patient's face.

BOX 10.5 ■ The Key to Initial Resuscitation

- Airway control: head tilt, chin lift and jaw thrust
- Effective use of a Laerdal mask or a bag and reservoir
- Effective bagging needs two people
- If gurgling: suction must be used (Yankauer) but only to the oropharynx

---

11. Continue resuscitation until the cardiac arrest team arrives to assist. Do not stop CPR to check the patient unless the patient starts to regain consciousness and shows clear signs of breathing normally again.

Notes on techniques of BLS Box 10.5 summarises the key to initial resuscitation.

- Only a small amount of resistance to breathing should be felt during rescue breathing, and each inflation should take about 1 s.
- The tidal volume to be achieved is about 600–700 mL in an adult, which is the amount normally required to produce visible lifting of the chest.
- The rescuer should wait for the chest to fall fully during expiration before giving another breath. This should normally take about 1 s.
- Once the airway is secured with an endotracheal tube or similar the lungs are ventilated at 10 breaths/min without any pause in chest compression.

Chest Compression

- *Any interruptions in chest compression lessen the chance of recovery and must be kept to an absolute minimum.*
- In an adult, the aim should be to press down approximately 5–6 cm and apply only enough pressure to achieve this.
- At all times the pressure should be firm, controlled and applied vertically. Erratic or violent action is dangerous.
- The recommended rate of compression is a rate, and not the number of compressions that are to be given in a minute; this will depend upon interruptions for rescue breathing.
- About the same time should be spent in the compression phase as in the release phase.
- As the chances are remote that effective spontaneous cardiac action will be restored by BLS without other techniques of ALS (including defibrillation), time should not be wasted by further checks for the presence of a pulse. Even short interruptions to chest compression have very adverse effects on the outcome so compression should not be interrupted.
- The presence of dilated pupils has, in the past, been variously used as a sign of cardiac arrest, failure of circulation during resuscitation and the presence of established brain damage. This sign is unreliable and should not be used to influence management decisions before, during or after CPR.

Recovery position. When circulation and breathing have been restored, it is important to maintain a good airway and ensure that the tongue does not cause obstruction. It is also important to minimise the risk of inhalation of gastric contents.

For this reason, the patient should be placed in the recovery position (Fig. 10.12). This allows the tongue to fall forward, keeping the airway clear.

- Remove the patient's spectacles.
- Kneel beside the patient and make sure that the patient's legs are straight.

FIGURE 10.12   The recovery position. Three movements (A, B and C) to reach this position.

- Open the airway by tilting the head and lifting the chin.
- Place the arm nearest you out at right angles to the patient's body, elbow bent, with the palm of the hand uppermost.
- Bring the patient's far arm across the chest and hold the back of the hand against the patient's nearest cheek.
- With your other hand, grasp the far leg just above the knee and pull it up, keeping the foot on the ground.
- Keeping the patient's hand pressed against the patient's cheek, pull on the leg to roll the patient towards you onto the patient's side.
- Adjust the upper leg so that both the hip and knee are bent at right angles.
- Tilt the head back to make sure the airway remains open.
- Adjust the hand under the cheek, if necessary, to keep the head tilted and facing downwards to allow liquid to drain from the mouth.
- Check breathing regularly and ensure that oxygen is being administered.

What the team leader of an arrest team should want to know from the ward team:

- How, when and where the arrest occurred? (use a common structured communication tool)
- Was there a witnessed account?
- What was the time from collapse to BLS?
- What was the initial rhythm?
- What was the time from arrest to defibrillation?
- Were there any special circumstances, for example, tricyclic overdose/hypothermia?
- What is the 'Do Not Attempt CardioPulmonary Resuscitation' (DNACPR) status?
- Is there a ReSPECT form in the hospital notes?
- Is there any equipment malfunction?
- Are the notes available for review?

Problems to avoid and look for during cardiopulmonary resuscitation

- Ensure suction and wide-bore rigid suckers (Yankauer) are available.
- Correct ampoules and drug doses.
- Ensure there are good IV lines that will not 'tissue', especially with sodium bicarbonate (all IV drug boluses should be followed by a 20 mL N saline flush).
- Avoid letting fluids 'run through'.
- Avoid injury to the patient's limbs and eyes from malposition and spillage.
- Avoid staff electrocution.
- Avoid burns to the patient during defibrillation—move oxygen masks or nasal cannulae at least a metre away from the patient's chest. High-flow nasal oxygen (HFNO) as used in COVID-19 patients saturates the surrounding area with oxygen.
- Ensure effective chest compression by changing the operator every 2 min.

One member of staff should be recording the events:
- timing of events
- number of shocks and strength
- administered drugs—dose and timing
- equipment problems

AFTER BASIC LIFE SUPPORT

Although BLS is a holding measure that keeps the patient alive, it must be continued throughout the resuscitation attempt, except when a patient is undergoing defibrillation. Once the arrest team arrives the situation can be reviewed, with the first priority being to analyse the heart rhythm from the ECG monitor or, more rapidly, via the self-adhesive defibrillation pads.

In a cardiac arrest, the heart rhythm falls into one of two categories:

1. Shockable rhythms: ventricular fibrillation and pulseless ventricular tachycardia (VF/VT). Patients in this group need immediate defibrillation.
2. Non-shockable rhythms: asystole (a straight line) and electric complexes, but with no palpable pulse (PEA, previously known as electromechanical dissociation). This group needs emergency drugs and continuing CPR.

Defibrillation Strategy

Once VF/VT is recognised, immediately give one shock (150–200 J bi-phasic defibrillator or 360 J monophasic defibrillator). Minimise the disruption to CPR by the delivery of the shock—with a manual defibrillator the time between stopping and restarting CPR should be less than 5 s.

Do not wait to check the rhythm or feel for a pulse but immediately restart chest compression.

Continue CPR for 2 min in the ratio 30:2 and then check the monitor.

If there is still VF/VT, give a second shock (150–360 biphasic) and restart CPR immediately.

After 2 min recheck the monitor and if there is still VF/VT give a third shock and restart CPR immediately—while CPR is proceeding give 1 mg of adrenaline (epinephrine) IV every 3–5 min and 300 mg of IV amiodarone after three shocks. There must be no unnecessary interruption to chest compression (plan the next steps and recharge the defibrillator during CPR).

Regardless of the rhythm, adrenaline (epinephrine) is given every 3–5 min (i.e., immediately after alternate shocks) until there is return of a spontaneous circulation. If, during CPR, the patient shows signs of life and the monitor shows an organised rhythm—check the pulse and if it is present start postresuscitation care, if not, continue CPR. Do not interrupt a 2-min spell of CPR if there is an organised rhythm but no signs of life—continue CPR and only check the pulse at the end of the 2 min.

Technical points in defibrillation. For maximum success, the shocks must be applied without delay. If left, VF deteriorates into asystole or PEA, which have a much worse prognosis. Effectively, defibrillation 'stuns' the heart, stops all electric activity and, if successful, the heart restarts with the natural pacemaker taking over to produce a normal rhythm. During CPR the time between stopping chest compression and administering the shock must be cut to the absolute minimum to maximise the chance of success. Self-adhesive pads are much preferred to defibrillator paddles.

The correct defibrillation electrode (or paddle) positioning is critical—one is placed to the right of the upper sternum below the clavicle, while the other is placed in the mid-axillary line approximately level with V6 ECG lead—avoiding breast tissue in a female (Fig. 10.13).

Automated External Defibrillators

Early defibrillation after the recognition of cardiac arrest and the immediate institution of BLS is the key to improved survival. This has been facilitated by the introduction of the automated external defibrillator (AED), which can:

- Analyse the heart rhythm and either advise a shock or the resumption of 30:2 CPR
- Provide spoken or visual directions on administering a shock or deliver a shock automatically
- Prompt immediate resumption of CPR after the shock. Do not stop CPR to check the patient unless the patient starts to breathe normally (not just agonal gasps which are common during CPR) or shows clear signs of coming back to life
- Time the 2-min CPR cycle and then prompt to assess the rhythm, respiration and pulse

FIGURE 10.13 The paddle/self-adhesive pad positions for defibrillation.

AEDs have played a major role in increasing the speed of response to cardiac arrest and increasing the number of people who can now successfully perform defibrillation.

Asystole and PEA. These non-shockable rhythms are treated with CPR, initially 30:2 but once the airway is secure continuous compressions at 100 per minute without pausing during ventilation at 10 breaths/min. Adrenaline (epinephrine) 1 mg is given as soon as there is IV access and continued every 3–5 min of CPR. Atropine is no longer recommended for PEA.

It is possible to make an erroneous diagnosis of asystole if the monitoring equipment fails or a lead becomes disconnected. Of equal importance is the risk of diagnosing spurious asystole after unsuccessful defibrillation when monitoring is performed through the defibrillator paddles. The shock can adversely affect the conducting properties of the gel pads so that the monitor shows a straight line (which can be misinterpreted as asystole) for sufficient time to critically delay the next shock. Rather than rely on 'through the paddles' monitoring, chest leads and a monitor are the preferred ways to assess the response to each shock. The value of 'through the paddles' monitoring is to obtain a rapid look at the rhythm that is present when the arrest team first arrives on the scene.

Fine VF or asystole?

If there is doubt about whether the rhythm is asystole or fine VF, manage the patient as a non-shockable rhythm. Do not attempt defibrillation—continue chest compression and ventilation.

Precordial thump?

A single precordial thump can be tried in a witnessed and monitored cardiac arrest but is only likely to be successful in the first few seconds after collapse, particularly in VT and occasionally in VF. The bottom edge of a fist is brought down sharply from about 20 cm above the lower half of the sternum.

The uses of adrenaline (epinephrine) in the collapsed patient. Adrenaline (epinephrine) is used in cardiac resuscitation and in the treatment of acute anaphylaxis. It increases the efficiency of resuscitation by:

- Increasing the flow of blood in the heart muscle
- Increasing the flow of blood through the brain
- Sustaining a falling blood pressure

There are two strengths of adrenaline (epinephrine): 1:1000 for intramuscular administration in anaphylaxis and 1:10,000, 10 times weaker, for IV administration in cardiac resuscitation and in severe unresponsive anaphylaxis. Details of adrenaline (epinephrine) administration are given in Table 10.4. Figure 10.14 shows the ALS algorithm.

TREATABLE CAUSES OF CARDIAC ARREST: 4H AND 4T

During cardiac resuscitation, it is vital that the team consider and correct any reversible causes of the cardiac arrest. For example, a patient with acute asthma may suffer an acute

TABLE 10.4 ■ **Administration of Adrenaline (Epinephrine)**

	Strength	
	1:10,000	**1:1000**
Concentration	1 g in 10,000 mL	1 g in 1000 mL
	1 mg in 10 mL	1 mg in 1 mL
Indications	Cardiac arrest	Acute anaphylaxis
Route	Intravenous	Intramuscular
Dose	1 mg (10 mL)	0.5 mg (0.5 mL)
If repeated:	Every 3–5 min	At 5 min

cardiorespiratory arrest during an attack as a result of a tension pneumothorax. A patient with a huge gastrointestinal bleed may arrest due to sudden hypovolaemia—in addition to BLS, this patient will need emergency fluid replacement.

Hypoxia. Hypoxia is the most easily preventable cause of cardiac arrest. The aim in any acutely ill patient is to monitor the oxygen saturation and keep the oxygen saturation above 90%. In the patient with COPD who has collapsed, the issue of controlled oxygen therapy is now irrelevant—in the emergency situation, high concentrations of oxygen are needed as an immediate life-saving measure.

Hypovolaemia. Sudden, severe fluid loss in the form of blood (gastrointestinal bleed or massive haemoptysis) or body fluid (diarrhoea or DKA) will lead to hypotension and cardiac arrest. The key is to recognise that the low blood pressure is due to fluid depletion rather than a problem with a sick heart and take appropriate action.

Hypothermia. Cardiac arrest can complicate severe hypothermia. CPR must be continued until the patient's temperature is brought back up above 35°C or the efforts are judged by a senior medical member of the team to be fruitless.

Hyperkalaemia and hypokalemia. A very high serum potassium, characteristically complicating acute renal failure, and a very low potassium, as may be seen in excessive diuretic treatment, can lead to cardiac arrest and must be addressed urgently. Intravenous calcium chloride is used for hyperkalaemia, for hypocalcaemia and in overdose with calcium channel blockers (e.g., nifedipine). Intravenous magnesium can be life saving in serious arrhythmias due to magnesium deficiency—seen in overdiuresis and with some chemotherapy regimes.

Tension pneumothorax. Characteristically, this gives a picture of PEA: a rhythm on the monitor but no palpable pulse. Unless the pneumothorax is recognised and treated, resuscitation will be unsuccessful.

Therapeutic accident. The common cause in this category is tricyclic poisoning after self-harm. Even very protracted resuscitation can be successful, and it is one of the few situations in which IV sodium bicarbonate can have a life-saving effect.

Tamponade. Cardiac tamponade occurs when there is a buildup of fluid under pressure in the pericardial sac—it compresses the heart and drastically reduces the cardiac

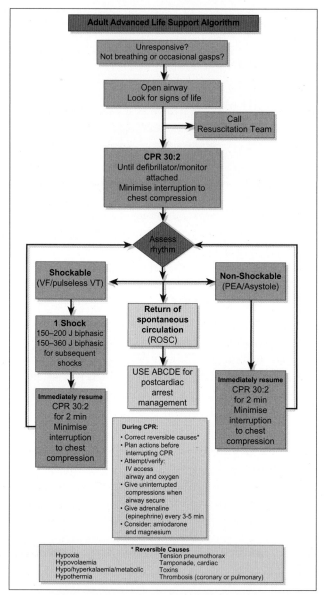

FIGURE 10.14 The ALS algorithm. *ALS,* Advanced life support; *CPR,* cardiopulmonary resuscitation; *PEA,* pulseless electrical activity; *VF,* ventricular fibrillation; *VT,* ventricular tachycardia. *(Reproduced with the kind permission of Resuscitation Council UK.)*

output to the extent that it can lead to sudden PEA. Resuscitation will be unsuccessful unless the fluid is also drained off.

Thromboembolism (pulmonary embolism). The classic cause of sudden death on the medical ward, massive pulmonary embolus can, in fact, be a reversible cause of cardiac arrest. It is likely that, in patients who survive, the cardiac massage acts to break up or dislodge a clot that is sitting in the pulmonary artery and preventing blood from leaving the right side of the heart.

ADVANCED AIRWAY MANAGEMENT

Effective uninterrupted chest compression and early defibrillation are the keys to surviving a cardiac arrest. Chin lift with bag-valved-mask ventilations are used in most in-hospital arrests until advanced airway techniques can be deployed (with no interruption to chest compression). This will either be endotracheal intubation or the easier supra-glottic airway (commonly the 'I-gel'), which sits above the vocal cords. Increasingly, the level of carbon dioxide in the expired breath is being monitored ('waveform capnography') during cardiac arrests to assess the effectiveness of chest compression (effective compression mimics the heart's normal action of bringing carbon dioxide back to the lungs) and to identify the return of normal circulation.

WHEN TO STOP THE RESUSCITATION PROCEDURE

Legally, the most senior doctor present has this responsibility. However, this doctor should consider other views within the team. Survival becomes less likely with time, but many patients have recovered from prolonged resuscitation, particularly after:

- Drowning
- Electrocution
- Hypothermia
- Tricyclic drug overdose

It is almost impossible to predict brain damage from the state of the patient during the arrest and, in particular, fixed dilated pupils are not a reliable guide. If the patient is oxygenated and undergoing efficient BLS, the repeated failure of defibrillation and appropriate cardiac drugs will eventually form the basis of the decision to stop resuscitation.

Dealing With the Relatives of a Victim of Cardiac Arrest

This is a task for an experienced member of the ward team, preferably the clinician who was with the patient nearest to the time of the arrest. No matter how distressed and distracted the relatives appear, it is likely that every detail of the day's events will be etched on their minds forever.

Find out whom you are addressing and if any key member such as a spouse is missing. You may need to gather clinical information from the relatives as well as provide them with news. Explain the situation in straightforward terms and do not be embarrassed if your comments sound like platitudes—it is far better to use everyday language that is clear and unambiguous than revert to medical jargon.

Thirty minutes ago John's heart suddenly stopped, and we put out an emergency call. The doctors and nurses are doing everything they can to try and get it started again. The situation is critical and we do not know if he is going to survive.

I am really sorry to have to give you this terrible news: John's heart stopped suddenly at 5:00 p.m. We were there within seconds and tried everything we could to get it started again. We worked on him for an hour, but it was absolutely hopeless; we could not get a heartbeat back and he died at 6.15 p.m. It happened with no warning and from the moment his heart stopped John will have known nothing about it. In the end it was very peaceful, and I am sure that he did not suffer.

You must let and encourage the family to see the body. Try not to have the family, however well-intentioned, 'protect' a wife or husband from seeing the body—it may be their last chance to say goodbye and they will come to value that moment. They must be allowed the chance to say an unhurried goodbye, to touch the body, to show their distress and to express their grief.

It is unlikely that you will know what to say, and silence is often as good as anything. Keep in mind that, to the ward staff, this is another episode on a very crowded day—but to the family, it is a life-changing event.

Answering Relatives' Questions in Cardiac Arrest

What has happened? The heart suddenly stopped beating, but we have been able to 'kick start' it using a small electric shock. The episode was short-lived and we were able to restore a normal heartbeat, probably before any further damage could be caused. The bruising or red marks on the chest are due to manoeuvres we had to perform to keep the blood pumping during the period when the heart had stopped. There will be pain and tenderness in this area for a few days.

Has the heart been damaged? It is too early to judge the extent of the damage. Good signs will be a return of the blood pressure to normal and successful withdrawal of all the intravenous drips and drugs.

Has there been a heart attack? We will only know from tests on the heart and blood, which we will get back once the patient has recovered. It is possible to have a cardiac arrest from a sudden electric fault without having an actual heart attack.

Has there been any brain damage? We cannot tell at present. The confusion/drowsiness/coma is not uncommon after a cardiac arrest and does not necessarily mean there is any permanent damage. The brain can go through a short-lived period of 'hibernation' after a cardiac arrest and still recover completely. We will only know if this is the case here after a period of time has elapsed (usually at least 24 and often up to 72 h).

Is the patient on a life-support machine? The mask gives extra oxygen and must be kept in position for the next 24 h. If the condition deteriorates and the oxygen mask alone is insufficient, we can use a life-support machine. This will take over all the breathing functions and pump air directly into the patient's lungs through a tube. If this is needed, the patients are moved to the ITU, put to sleep and then kept heavily sedated while they are on the machine.

The Aftercare of Patients Who Undergo Successful CPR

Post cardiac arrest syndrome. In some patients the period immediately after a cardiac arrest is characterised by a combination of cerebral dysfunction, cardiac instability and a sepsis-like inflammatory response. The clinical picture varies from coma to recurrent seizures and multiorgan failure. Their initial care is based on the ABCDE principle maintaining, for example, oxygen saturations at 94%–98% and blood sugars at less than 10. Most of these patients will then require intensive care where interventions such as therapeutic hypothermia and emergency coronary angioplasty have been shown to improve outcomes.

Some patients are traumatised by the events associated with successful CPR. The physical effects—chest bruising, defibrillation burns and even rib fractures—require simple explanation and symptomatic treatment. The psychological effects are more enduring:

- 'Near-death experiences'
- Acute anxiety
- Loss of confidence
- Fear of a second arrest
- Recurrent nightmares

For the first time in their life, the patient has become aware of their own mortality. The key to their immediate management is to:

- Give an honest account and explanation of the events that took place.
- Listen to the patient's concerns.
- Give firm reassurance.
- Consider offering other forms of help—discussion with the doctors, the priest and the clinical psychologist.

Do Not Attempt Cardiopulmonary Resuscitation (DNACPR)

It is important to try and differentiate between the natural process of dying and a sudden cardiorespiratory arrest from which a patient can be rescued. If the patient has a physical illness from which there is no likelihood of recovery and if it is clear that before admission the patient's life was nearing its end, then resuscitation would seem futile. Common examples of the latter include patients with cancer who are bedbound and can no longer take oral medication and patients with worsening heart failure despite repeated admissions and optimisation of their drug regimen. Conversely, cardiac arrest as an early complication of an acute myocardial infarction is worth an attempt at resuscitation in virtually all situations.

The distinction may not be obvious in every case, and so it is important that decisions concerning resuscitation are made by a senior member of the medical team—ideally, but not always, the consultant. It is also essential to understand that a mentally competent adult can refuse consent to medical treatment (including resuscitation), even if that decision would lead to the person's death.

COMMUNICATION AND EXPLANATION

Communication is of paramount importance in this area. Patients must be involved in DNACPR decisions unless the discussion would cause them physical or mental harm. If CPR would not be successful, it must be explained to the patient why this is so and why it is the reason for a DNACPR decision. Discussions must be held with all the relevant parties. It is important to provide patients with a realistic assessment of the likely outcome of a cardiac arrest (the benefits vs. the burdens). Many patients, for example, would decline resuscitation if they were given a 50% chance that the outcome would include severe cognitive or functional impairment. DNACPR decisions must be clearly documented, with the underlying reasons, in the nursing and medical notes, and the status of each patient on the ward communicated at handover (Case Study 10.8). Where a patient lacks capacity and where there is no advanced directive or power of attorney, decisions are made by senior medical staff which, while taking into consideration those close to the patient, are in the patient's best interests.

The on-call team must be included in the communication. There is little point in having a detailed discussion at 5:00 p.m., only for the arrest team to attend at 3:00 a.m. and be faced with a ward team who are not aware of the resuscitation status of their patients.

When in doubt: resuscitate.

A DNACPR PROTOCOL

It is important to work to a protocol. There should be a standard way to review and record DNACPR decisions in the notes. Any DNACPR notice that has been posted

CASE STUDY 10.8	A 5-Year-old Male Who Declines Resuscitation and Dies Peacefully

A 55-year-old male with lung cancer had undergone palliative chemotherapy and came in with marrow failure and septicaemia. Despite antibiotics, he deteriorated. He asked the staff, in the presence of his family, to have no more tests or any 'messing about'. Although weak and drowsy he understood the situation exactly. Subcutaneous morphine and haloperidol were used to control his pain and breathlessness. The decision not to resuscitate was formally posted in his nursing and medical notes. He died peacefully.

should be kept under regular review, as the status of the patient may alter as their medical condition changes.

When a DNACPR decision is appropriate

- When resuscitation would not be successful
- When resuscitation is against the patient's wishes (expressed when the patient was competent to do so)
- When resuscitation would not be in accord with an advanced directive
- Where successful resuscitation is likely to be followed by a length and quality of life that would be an intolerable burden to the patient. This is the most common reason for not performing resuscitation and is the most difficult area in which to make decisions. As an example, a family looking after a severely disabled young adult would have a vital role in expressing what to them (and the patient) is and is not an acceptable quality of life.

IMPORTANT POINTS ABOUT DNACPR

- In any discussions, do not exclude close friends and family members. Particularly in the case of patients with learning disorders and the young chronic sick, the professional carers from long-stay institutions and nursing homes may consider themselves as 'family' and must be included in the discussions.
- It can be helpful to 'anticipate' cardiac arrests or sudden deterioration so that some early discussion can be had with relatives. Patients with advanced disease, say with COPD or severe cardiac failure, who survive 'near misses', can be asked if they want to be involved in future discussions concerning resuscitation should the same thing happen again.
- It should be made clear to everyone—staff, patients and relatives—that a DNACPR decision is *not* the same as withdrawing all forms of care. The priority in these patients remains medical treatment, nursing care and, if the situation deteriorates, ensuring the patient is kept comfortable, dignified and free of pain.

THE RESPECT FORM

The widespread introduction of the Recommended Summary Plan for Emergency Care (ReSPECT) has been an important advance in the appropriate use of CPR. The form is completed after a detailed discussion between the patient and their senior clinician. It acknowledges a shared understanding of the patient's health and likely care needs—documenting any existing Advanced Care Plans or an Advanced Decision to Refuse Treatment (which imposes a legal obligation on the health professionals). A section of the form characterises the patient's emergency treatment choice in terms of what outcome would be most valued and what would be most feared. There follows a section from the clinician on specific recommendations and realistic limits to the emergency care that includes whether or not to attempt CPR.

Answering Relatives' Questions About 'Do Not Resuscitate' Decisions

Does this decision mean that all treatment will now be withdrawn? No, it does not mean this at all. Resuscitation means starting urgent life-support measures if the heart stops—the aim is to restore a normal heartbeat. We do this if there is a reasonable chance of restoring the patient to the patient's previous health without suffering side effects or damage as a result of the cardiac arrest and subsequent resuscitation. After considering this, and as a result of our discussions with you, we have decided that either resuscitation would not work or it would leave the patient in an intolerable situation. However, we can still treat other complications apart from a cardiac arrest—infection, congested lungs, low blood pressure—and we can still ensure effective symptom control if there is pain, distress or breathlessness.

Bereavement on the Acute Medical Unit

Bereavement on the AMU is an important and difficult problem:
- The deaths will be sudden.
- The relatives will have had little warning.
- The ward will be busy and staff time will be at a premium.

However, if bereavements are handled sensitively, relatives are more likely to come to terms with their loss and the risks of subsequent abnormal grief reactions will be reduced. Two examples of the common problems encountered after bereavement are given in Case Study 10.9.

There are a number of problems surrounding sudden death in hospitals, particularly regarding the actual sequence of events. Relatives need to know what went on, who was present, whether the patient asked for their next of kin, whether there were any nurses present and whether the doctors had been called. It is extremely important that the actual events are covered in detail at the time of the death because only then can the relatives start to come to terms with the situation. It is common for relatives to mull over the events surrounding the death. Even months later, they may have several unanswered questions.

CRITICAL TASKS WHEN DEALING WITH THE BEREAVED

Ensure effective communication with relatives. Ensure that communication with the relatives of very sick patients remains the utmost priority in the ward.

Make sure the facts are correct
- Make absolutely sure that you have the facts correct:
  - That the patient in question has died

CASE STUDY 10.9	**Bereavement**

CASE 1

A 75-year-old female with known ischaemic heart disease, severe airflow obstruction and myelodysplasia was diagnosed as having an advanced squamous carcinoma of the lung. There had been full involvement by a consultant chest physician and the lung cancer specialist nurse. The patient had her own patient-held record.

The patient was admitted after a period of deterioration with dehydration and sepsis. She initially responded to IV antibiotics. Unfortunately, at 3:00 a.m. the patient became acutely distressed, hypotensive and confused. She died over a period of 20 min. The relatives came to the ward after the patient had died.

Several months after the event, despite extensive counselling, the daughter was still extremely distressed. She felt guilty, having promised that her mother would die at home and that, if it was necessary, she would take her out of hospital. Previous members of the family had died in unexpected circumstances on their own. In addition, she had 'chivvied' her mother along during her final illness to encourage her not to give up. She felt guilty about this.

CASE 2

A 55-year-old female with known advanced breast cancer previously treated with chemotherapy and radiotherapy was admitted for 'terminal care'. The lesion was fungating, she had a pleural effusion and could not move at all in bed without the help of two nurses. Her husband did not leave her side. She was started on subcutaneous opiates and moved onto another ward which, in the information sheet for the AMU, is described as a 'recovery ward'. She died suddenly from a pulmonary embolus at 5:00 a.m. a few days later. Weeks later, her husband came back to the hospital with a number of complaints.

- He had not realised that she was dying.
- If she was dying, why had she been moved to a 'recovery ward'?
- When was she last seen alive and by whom?
- Why was her usual medication cut down?
- Did she die alone, and why was he not called in?

We had talked to the husband on several occasions at the bedside. We had not appreciated that, in his distress, he had not taken in the most fundamental issue about his wife's illness. He needed to know everything about the final few hours when he was not there with her. He was still inconsolable months later because of the way in which we had failed to communicate effectively with him.

- That you are dealing with that patient's relatives
- That you know their names and relationships
- That the relatives you are talking to include the next of kin

Find out the likely cause and mode of death

- Find out from the doctors the likely cause of death.
- Speak to those who were with the patient in the final moments: the relatives will need to know these details. Sometimes relatives will ask to speak to the night shift who were involved.

Give the relatives time with the deceased

- Ensure the relatives have an unhurried and private time with the deceased.
- Give the relatives enough time:
  - To absorb the news and recover from the initial shock

- To express their distress
- To ask questions

CRITICAL TASKS WHEN DEALING WITH THE BEREAVED

- Ensure effective communication with relatives
- Make sure the facts are correct
- Find out the likely cause and mode of death
- Give the relatives time with the deceased
- Ensure liaison with the patient's GP

Ensure liaison with the patient's GP. Ensure that the ward lets the patient's GP know of the death.

IMPORTANT TASKS WHEN DEALING WITH THE BEREAVED

Establish the need for coroner involvement or postmortem. Establish from the doctors whether they:

- Will need to inform the coroner/procurator fiscal
- Would like to seek permission for a postmortem

Help the relatives with practical details. Ensure the relatives understand the process of:

- Death certification
- Handling the deceased patient's possessions
- The help that bereavement officers and the undertakers will give

Understand the role of the coroner and death certification. Make sure you understand the role of the coroner and know before dealing with the relatives whether (and when) a death certificate can be issued.

Be sensitive to distress among staff. Be sensitive to distress among junior members of the nursing and medical team after a bereavement. For staff, a series of deaths and the associated feelings of inadequacy/failure that they engender may leave them vulnerable and stressed.

IMPORTANT TASKS WHEN DEALING WITH THE BEREAVED

- Establish the need for coroner involvement or postmortem
- Help the relatives with practical details
- Understand the role of the coroner and death certification
- Be sensitive to distress among staff

Further Reading

Royal College of Physicians, 2017. National Early Warning Score (NEWS) 2: Standardising the Assessment of Acute-Illness Severity in the NHS Updated Report of a Working Party. RCP, London.

Oxygen Therapy

BTS guideline for oxygen use in adults in healthcare and emergency settings. Thorax (Suppl.1), 2017.

Sepsis

Rhodes, A., et al., 2017. Surviving sepsis campaign: international guidelines for management of sepsis and septic shock. Critical Care Medicine 45, 486–552.
Gildea A, Mulvihill C, McFarlane E, Gray A, Singer M, Recognition, diagnosis, and early management of suspected sepsis: summary of updated NICE guidance. BMJ, 385, 2024, q1173. https://doi.org/10.1136/bmj.q1173.

Transfusion

Acute Kidney Injury: Prevention, Detection, Management. 2019 NICE Clinical Guideline (NG148). https://www.nice.org/guidance/NG148.
British Committee for Standards in Haematology, Blood Transfusion Task Force, 2012. Guideline: The Administration of Blood and Blood Components and the Management of Transfused Patients. www.b-s-h.org.uk/media/5152/admin_blood_components-bcsh-05012010.pdf.

Resuscitation

Resuscitation Guidelines, 2021. https://www.resus.org.uk/library/2021-resuscitation-guidelines.

CHAPTER 11

Emerging Problems: Outbreaks and Deliberate Releases — SARS and COVID-19, Toxins and Biologic Agents

Introduction

This chapter considers the possibility that the acute medical unit (AMU) has to deal with the outbreak of an infectious disease or with an act of bioterrorism—the deliberate release of a biological agent or toxin. Such an occurrence, although unlikely, has very serious implications for the personal safety of the hospital staff. Despite infection control measures, many of the fatalities in the severe acute respiratory syndrome (SARS) outbreak were among the nursing and medical staff on the acute units. SARS is a typical example of spread by airborne transmission for which specific protective measures are required as soon as a suspected case occurs.

How Infection Spreads

- Close contact with unrecognised infected persons
- Infectious respiratory secretions—cough and sneeze
- True airborne transmission ('aerosol')
- Faecal and oral transmission
- Contact with body fluids, organs and blood
- Contact with contaminated body surface (shaking hands)
- Touching contaminated external surfaces

The possibility of an outbreak of an unfamiliar infection or disease caused by bioterrorism cannot deflect the ward staff from basing all their initial management of seriously ill patients on the principle of probability: common things occur commonly. Thus an outbreak of severe pneumonic illness is more likely due to *Legionella* from, say, a faulty cooling tower (as in a 2003 outbreak in Montpellier) than from SARS or an airborne terrorist release of plague. A patient with progressive paralysis is far more likely to be suffering from Guillain-Barré syndrome than from botulism, and a haemorrhagic rash is more likely to be meningococcal septicaemia than the Ebola virus.

Nonetheless, there is an issue of early recognition because, in their initial stages, these rare infections and toxins share clinical features with more commonplace conditions. The fact that deliberate infections and mass poisonings have taken place in recent years means further attacks are likely. Staff should therefore remain vigilant, and plans must be in place. Previously, the responses to outbreaks and toxic releases have been characterised by:

- Inadequate preparations
- Late recognition
- Poor communications

It is critical that the most up-to-date information is on hand. Local expertise will be limited, although there is increasing experience with strict respiratory protection through its use in multidrug-resistant tuberculosis (MDTB). Fortunately, international experience and guidelines are freely available electronically through several important websites.

The minimum knowledge that is required is:

- How to recognise an outbreak alert (using SARS or COVID-19 as examples).
- The broad nature of the most likely bioterrorist threats (anthrax, botulism, plague, smallpox, tularaemia, viral haemorrhagic fevers [VHFs] and the nerve gas sarin).
- How to protect the health of the staff.

There are several basic principles involved:

- Awareness of new threats and the emergence of novel infections/agents.
- An appreciation that there may be no previous personal experience with cases.
- The need for immediate, up-to-date information from the Internet.
- The need to review protocols and procedures in light of new information.

- The skills of infection control in highly contagious patients.
- The need for timely communication.
- The rapid involvement of designated staff and resources.

SARS-CoV-2 and COVID-19

In December 2019, a cluster of unusual cases of severe pneumonia was identified in Wuhan City in China. In January 2020, the cause was identified as a novel virus, SARS-CoV-2, which had probably crossed from a bat population to humans. The virus was highly contagious, and on the 11th of March 2020, the World Health Organization (WHO) declared that the disease, by then known as COVID-19, had become a global pandemic. COVID-19 subsequently overwhelmed healthcare systems worldwide and reached every continent, including Antarctica. Estimates are that by February 2023, COVID-19 had killed 6.5 million people, and in the United Kingdom at least 70% of the population has had COVID-19, of whom 180,000 had died.

In its original form, the virus caused serious illness with high mortality. As the population has developed natural resistance and as public health strategies have been introduced (notably the SARS-CoV-2 vaccination programmes), the virus, which has evolved through several mutations, has become more infectious but less virulent.

The highly infectious nature of SARS-CoV-19 (from 2 days before symptoms start for a minimum of a week) has been a major challenge. Person-to-person spread is by droplets from the upper airways (sneezing, coughing, singing), by aerosol—small virus-containing particles suspended in the air (speaking, breathing, particularly during any exertion) and by direct contact with contaminated surfaces, including those of the patient. Aerosol-generating activities such as nebulisation, suction, chest physiotherapy and high-flow nasal oxygen add to the risk of spread. Special isolation measures have had to be developed based on cohorting suspected cases ("Red" wards and "Green" wards), negative pressure rooms with improved ventilation, minimising social contact and, most importantly, the use of effective personal protective equipment (PPE).

Full PPE consists of a fluid-resistant surgical gown, cap, visor, goggles, gloves and an FFP3 mask (FFP stands for Filtering Face Piece and the higher the number, the more effective the filter). It is mandatory that health professionals be familiar with donning and doffing PPE and that they have been fit tested with the appropriate mask. There are instructional videos on the UK Health Security Agency website.

Principles of treatment
- Maintain a high suspicion of a COVID-19 diagnosis (atypical features include unexplained confusion)
- Assess risk factors associated with deterioration
  - Age
  - Ethnicity
  - Body mass index

- Comorbidity
- Immune suppression
- Learning disorder
- Suboptimal COVID-19 vaccination history
- No previous COVID-19 infection
- High National Early Warning Score 2 (NEWS2) on admission
- In the elderly, also use the Clinical Frailty Scale
- Formulate an escalation plan, ceiling of care and DNACPR (do not attempt cardiopulmonary resuscitation) status (has the ReSPECT form been reviewed?)
- Patient to be cared for in an appropriate environment (emergency assessment unit [EAU], respiratory support unit [RSU], intensive therapy unit [ITU]?)
- Correct hypoxia (standard oxygen administration, continuous positive airway pressure [CPAP], high-flow nasal oxygen [HFNO], ITU ventilation)
- Optimise comorbidities (e.g., asthma, diabetes)
- Administer definitive treatment: antivirals, neutralising antibodies, dexamethasone
- Ongoing liaison with the ITU outreach and RSU teams
- Keep abreast of the rapidly changing COVID-19 guidelines

Overcoming Communication Barriers in COVID-19

There are obvious reasons why communication is particularly challenging for patients isolated with COVID-19. PPE inhibits the usual communication skills of non-verbal language, physical contact with the patient and the use of a clear, audible voice. This can be compounded by confusion, isolation, disorientation and, in the elderly, delirium. These barriers are combined with the unfortunate reality that the conversation may have to impart very bad news. These points may be helpful in improving communication in these very challenging situations:

- Plan the aims of the proposed encounter.
- Talk slowly in a loud and low voice.
- Approach from the front of the patient and position yourself at eye level.
- Introduce yourself and your role, and if necessary repeat this frequently.
- Identify yourself clearly; for example, first name and role written on your visor.
- Explain the need for PPE.
- Use gestures and body language more than you would normally.
- Engage family members in the conversation, for example, using Skype.
- COVID-19 delirium may require specialist management and is covered in Chapter 9.

A summary of the PPE requirements in COVID-19:

- Neck-to-heel gowns and gloves—to be left in the room before leaving.
- A respirator mask conforming to EN149:2001 FFP3, such as the 3M mask: 1873 V.
- Staff using an FFP3 mask must be fit tested.
- The mask must be left on until out of the room.

- Cap and goggles or visor—to be removed and left in the room.
- Boots.
- Strict handwashing in alcohol—before and after leaving the room.

SURGICAL MASKS VERSUS PARTICULATE RESPIRATORS (FFP MASKS)

Surgical face masks are designed to prevent droplet emission and act as a barrier to splashes of liquid. They will capture microorganisms in the exhaled breath but do not protect against airborne infection; for this, an appropriate respirator is needed. *Respirators* are high-filtration masks that prevent inhalation of submicron-sized particles. They do not filter the wearer's expired air. To be used safely and to maintain a high filtering efficiency, the respirator must be fitted correctly, with a less than 10% leak. Healthcare workers on COVID-19 wards who wear FFP3 masks are at a much-reduced risk of infection compared to those using surgical masks—they therefore should be freely available and used routinely.

Fig. 11.1 gives an overview of the initial pathway for a potential case of SARS-CoV-2. Fig. 11.2 summarises the strict infection control measures that are required.

TARGETED TREATMENT OF COVID-19

The treatment recommendations are evolving rapidly but all have the same aims:
- Reduce disease severity (hospital admissions and death)
- To be effective in high-risk, vulnerable patients
- Reduce the risk of long-term COVID-19
- Reduce transmissibility

The principles are to reduce the viral load (antiviral drugs such as remdesivir and synthetic antiviral antibodies such as sotrovimab)—to reduce the body's exaggerated inflammatory response (dexamethasone) and to neutralise the self-harming mediators released by the body in response to the infection (such as baricitanib and tocilizumab). The exact combination depends on the stage and severity of the infection.

OTHER EMERGING INFECTIONS

COVID-19 is only one example of a new infectious disease that has profound implications for Public Health. In August 1999, eight similar cases of encephalitis were admitted to hospitals in the Northern Queens district of New York. Four of the individuals were paralysed and needed ventilation. All eight usually spent their evenings out of doors in the vicinity of breeding sites for *Culex* mosquitoes, which were suspected to be spreading a virus. Subsequent investigations of a substantial number of bird deaths in the area and of the patients identified the offending organism: West Nile virus. The lessons from the successful recognition of this disease include:

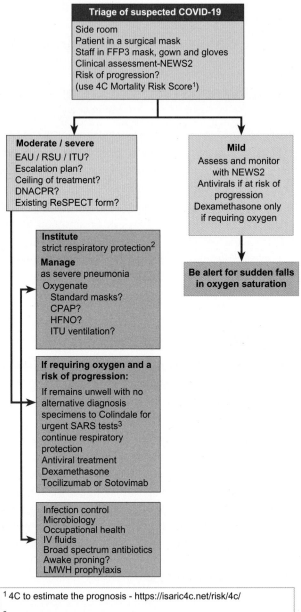

Triage of suspected COVID-19

Side room
Patient in a surgical mask
Staff in FFP3 mask, gown and gloves
Clinical assessment-NEWS2
Risk of progression?
(use 4C Mortality Risk Score[1])

Moderate / severe
EAU / RSU / ITU?
Escalation plan?
Ceiling of treatment?
DNACPR?
Existing ReSPECT form?

Mild
Assess and monitor
with NEWS2
Antivirals if at risk of
progression
Dexamethasone only
if requiring oxygen

Institute
strict respiratory protection[2]
Manage
as severe pneumonia
Oxygenate
Standard masks?
CPAP?
HFNO?
ITU ventilation?

**Be alert for sudden falls
in oxygen saturation**

**If requiring oxygen and a
risk of progression:**
If remains unwell with no
alternative diagnosis
specimens to Colindale for
urgent SARS tests[3]
continue respiratory
protection
Antiviral treatment
Dexamethasone
Tocilizumab or Sotovimab

Infection control
Microbiology
Occupational health
IV fluids
Broad spectrum antibiotics
Awake proning?
LMWH prophylaxis

[1] 4C to estimate the prognosis - https://isaric4c.net/risk/4c/

[2] Negative pressure room, high-filtration mask (FFP3), cap, gown,
gloves and eye protection

[3] Sputum, urine (20–30 mL), stool, EDTA blood (5 mL), acute serology

FIGURE 11.1 The initial pathway for a potential case of the severe acute respiratory syndrome (SARS). *CPAP*, Continuous positive airway pressure; *DNACPR*, do not attempt cardiopulmonary resuscitation; *EAU*, emergency assessment unit; *EDTA*, ethylenediaminetetraacetic acid; *HFNO*, high-flow nasal oxygen; *ITU*, intensive therapy unit; *LMWH*, low-molecular-weight heparin; *NEWS2*, National Early Warning Score 2; *RSU*, respiratory support unit.

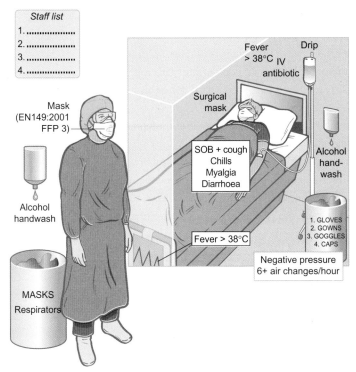

FIGURE 11.2 The strict infection control measures required for a potential case of severe acute respiratory syndrome. *SOB,* Shortness of breath. Gloves, then gown, then eye protection are removed and discarded in the patient's room. The respirator / mask is only removed after leaving the room and closing the door.

- An awareness of the importance of clustering of cases
- The value of good communication
- Excellent cross-professional working

More recently, in 2003, a virulent avian flu virus broke out in Southeast Asia. The virus, the H5N1 strain of bird flu, crossed the species barrier from domestic ducks to human and killed 20 people in Thailand and Vietnam. There have been 450 cases of human H5N1 since 2003. The recent pandemic among the bird population has raised concerns that there will be more human cases, including person-to-person spread. Many believe that a major flu pandemic from this type of source is inevitable. COVID-19 and influenza spread in the same way, so similar infection control measures would be required.

H1N1 2009 INFLUENZA (SWINE FLU)

The 2009 swine flu pandemic typified the challenges of a new viral threat:

- The possibility of an overwhelming number of seriously ill cases. In fact, in England, between June and November 2009, there were 540,000 cases but only 138 deaths.
- The emergence of at-risk populations with a higher mortality rate includes those over 20 weeks pregnant, those with comorbidity, especially asthma, the morbidly obese and the elderly.
- The need to apply assiduously in-patient infection control measures appropriate to a droplet-spread infectious disease.
- To ensure that there is early isolation and treatment, but not at the expense of ignoring the possibility of other diagnostic possibilities: community-acquired pneumonia, bacterial meningitis and septicaemia.
- The role of antiviral and anti-inflammatory medications.

VIRAL HAEMORRHAGIC FEVERS: EBOLA, LASSA, MARBURG AND CRIMEAN-CONGO

These VHFs:

- Require early diagnosis and effective isolation
- Are difficult to recognise at their onset
- Spread rapidly by contact with body fluids
- Are often fatal
- Often have no effective treatment

The assessment of a patient with a fever arriving back from an affected area must follow national protocols and includes exposure (infected patients—any VHF; fruit bats—Marburg; tick bites—Crimean-Congo fever; rats—Lassa fever), clinical features (bruising and mucous membrane bleeding, joint pain, severe diarrhoea) and exclusion of malaria and typhoid. High-risk cases require enhanced local infection control measures pending potential transfer to a high-level isolation unit. Definitive treatment may involve early antivirals (ribavirin in Lassa fever) and supportive care—IV fluids, oxygen and appropriate blood products to treat clotting abnormalities and haemorrhage.

Unusual Illnesses—Deliberate Release of Infectious and Chemical Agents

In 1979, at least 66 Russian people downwind from a weapons research facility died of inhalation anthrax after an accidental release of anthrax spores into the atmosphere. Iraq has admitted deploying anthrax in missiles, and in the United States in 2001, there were 11 cases of inhalational anthrax, including five deaths after malicious dissemination of anthrax spores via the postal service.

In 1994 and 1995, the Aum Shinrikyo religious cult released the neurotoxin sarin gas in terrorist attacks in Japan. The second attack was in the Tokyo subway, where plastic bags of dilute sarin were punctured with umbrella tips. The released vapour was directly absorbed through the skin and lungs; other people were then indirectly exposed from the initial victims' contaminated clothing. In total, 1000 passengers were injured, 12 of whom died. The hospitals were overwhelmed: many staff members were secondarily exposed because there was no chemical-resistant personnel equipment (butyl rubber gloves and boots), there were no decontamination facilities, and ventilation in the treatment areas was poor. The antidotes, atropine and pralidoxime, were soon exhausted. Another 4000 people reported to hospital—many had nothing wrong with them and were not actually exposed.

In 2018 in an act of international terrorism, two Russian nationals were deliberately poisoned with liquid Novichok, a highly potent neurotoxin, smeared on the door handles of their house in the English city of Salisbury. Fortunately, they were diagnosed quickly and responded to intensive treatment with pralidoxime and atropine after being admitted unconscious and severely ill. Sadly, 3 months later, some of the discarded poison led to the death of a third local person who was inadvertently exposed.

Deliberate Release of Infectious Agents

GENERAL PRINCIPLES

The effects of a deliberate release of an infectious or biological agent may be recognised only when cases of *unusual illness* appear on the AMU. This is particularly likely after a covert release, as there will be no mass Emergency Service response and the presentation of the cases may have a less obvious pattern—the connection between them may not be immediately apparent.

An unusual illness may present in three ways:

- A diagnostic puzzle
- An illness 'out of place'—such as a tropical disease with no travel history
- The failure of a 'conventional' illness to respond to usual treatment

Obviously, an outbreak or clustering of such cases has much more significance than a single incident, but in covert deliberate release, the cases may be admitted to hospital with no immediately obvious pattern. Ideally, vigilance and awareness should be high at all times, but the likelihood of a deliberate release remains so low that there is a danger that, over time, the possibility is forgotten.

It may therefore be advisable to have named members of the ward staff whose responsibility is to keep themselves updated on current risks and infection control measures, to liaise with other appropriate departments and to maintain a file of information on the ward giving relevant protocols, contact details and websites.

There are four important areas in the management of potential cases:

1. Awareness and recognition
2. Communication
3. Decontamination and containment
4. Early advice

AWARENESS AND RECOGNITION

Cases will not necessarily come in well-defined clusters, even if there is common exposure. Their presentation may be staggered or delayed from the time of exposure.

There are several warning signs of a potential outbreak:

- The receipt of a prior warning or threat
- People with a similar disease or syndrome presenting at the same time
- A number of cases of unexplained disease or death
- A familiar illness occurring in an unusual setting within a community
- An illness affecting a key sector of the community
- A familiar disease with an unusually high death rate
- A disease with an unusual geographic or seasonal distribution
- An unusual, atypical, genetically engineered or antiquated strain of agent
- Simultaneous outbreaks of similar illnesses in separate areas
- Unusual transmission routes, for example, by aerosol, food or water
- Animal deaths or illnesses that precede or accompany human illnesses or deaths
- An illness only among people in proximity to common ventilation systems

Taking the correct samples for screening for infections and toxins. The samples for screening for infectious diseases should contain at least two sets of blood cultures. Two 10-mL samples of clotted blood are also required for serology and biotoxin measurements. Two 10-mL EDTA blood samples are needed for sophisticated molecular identification studies. A 20-mL sample of urine in a preservative-free bottle should also be sent.

To identify chemical toxins from high-risk cases, 'Toxiboxes' are situated in the accident and emergency department and should be used for handling and transporting samples to the laboratory. The Toxibox has the containers and packaging to send these samples:

1. 10 mL of blood in a plastic lithium tube
2. 5 mL of blood in a glass lithium tube
3. 4 mL of blood in an EDTA tube
4. 300 mL of urine in a preservative-free bottle

The samples require careful handling and they need to be marked 'high risk'. Each bottle is bagged separately. Blood forms, in separate bags, are attached to each matching bottle. Once the laboratories have been alerted, the samples are delivered urgently, by hand.

COMMUNICATION

There will have to be excellent lines of communication locally with Occupational Health, Control of Infection, Laboratory Service and, if an outbreak is confirmed, with regional and national bodies. There will inevitably be health and safety priorities that will be the responsibility of the local occupational health department. The local Health Protection Unit, which is part of the National Health Protection Agency, will coordinate other aspects of management. This will include informing the police of a suspected outbreak, obtaining expert medical opinions and overall incident control.

DECONTAMINATION AND CONTAINMENT

The principles are to prevent further harm, to optimise treatment and, of paramount importance, to protect the healthcare staff from harm (*if there is any doubt, action must always be taken to protect the staff*). For outbreaks in which *biological* agents are involved, the principle is the adoption of infection control—single rooms, the use of Universal Precautions and, when suspicion is high, specialised respiratory protection.

Universal Precautions. It is not always possible to identify people who may spread infection to others; therefore precautions to prevent the spread of infection must be followed at all times. The following routine procedures are usually called 'Universal Precautions' and are designed to prevent exposure to potentially infectious blood and body fluids and to avoid injury by sharp objects:
- Practice good basic hygiene with regular handwashing.
- Cover wounds or skin lesions with waterproof dressings.
- Avoid contamination of people and clothing with blood/body fluids.
- Disposable gloves and aprons should be worn when attending to dressings, performing aseptic techniques or dealing with blood/body fluids.
- Handle and dispose of sharps safely.
- Avoid puncture wounds, cuts and abrasions in the presence of blood.
- Avoid using sharps if possible.
- Protect eyes, mouth and nose from blood splashes.
- Know what to do if there is a sharps injury or blood splash incident.
- Clear up blood spillages promptly and disinfect surfaces.
- Dispose of contaminated waste safely.
- Know how to deal with soiled linen.
- Clean, disinfect and sterilise equipment as appropriate.

Specialised respiratory protection. Where there is a risk of the airborne spread of serious infection (e.g., MDTB, SARS, VHF), strict respiratory precautions are needed to minimise the risk to staff:
- Negative pressure rooms with 6 to 9 air exchanges per hour
- Staff wearing gloves, disposable gowns, caps, boots and eye protection
- High-specification masks
- Ammonia, phenol and alcohol-based disinfectants
- Hourly surface and floor wipes with diluted bleach (1 in 49 dilution of 5.25% sodium hypochlorite)
- Alcohol-based handwashes

- Initial visiting restrictions
- All gowning and de-gowning carefully supervised:
  - Gloves, gowns, eye protection and caps must be left inside the room.
  - Masks/respirators must not be removed and discarded once outside of the room with the door closed.

For outbreaks in which *chemical* exposure is involved, the initial management is centred on initial decontamination, which is the responsibility of the ambulance service and will take place in a designated area. It would be highly unusual for decontamination to take place on a ward, as it is a highly specialised and hazardous operation.

SEEK EARLY ADVICE

It is of critical importance to maintain a list of up-to-date websites and contact telephone numbers on the AMU.

Poisoning With Biological Agents
EXAMPLES OF POTENTIAL PATHOGENS AND INITIAL SYMPTOMS

This section gives a brief clinical overview of what experts believe to be the most likely terrorist agents. Websites are available for more detailed information.

Anthrax. Influenza-like symptoms, followed 2 to 4 days later by the rapid development and progression of severe respiratory failure and shock. Mortality rates in inhalation anthrax are extremely high, but specific treatment combines ciprofloxacin, vancomycin and rifampicin. Steroids may also help.

Plague. Severe myalgia, sore throat and headache merge into a severe pneumonic illness with copious bloody sputum. Specific treatment is with gentamicin, ciprofloxacin and doxycycline.

Botulism. The patient remains alert, with no sensory loss but develops rapidly descending flaccid paralysis due to blockage of nerve impulses to the muscles. There is no fever. Specific treatment is with an antitoxin, but the key is supportive care, which often includes ventilation.

Smallpox. Two to three days of severe fever, headache and malaise followed by a deeply seated rash spreading and progressing from the mouth and face to the trunk, limbs, palms and soles. Treatment is supportive. Specific treatment is probably ineffective, but the antiviral drug cidofovir can be tried.

Tularaemia. A pneumonic illness with flu-like features or a septicaemic illness with severe shock. Specific treatment is with gentamicin.

Ebola virus. Fever, abdominal pain and bloody diarrhoea followed by bleeding from the nose, the gastrointestinal tract and into the skin. Treatment is supportive.

Lassa fever. Fevers, shivering attacks and severe tonsillitis followed by a disturbed conscious level, respiratory distress and abdominal distension. Treatment is supportive.

Table 11.1 summarises the features of and responses to poisoning with biological agents.

Poisoning With Nerve Agents

There are five organophosphorous nerve agents, but there is most experience with sarin, which is a highly volatile vapour that acts predominantly after inhalation but is also absorbed through the skin. In the event of a deliberate release, victims should arrive at the hospital having already been decontaminated so that only standard hospital precautions would be necessary for personal staff protection. The AMU would be receiving moderately ill patients, not those in need of immediate ITU care, for whom the main objectives will be antidote administration and the treatment and monitoring of any respiratory difficulties.

Nerve agents act by blocking the enzyme, acetylcholinesterase, which normally works as a break on nerve impulse transmission. The clinical effects are therefore due to an overload of nerve traffic throughout the nervous system. The antidotes—atropine and related drugs—act by unblocking the enzyme and reducing the flow of traffic.

For clinical purposes, the three important effects are due to overactivity in the parasympathetic nerves—the nerves that oppose the sympathetic nervous system—and hence the signs of nerve agent poisoning are the 'opposite' of the fight or flight reaction:

*B*radycardia—pulse rate of less than 40 beats/min

*B*ronchospasm—severe wheeze

*B*ronchorrhea—excessive airway and lung secretions

This overactivity is reversed by atropine and two related drugs: pralidoxime and obidoxime. Their effectiveness as antidotes can be monitored by the improvement in these three features.

- Overactivity in the nerves to the respiratory muscles leads to respiratory distress and, ultimately, respiratory arrest.
- Overactivity in the brain leads to coma and convulsions. Convulsions can be prevented with diazepam.

The management after initial decontamination can be summarised by ABC:

1. Antidote administration
2. Breathing support
3. Coma and convulsion care

ANTIDOTE ADMINISTRATION

Atropine is an effective but short-lived antidote that is given intramuscularly every 5 min until the pulse rate increases above 80 beats/min. Pralidoxime and obidoxime have a slower onset but are long-acting. When given IV, they are effective for around 4h. Intravenous diazepam prevents convulsions and other signs of muscular overactivity, particularly muscular twitching.

TABLE 11.1 ■ Poisoning With Biological Agents

Disease	First Symptom	Severe Pneumonia	Clinical Picture	Rash	Staff Prophylaxis	Control of Infection
Anthrax	Fever	Yes	Rapid deterioration over 1–6 days	Yes	Antibiotics	No isolation, G, A, HW
Plague	Fever	Yes	Rapid deterioration over 1–6 days	Yes (H)	Ciprofloxacin	SR, G, GN, E, HW, FFP3
Botulism	No	No	Sudden descending flaccid paralysis	No	Not needed	No isolation, G, A, HW
Smallpox	Fever	No	Fever++, systemic symptoms++, abdominal pain	Yes (H)	Immediate vaccination	SR*, G, GN, E, HW, FFP3
Tularaemia	Fever	Yes	Variable rate of deterioration	Yes	Not needed	SR, G, GN, E, HW, FFP3
VHF	Fever	No	Rapid deterioration, abdominal pain, diarrhoea	Yes (H)	Nil	SR*, G, GN, E, HW, FFP3

A, apron; E, (eye protection) goggles; FFP3, particulate filter respirator for staff/surgical mask for the patient; G, gloves; GN, fluid-resistant gown; H, haemorrhagic rash; HW, handwashing++(alcohol); SR, side room; SR*, side room in a designated centre; VHFs, viral haemorrhagic fevers (Lassa fever, Ebola, etc.).

The frontline emergency services may have already administered antidotes using the *Autoject (Combo Pen) L4 A1*, which contains a single-dose combination of atropine, pralidoxime and a form of diazepam. It is given intramuscularly into the lateral aspect of the thigh every 5 to 15 minutes, depending on the improvement in the '3 Bs', to a maximum of three doses.

BREATHING SUPPORT

Death from nerve agent poisoning is usually due to respiratory failure. The mainstay of management is based on high concentrations of oxygen and nasopharyngeal suction to keep the upper airway clear of excessive secretions.

Signs of improvement will be:
- Less wheezing
- An increasing pulse rate
- Reduced airway and nasopharyngeal secretions

COMA AND CONVULSION CARE

This comprises the standard management and monitoring of a reduced level of consciousness and the immediate treatment of any convulsions with IV diazepam.

Key Clinical Skills in Outbreaks and Deliberate Releases

- Core skills in infection control:
  - Understanding the routes by which infection spreads
  - Strict adherence to and proper use of Universal Precautions
  - Supervision of twice-daily cleaning and disinfection of rooms (particularly touched surfaces, e.g., bed rails, TV controls)
- Advanced skills in the use of PPE:
  - The use of high-filtration respirator masks, including the use of a fit test
  - Ensuring there is consistency in the use of PPE by all team members
- Core Clinical skills in the assessment of critically ill patients:
  - Initial assessment using the generic ABCDE approach
  - Monitoring of the critically ill with impending respiratory failure
  - Supporting the patient and their family
- Advanced communication skills for the care of patients in isolation:
  - Dealing with fear and anxiety in a victim of a 'dreaded' illness
  - Minimising the bars to communication imposed by protective clothing
  - Minimising the impact of the illness on the patient's well-being

- Disease-specific clinical problems:
  - Ensuring that a system exists for early recognition and immediate infection control
  - Minimising high-risk procedures
  - Reducing possible transmission from the time of the first clinical encounter
  - Designating 'clean' and 'dirty' areas for isolation materials
- Dealing with the individual threat to personal health:
  - The issue of 'working quarantine'
  - The concept of 'cohort care'—logging healthcare personnel
  - Limiting and educating visitors
- Participating in a strong management system:
  - The best systems for controlling an outbreak are those that have been tested.
- Using information systems on the Internet
- The supervision and protection of relatives and visitors

Conclusion

From the personal testimony of healthcare professionals involved with the global COVID-19 pandemic, it is clear that caring for large numbers of critically ill patients with a highly infectious disease places a major burden on the healthcare system. It also presents a huge personal challenge to individual staff. Inevitably, if the problem recurs, the AMUs will be on the front line and will have to cope. It is the responsibility of acute unit staff to be aware of the current threats and to be up to date on their management: to understand the issues of effective infection control, to institute them instantly when any suspicion is raised and to ensure that health personnel are not put at unnecessary risk. There are many sources of advice once the diagnosis is made, but the key is a high index of suspicion and appropriate levels of vigilance.

Further Reading

Fink, D., et al., 2018. Fever in the returning traveller. British Medical Journal 360, j5773.
Initial investigation and management of outbreaks and incidents of unusual illnesses. Health Protection Agency. https://webarchive.nationalarchives.gov.uk/ukgwa/20140714084352/http://www.hpa.org.uk/webc/HPAwebFile/HPAweb_C/1201265888951

COVID-19 Rapid Guideline: Managing COVID-19

NICE guideline [NG191]. Published: 23 March 2021. Last updated: 22 June 2023. https://www.nice.org.uk/guidance/NG191
COVID-19: information and advice for health and care professionals - GOV.UK. (www.gov.uk) https://www.gov.uk/guidance/covid-19-information-and-advice-for-health-and-care-professionals
Guidance: viral haemorrhagic fevers: origins, reservoirs, transmission and guidelines 2018. https://www.gov.uk/government/publications/viral-haemorrhagic-fever-algorithmandguidance-on-management-of-patients

INDEX

Note: Page numbers followed by *f* indicate figures, *t* indicate tables and *b* indicate boxes.